Yoga Therapy Across the Cancer Care Continuum

CONTRIBUTORS

Karen Apostolina • Marsha D. Banks-Harold • Cheryl Fenner Brown
Marianne Woods Cirone • Amelia Coffaro • Nischala Joy Devi
Christa Eppinghaus • Teri Gandy-Richardson • Chandrika Gibson
Sandra Susheela Gilbert • Sadie Grossman • Suveena Guglani
Kate Holcombe • Sharon Holly • Kelsey Kraemer
Tonia Kulp • Johanne Lauktien • Jennie Lee
Annette Loudon • Lee Majewski • Smitha Mallaiah
Sanmay Mukhopadhyay • Bhavani Munamarty • Lórien Neargarder
Charlotte Nuessle • Maryam Ovissi • Miriam Patterson
Tina Paul • Tari Prinster • Lois Ramondetta • Kiran Shenoy
Stella Snyder • Doreen Stein-Seroussi • Michelle Stortz
Jennifer Collins Taylor • Robyn Tiger • Satyam Tripathi • Tina Walter

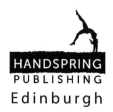

HANDSPRING
PUBLISHING
Edinburgh

Yoga Therapy Across the Cancer Care Continuum

Leigh Leibel ◆ Anne Pitman

Foreword Lorenzo Cohen

First published in Great Britain in 2023 by Handspring Publishing, an imprint of Jessica Kingsley Publishers
An imprint of Hodder & Stoughton Ltd
An Hachette UK Company

2

A CIP catalogue record for this title is available from the British Library and the Library of Congress
ISBN 978-1-912085-91-0
ISBN (Kindle ebook) 978-1-912085-92-7

Printed and bound by CPI Group (UK) Ltd, Croydon, CR0 4YY

Jessica Kingsley Publishers' policy is to use papers that are natural, renewable, and recyclable products and made from wood grown in sustainable forests. The logging and manufacturing processes are expected to conform to the environmental regulations of the country of origin.

Handspring Publishing
Carmelite House
50 Victoria Embankment
London EC4Y 0DZ

www.handspringpublishing.com

CONTENTS

ABOUT THE AUTHORS/EDITORS

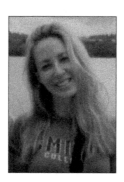

Leigh Leibel, PhD student, MSc, ACSM/ACS-CET, C-IAYT

Leigh Leibel (she/her) is an integrative oncology specialist and health journalist based in New York City. Since 2015, she has had a clinical practice in the Division of Hematology/Oncology, Columbia University Irving Medical Center, where she designs evidence-based mind-body interventions and healthy lifestyle programs for people with cancer to mitigate adverse treatment side effects and improve clinical outcomes. In addition, Ms Leibel is co-founder of the Center for Global Health Equity and Empowerment (GHEE) where she advocates for cancer risk reduction and patient-centered care worldwide, and works with an international team of specialists to develop equity-based cancer prevention interventions delivered during community health fairs in Abuja, Nigeria, and other low-middle-income countries (LMICs).

Ms Leibel completed a summer fellowship in cancer prevention and control at the National Institutes of Health/ National Cancer Institute (NIH/NCI) and holds a Master of Science in Yoga Therapy (Honors) from S-Vyasa University, Bengaluru, India, and is pursuing her PhD in Yoga. Currently, she serves on the Board of Trustees of the Society for Integrative Oncology (SIO), co-chairs both the SIO Yoga Special Interest Group and the SIO Committee on Best Practices in Yoga/Yoga Therapy in Cancer Care, and is a member of the Advisory Board of Cancer Health magazine. Formerly with CNN, she was founding executive producer of CNN Accent Health, a leading patient-education media network in physician offices that reached 173 million patients annually.

Find her @leighleibel and www.leighleibel.com

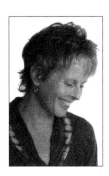

Anne Pitman, MSc, E-RYT 500, RPYT, C-IAYT, Pain Care Certified

Anne Pitman (she/her) holds a Masters in Kinesiology and is the Director of the School of Embodied Yoga Therapy (www.embodiedyogatherapy.com), accredited with the International Association of Yoga Therapists (www.iayt.org). She has over 35 years of experience in educating movement teachers, teaching embodied yoga and pioneering yoga therapy in Canada. Trained in functional biomechanics and Scaravelli-inspired yoga, Anne is also informed by the world of somatics (Feldenkrais, Body Mind Centering, Continuum, Trager) and is a continuing scholar at the Orphan Wisdom School (www.orphanwisdom.com), an apprenticeship in grief literacy and the skills of living and dying well. As a practicing yoga therapist at the Ottawa Integrative Cancer Centre (www.thechi.ca), Anne sees people, one-on-one, who are facing cancer with concomitant shock, trauma, anxiety, depression, and pain. In clinic, she is an Integration, Research and Programming Consultant, designing yoga interventions for cross-disciplinary research (with the Ottawa Hospital and University of Ottawa) and creating popular, evidence-informed cancer programs such as Head Start (for those facing breast cancer) and Inspire Now! (for those living with lung cancer). Her yoga therapy retreat, Informed by Cancer, gathers people into welcome community after treatment, addressing nervous system impact, lingering side effects and the ongoing fear of recurrence and death. In a continued attempt to thwart ageism and death phobia, she facilitates A Year to Breathe, a year-long meditation program, inviting yoga and healthcare practitioners to befriend and practice toward their own dying time, resourcing a love of life and authenticity in professional practice. In private practice at Bad Dog Studio (www.annepitman.ca), Anne offers a slow, non-insistent, inquiry-based, co-regulated compassionate yoga therapy care for the multitude of life's shatterings, in troubled and uncertain times. A champion for healthcare integration, she regularly speaks at medical and yoga therapy conferences on diagnosis shock, the unrecognized grief of cancer, and the tender practice of accompanying people facing their dying days. She enjoys life with her husband, sons and their families amongst the beauty of Ottawa, Canada.

CONTRIBUTING AUTHORS

Karen Apostolina (E-RYT 500)
Karen is a yoga4cancer-certified teacher and mentor and a Relax and Renew-certified trainer. Karen works with cancer patients and survivors to strengthen immunity, relax the nervous system, and activate the body's natural capacity for healing. She graduated from the Loyola Marymount University Yoga Therapy RX Program, has a BA in Journalism from California State University, Northridge, and received the Edward R. Murrow Award for Short Feature Reporting. She wrote for the *LA Times*, was a freelance feature reporter for KPCC in Pasadena, California, and the editor of *Verdugo Monthly Magazine*.
Website: www.karenapostolinayoga.com

Marsha D. Banks-Harold (BSEE, TCTSY-F, E-RYT 500, YACEP, RPYT, RCYT, C-IAYT)
Marsha is Director of PIES Fitness Holistic Yoga Therapy and Teacher Training Programs, owner of PIES Fitness Yoga Studio, creator of "My Body Don't Bend That Way" yoga, an executive electrical engineering leader, co-founder of Awakening Yoga Spaces, and a Trauma Center Trauma Sensitive Yoga facilitator and mentor through the Center for Trauma and Embodiment. She is an IAYT-certified Yoga Therapist, experienced workshop leader, public speaker, and a contributing author to *Yoga Therapy Foundations, Tools, and Practice: A Comprehensive Textbook* and *Yoga Therapy Today*. Marsha blossoms in creating supportive, inclusive, diverse, adaptive, and accessible yoga and yoga therapy experiences for all.
Website: www.piesfitnessyoga.com

Cheryl Fenner Brown (E-RYT 500, YACEP, C-IAYT)
Cheryl became instantly enchanted when she found yoga and the subtle connections between the breath, body, mind, and emotions. Her classes weave anatomy, philosophy, *āsana, mudrā*, chanting, *prāṇāyāma* and *yoganidrā* together for a well-rounded, compassionate experience. Cheryl encourages each student to honor where they are in their bodies every time they step onto the mat, so deep healing and transformation can take place. Cheryl is an IAYT-certified Yoga Therapist specializing in yoga for cancer, older adults, and structural difficulties, and offers teacher trainings on these techniques across the country.
Website: www.yogacheryl.com

Marianne Woods Cirone (MS, MFA, CYT 500)
Marianne is a writer, yoga and wellness educator, teacher, and advocate for people affected by cancer. She is the co-author of *From Alignment to Enlightenment: Using Props to Achieve Stability and Ease in Yoga Poses* and founder of the *Integrative Cancer Review* that promotes safe, effective, and accessible integrative therapies for people affected by cancer. At the Living Well Cancer Resource Center, a division of Northwestern Medicine, Marianne developed safety protocols and managed thousands of wellness visits each year. She has received certifications from the Temple of Kriya Yoga, Moksha Yoga, Atma Yoga, yoga4cancer, the Cancer Exercise Training Institute, and holds a Master of Health Systems Management degree, and an MFA in Creative Writing.
Website: www.integrativecancer.org

Amelia Coffaro (BA, RYT 500, C-IAYT)
Amelia is an IAYT-certified Yoga Therapist who practices in the infusion center at Ascension Columbia St Mary's Cancer Center in Milwaukee, Wisconsin. She is a member of the SIO Yoga Special Interest Group and the SIO Patient Advocate Committee, and the Project Manager for the Bounce Back Study Stakeholder Group, a stress management program for adolescent and young adult cancer survivors. After experiencing a rare and aggressive form of breast cancer at age 27, she dedicated her work to meeting the unique needs of people with cancer. She is passionate about creating accessible, inclusive, and holistic healing communities for young adults with cancer and chronic illness, and using mind-body medicine to empower young people in their health and healing.
Website: www.ameliacoffaro.com

Nischala Joy Devi (C-IAYT)
Nischala is an IAYT-certified Yoga Therapist who serves on the IAYT Advisory Council and is the author of numerous books: *The Healing Path of Yoga; The Secret Power of Yoga; A Woman's Guide to the Heart and Spirit of the Yoga Sutras; The Namaste Effect*; and *Meditation in the Yoga Tradition*. Her teachings reflect a heart-centered perspective of

spirituality and scripture. Educated by masters in India and worldwide, she was a monastic disciple of Sri Swami Satchidanandaji. She conducted landmark research in pioneering yoga for life-threatening diseases, Dean Ornish's Program for Reversing Heart Disease. Nischala Devi co-founded the Commonweal Cancer Help Program and has dedicated many years to helping people live vital lives while living with cancer.
Website: www.abundantwellbeing.com

Christa Eppinghaus (MSc, PT, CLT, C-IAYT)
Christa holds a Master of Science in Yoga Therapy from Maryland University of Integrative Health and is a physical therapist and IAYT-certified Yoga Therapist working in a variety of settings: trauma/acute care, orthopedics/sports medicine, cardiopulmonary rehabilitation, acute/LTC rehabilitation, and most recently in oncology/lymphedema as a lymphedema therapist. In addition, Christa is a Healing Touch Therapist and Vipassana Mindfulness Meditation Teacher. The diversity of her professional training allows for a cross-pollination of her skills between traditional medicine and integrative care. She treats the whole person; mind, body, and spirit, with a deep respect, allowing joyfulness and peace to unfold in her clients' lives.
Business: Inner Wisdom Yoga and Meditation.

Teri Gandy-Richardson (RYT 500)
Teri is a yoga teacher who trained in yoga4cancer oncology yoga after her own diagnosis of cancer and experience of bilateral mastectomy. As an African American woman, she well understands health disparity and statistics, and is a walking example of the power of having had a previous yoga practice AND implementing oncology yoga in addressing side effects of treatment. She believes opportunity and access is key! Teri empowers people with yoga and applied philosophy to embrace life's struggles as a path to having more impact, stability, and calm in their lives.
Website: www.terigandyrichardson.com

Chandrika Gibson (ND, PhD, MWell, E-RYT 500, C-IAYT)
Chandrika is an Australian scholar-practitioner and IAYT-certified Yoga Therapist who is a recognized leader in the fields of integrative oncology and mind-body medicine. She has worked extensively with people diagnosed with cancer in her roles at the Cancer Council Western Australia, Solaris Cancer Care, and Breast Cancer Care Western Australia. Chandrika's Master's research explored the impact of yoga on psychological and physiological stress and relaxation responses in breast cancer survivors, and her PhD investigated the psychosocial education and support needs of people diagnosed with head and neck cancer. Her research has been published in high-impact peer reviewed journals. Chandrika owns Surya Health and is a co-founder of Wisdom Yoga Institute where she trains yoga teachers to become evidence-informed yoga therapists.
Website: www.wisdomyogainstitute.org

Sandra Susheela Gilbert (BA, E-RYT 500, C-IAYT)
Sandra began her career as an IAYT-certified Yoga Therapist in oncology, first with family members at end of life and then in the Orthodox Jewish community in Brooklyn, New York. She was one of the first Urban Zen integrative therapists at Beth Israel Hospital and piloted yoga and oncology programs at Mt Sinai and Lenox Hill hospitals in New York City. Sandra trains yoga teachers and therapists to work with people with cancer and chronic illness through the Integral Yoga tradition and her YCat (Yoga Therapy in Cancer and Chronic Illness Teacher Training) program, leads workshops and retreats, consults, and teaches in yoga research at Vanderbilt University School of Nursing, and maintains a private yoga therapy practice.
Website: www.ycatyogaincancer.com

Sadie Grossman (MS, E-RYT 500, C-IAYT)
Sadie holds a Master of Science in Yoga Therapy from Maryland University of Integrative Health and is an IAYT-certified Yoga Therapist. She is the on-site meditation and mindfulness provider for University of Pittsburgh Medical Center Hillman Cancer Center, Wellness and Integrative Oncology Program, where she participates in trainings for oncology nurses and sees clients privately, contributes to seminars, and speaks publicly on her

work as a yoga therapist. As a senior teacher for One Point One Yoga, she co-leads advanced and 200-hour teacher trainings.
Website: www.sadiegrossman.com

Suveena Guglani (PhD student, MSc, C-IAYT)
Suveena is an IAYT-certified Yoga Therapist and a Radiation Physicist, working with cancer patients undergoing radiotherapy. Pursuing her passion for Yoga, and in the pursuit of *Jñana* Yoga, she completed her Master of Science in Yoga Therapy from S-VYASA University, Bengaluru, India and is pursuing her PhD Yoga. She actively volunteers with Hindu Temple of the Woodlands where she currently serves as President of the Executive Committee. Suveena works with clients with many different ailments, but predominantly in the field of oncology, in private clinic, and as a faculty/mentor at S-VYASA-USA, Houston.
Website: www.vyasahouston.org

Kate Holcombe (MFA, E-RYT 500, C-IAYT)
Kate is an IAYT-certified Yoga Therapist and the founder and director of Healing Yoga Foundation, a non-profit project of Commonweal dedicated to supporting and empowering individuals through Yoga, regardless of ability, background, experience, or financial means. Kate was a student of T.K.V. Desikachar in Chennai, India, studied Sanskrit at UC Berkeley and Kuppuswami Sastri Research Institute, Chennai, and is a guest lecturer for the University of San Francisco, Department of Philosophy. She is most passionate about the practical application of *Patañjali-s Yoga Sūtra-s*. Kate has been profiled in *Yoga + Joyful Living (Yoga International)*, *Yoga Journal*, and the *San Francisco Chronicle*. She has served as the Yoga Coordinator and Lead Teacher at the Commonweal Cancer Help Program since 2007.
Website: www.healingyoga.org

Sharon Holly (YTRx-800c, E-RYT 500, YACEP, RCYT, C-IAYT)
Sharon is an IAYT-certified Yoga Therapist who specializes in yoga for cancer. After her own experience with breast cancer, teaching fellow surviving thrivers has become her life's purpose. Sharon graduated from the Loyola Marymount University Yoga Therapy Rx program, and has gained certification in the Optimal State of Living® Mental Health and Physical Program (where she is faculty), yoga4cancer, Amrit Yoga Nidra for Adults and Kids, and Level II iRest Yoga Nidra. In addition to private practice, Sharon teaches at psychological treatment centers, physical therapy offices, preschools, and cancer centers throughout Los Angeles, including Tower Cancer Research Foundation Magnolia House, Cedars-Sinai Cancer Center, Cancer Support Community, and the Foundation for Living Beauty where she leads retreats for women with cancer.
Website: www.sharonholly.com

Kelsey Kraemer (MS, E-RYT 500, C-IAYT)
Kelsey is a mother, IAYT-certified Yoga Therapist, and a Full Spectrum Birth Doula. Upon earning her Master of Science in Yoga Therapy from Maryland University of Integrative Health, she spent many years serving patients at Indiana University Health in the fields of oncology, chronic pain management, and women's health. Kelsey now guides women through a deeper understanding of spirituality, embodiment, and eco-feminism through women's yoga retreats and teacher trainings.
Website: www.kelseykraemeryoga.com

Tonia Kulp (MS, E-RYT 500, C-IAYT)
Tonia is an IAYT-certified Yoga Therapist practicing at Children's Hospital of Philadelphia, Pennsylvania. She holds a Master of Science in Yoga Therapy from Maryland University of Integrative Health, where she is also an adjunct faculty member. Tonia specializes in yoga therapy for pediatric oncology patients, working across various medical units to provide individualized yoga therapy for patients and caregivers. She is a Reiki Master Teacher, certified reflexologist, End of Life Doula, iRest Level 1 Teacher, and has completed specialized training in trauma-informed care, pain care, and behavioral health.
Website: www.chop.edu/administrative-staff/kulp-tonia-d

Johanne Lauktien (BA, RYT 500, C-IAYT)

Johanne is an IAYT-certified Yoga Therapist specializing in adult oncology. She is also certified in Yoga for Survivors and has two certifications with distinction from Upaya Zen Center in professional training for clinicians in Compassionate Care of the Seriously Ill and Dying and G.R.A.C.E. interventions based in Compassion-Based Interactions in the Clinician/Patient Encounter. She is the founder of Yoga Instruction & Healing for Cancer Survivors, with a mission to break down barriers in the medical community and bring the positive research-based benefits of yoga to cancer centers and more diverse populations, including Spanish-speaking communities. She educates, implements, and operates remedial yoga, specifically for a conventional clinical environment, for patients coping with cancer's debilitating side-effects.

Website: www.johannelauktien.com

Jennie Lee (E-RYT 500, YACEP, C-IAYT)

Jennie is a Nautilus Book Award-winning author of three books: *Spark Change: 108 Provocative Questions for Spiritual Evolution*; *True Yoga: Practicing with the Yoga Sutras for Happiness & Spiritual Fulfillment*; and *Breathing Love: Meditation in Action*. An IAYT-certified Yoga Therapist and spiritual coach, Jennie counsels private clients, facilitates international wellness retreats, and is a regular contributor to national magazines and other yoga-related books.

Website: www.jennieleeyogatherapy.com

Annette Loudon (MMedSc, AAYT, YA, Fitness Australia, ALA, C-IAYT)

Anette has worked therapeutically with yoga across a variety of populations in Australia where she resides, including remote and indigenous populations. She holds a Master of Medical Science degree. Her research interest is "Yoga for Secondary Lymphoedema from Breast Cancer Treatment" and she has six peer-reviewed journal articles and two DVDs on this topic. She speaks at yoga, yoga therapy, and medical conferences and teaches on several yoga therapy courses around Australia. She is a self-employed IAYT-certified Yoga Therapist and Pilates therapist.

Lee Majewski (MA, PGDYEd, C-IAYT)

Lee is an author, researcher, and IAYT-certified Yoga Therapist with expertise in cancer care and psychosomatic chronic disease. She is founding director of Yoga for Health Institute, a non-profit organization located in Toronto, Canada, and a visiting Senior Yoga Therapist at Kaivalyadhama Yoga Institute in India. Her own journey through cancer brought home the value of ancient yogic methods and resulted in creating a unique healing retreat, Beyond Cancer, residential and online. As a result of program effectiveness and being the first of its kind, Beyond Cancer has received an influx of international recognition. She is the co-author of *Yoga Therapy as a Whole Person Approach to Health*.

Website: www.yogaforhealth.institute

Smitha Mallaiah (PhD(c), MSc, C-IAYT)

Smitha is a Senior Mind-Body Intervention Specialist and IAYT-certified Yoga Therapist at the University of Texas MD Anderson Cancer Center's Integrative Medicine Program, Department of Palliative, Rehabilitative and Integrative Medicine. She works alongside other integrative medicine clinicians using yoga therapy with inpatients and outpatients going through cancer, from diagnosis through end of life. She is involved in developing and teaching yoga research interventions for various cancer populations. She has co-authored yoga publications and presented her work at national and international conferences on the efficacy of yoga in cancer care. She is the Program Director for the Yoga Therapy Training Program at S-VYASA-USA, Houston, where she actively mentors students. She holds a Master of Science in Yoga Therapy from S-VYASA University, Bengaluru, India, where she is working on her PhD Yoga.

Website: www.vyasahouston.org

Sanmay Mukhopadhyay (PhD student, BSc, BTech, MTech, MBA, MSc, PGDYT, C-IAYT)

Sanmay grew up in a yogic culture and was initiated into Yoga using Bisthu Ghosh's traditions, attending many yoga lineages such as Iyengar, Vinyasa, Hatha Yoga, Bikram and Patajali Yoga. He is an IAYT-certified Yoga Therapist and teaches yoga, health/wellness and

disease management, specializing in ancient scriptures to create the foundation for the yogic journey. He holds a Masters of Science in Yoga from S-Vyasa University, Bengaluru, India and is pursuing the PhD Yoga. Sanmay launched a major yoga-based disease management app (free of charge) called "Dr Yogi," using creative modification techniques. Proceeds from his yoga therapy and general sessions go to helping underserved people in USA and India. Sanmay also works with homeless people in the USA, as well as differently-abled people. He designs corporate programs on stress and anxiety, and collaborates with clinics and hospitals on pain management, lung diseases, and cancer. His YouTube channel is appropriately called "The Techie Takie Yogi."
YouTube channel: www.youtube.com/channel/UC2YyZglpD12GHxaVm1iZdFw?

Bhavani Munamarty (CYT 500, RYS 200)
Bhavani is a Yoga Therapist and Trainer. She started her yoga journey primarily to relieve the back pain and mental stress resulting from a corporate job in the United States. Having experienced the many benefits of Yoga, she trained as an instructor and yoga therapist to deepen her knowledge and learn more about the therapeutic benefits of Yoga. Bhavani currently lives in India.
Website: www.unionyogaayurveda.com.sg

Lórien Neargarder (BSME, E-RYT 500, C-IAYT)
Lórien is the author of *Cancer + Yoga: For People Living with Cancer and Their Yoga Teachers, Healthcare Providers and Caregivers*. She has experience teaching yoga in a pain management clinic, in psychiatric wards and has worked with people with cancer, survivors and their caregivers throughout the San Francisco Bay area, California, and in Brevard County, Florida. She is an IAYT-certified Yoga Therapist, holds two 500-hour yoga certifications, completed 200 hours of Qigong training, and has certificates in therapeutic yoga, yoga4cancer, and cancer exercise. Lórien co-founded Complementary Cancer Care, a nonprofit that offers non-medical complementary therapies, including yoga, to people dealing with cancer, free of charge.

Website: www.yogabylorien.com

Charlotte Nuessle (BSc, RYT 500, C-IAYT)
Charlotte is an IAYT-certified Yoga Therapist and was a consultant with Leila J. Eisenstein Cancer Center, Providence Medford Medical Center. She developed and delivered a body and mind support group for women with a breast cancer diagnosis that focused on physical and emotional survivorship skills, while promoting a social network of safe connection. She blends three wisdom approaches: strengthen inner resources of resilience; evidence-based understandings of our nervous system; and therapeutic yoga applications. Charlotte is a contributing author to the book *The Key to Cancer*.
Website: www.charlottenuessle.com

Maryam Ovissi (E-RYT 500, C-IAYT)
Maryam is an IAYT-certified Yoga Therapist and the author of *Care of the Whole Self: Yoga Inspired Tools to Befriend the Self*. She studied in the lineage of Sri Krishnamacharya through the Mohans and Svastha Yoga Therapy. Maryam began her yoga career working with a cancer survivor. This prompted her interest in inviting trauma-informed yoga to befriend the journey with cancer. She is a Clinical Yoga Therapist with Life with Cancer, INOVA, offering Bedside Yoga Therapy. Maryam is the founder and chief caregiver of Beloved Yoga (studio and school) in Northern Virginia, and has had the privilege to share her craft through group and private sessions, as well as in conferences and clinical settings. She co-founded Befriending the Journey with Cancer, a unique program that bridges yoga and nutrition.
Website: www.maryamovissi.com

Miriam Patterson (MAT, MSJIR, C-IAYT)
Miriam holds both a Master of Arts in Teaching and a Master of Social Justice and Inter-Cultural Relations, and is an IAYT-Certified Yoga Therapist. She received teacher training with the Sivananda Ashram in Val Morin, Quebec, and certified yoga therapy training at Yoga Therapy Toronto, informed by the teachings of Desikachar and his teacher Krishnamacharya. Her style and approach to yoga is also influenced by the

teachings of Zen Buddhist monk and teacher Thich Nhat Hanh. Miriam's own experience with cancer led her to her private practice, as well as working closely with the Canadian College of Naturopathic Medicine Cancer Clinic, and designing and facilitating cancer retreats, as the Programmer at the Abbey Retreat Center (ARC) in Haliburton, Canada.
Website: www.practicewithmiriam.com

Tina Paul (MS, E-RYT 500, C-IAYT)
Tina is an IAYT-certified Yoga Therapist practicing at Memorial Sloan Kettering Cancer Center Integrative Medicine Services in New York City with patients undergoing cancer treatment and recovering from cancer, and their caregivers and is involved in an NIH-funded clinical trial examining the effect of yoga on chemotherapy-induced peripheral neuropathy. Tina holds a Master of Science in Yoga Therapy from the Maryland University of Integrative Health where she serves as adjunct faculty. She has also completed yoga4cancer training. She grew up with the philosophy of Yoga as shared by her family and is grateful for the opportunity to share this wisdom practice with others. She offers customized workshops for employee wellness and stress reduction, and also uses therapeutic yoga for chronic pain management.
Website: www.yogawithtina.com

Tari Prinster (RYT, C-IAYT)
Tari is a cancer survivor, IAYT-certified Yoga Therapist, author, and founder of yoga4cancer – a specific, safe and effective Oncology Yoga method that uses well-researched principles of yoga and physiology to reduce the side effects of cancer and its treatments. Tari's organization has trained professionals worldwide and supports research to assess the contributions of yoga in oncology. Her book *Yoga for Cancer: A Guide to Managing Side Effects, Boosting Immunity, and Improving Recovery for Cancer Survivors* is an illustrated guide for cancer survivors available in English, Spanish, and Japanese.
Website: www.yoga4cancer.com

Lois Ramondetta (MD, RYT 500, C-IAYT)
Lois is a physician, IAYT-certified Yoga Therapist, Professor, University of Texas MD Anderson Cancer Center in Houston, and the co-author of *The Light Within: If Not Now, When?* She is actively involved in research evaluating the effects of yoga therapy on the psychologic and physiologic experience of chemotherapy and radiation for cervical cancer treatment. Lois looks for opportunities to use yoga philosophy and techniques to help others reduce anxiety and depression and to find meaning and a sense of peace during difficult experiences.
Website: www.faculty.mdanderson.org/profiles/lois_ramondetta.html

Kiran Shenoy (CYT 500, RYT 500, E-RYT 200)
Kiran is a Yoga Therapist, an experienced Senior Yoga Trainer, and a Clinical Researcher in yoga and allied sciences. She is co-author of a yoga book, and has completed the Ayurveda Foundation Course (AFC) in Singapore. She lectures, and conducts one-to-one and couples therapy sessions at Union Yoga Ayurveda, Singapore.
Website: www.unionyogaayurveda.com.sg

Stella Snyder (PhD student, MSc, C-IAYT)
Stella is an IAYT-certified Yoga Therapist and teaches yoga and meditation to cancer patients. She is trained through Integral Yoga's Yoga Therapy for Cancer and Chronic Illness certification (YCat) and the Pranayoga Institute of Yoga and Holistic Health. Stella works in Behavioral Science Research at MD Anderson Cancer Center in Houston, Texas, as a Mind-Body Intervention Specialist and a Clinical Studies Coordinator and is pursuing her PhD.
Website: www.iayt.org/member/stellasnyder

Doreen Stein-Seroussi (MPA, MA, E-RYT, C-IAYT)
Doreen holds two Master's degrees, is an IAYT-certified Yoga Therapist, and is on the Board of Trustees of the Society for Integrative Oncology. She has provided evidence-informed, mind-body practices in a variety of

settings to help alleviate the symptoms and stresses associated with cancer and its treatment. Her 18 years in oncology have included being a founding yoga teacher for the Cancer Support Program at the Lineberger Comprehensive Cancer Center (University of North Carolina), providing in-patient and out-patient yoga therapy. She also spent 11 years providing yoga support at the Cornucopia Cancer Support Center and was a Board member for New Life After Cancer.

Michelle Stortz (MFA, E-RYT 500, YACEP, C-IAYT)
Michelle is an IAYT-certified Yoga Therapist specializing in yoga for cancer and chronic illness. She has designed two virtual courses for cancer survivors: *Stronger After Cancer* and *Finding Your Ground: Thriving with Metastatic Cancer*. Michelle works for Abramson Cancer Center at Pennsylvania Hospital (Penn Medicine); Fox Chase Cancer Center; Unite for Her; and Cancer Support Community of Greater Philadelphia. She is in private practice, conducting classes, retreats, and private sessions. Michelle also teaches meditation, drawing on both the Buddhist tradition and the Mindfulness-Based Stress Reduction curriculum.
Website: www.michellestortz.com

Jennifer Collins Taylor (MSW, CMP)
Jennifer holds a Master of Social Work focused on end-of-life and hospice care. She has over 900 hours of yoga therapy training, and is a certified music practitioner, bringing harp music to the bedside of the seriously ill. She is the author of *Living Life Dying Death: A Guide to Healthy Conversations About Death and Dying to Inspire Life and Living*, and creator of an instrumental harp CD *Life Beyond Words*, a source of relaxation, peace, comfort, joy and inspiration. Jennifer conducts presentations on the value and power of open, compassionate, nonjudgmental communications surrounding matters of life and death.
Website: www.jennifercollinstaylor.com

Robyn Tiger (MD, C-IAYT)
Robyn is a physician and IAYT-certified Yoga Therapist on a mission to empower others with self-care tools backed by science and research. She uniquely combines her years as a diagnostic radiologist with certifications in yoga therapy, meditation, and life coaching in her innovative accredited courses, group sessions, private coaching, and podcast (StressFreeMD) that focus on complete physical, mental, and emotional well-being and resilience. She is deeply passionate about helping others relieve stress, elevate calm, and live their best lives. She is lead faculty and subject matter expert in stress management for the American College of Lifestyle Medicine (ACLM).
Website: www.stressfreemd.net

Satyam Tripathi (BAMS, MD [Yoga and Rehab], E-RYT 500, C-IAYT)
Satyam is an Ayurveda and yoga therapy consultant, clinical integrative medicine physician and researcher, IAYT-certified Yoga Therapist, author and teacher of yoga, Ayurveda and allied holistic health science at Union Yoga Ayurveda, Complementary and Traditional Clinic, Singapore. His research interest is in exploring the effectiveness of holistic and innovative new techniques. Satyam's recent case reports are published in the *Journal of Integrative Medicine Case Reports* (JIMCR), an international peer-reviewed, open-access journal.
Website: www.unionyogaayurveda.com.sg

Tina Walter (BA, C-IAYT)
Tina is a YCat-trained, IAYT-certified Yoga Therapist, providing interventions in both Cincinnati and Northern Kentucky hospitals while people receive outpatient chemotherapy and inpatient care. She teaches yoga and meditation for the Cancer Support Community and is a speaker and published writer on yoga therapy and cancer.
Website: www.therapevoyoga.com

FOREWORD *by Lorenzo Cohen*

We are at an unprecedented time in the history of cancer medicine. We have a profound understanding about the causes of cancer and the multiple biological processes that are necessary to allow that one original mutated cell to grow and thrive in the body. This knowledge has led to treatment responses never seen before. In particular, the new immunotherapy-based checkpoint inhibitors, unleashing the power of the immune system, have resulted in actual "cures" in people with advanced disease that historically had dismal outcomes. Learning more about the key drivers of the carcinogenic processes allows for more targeted treatments and, importantly, reinforces the importance of a behavioral approach to cancer prevention and control.

It is clear that how we lead our lives – what we eat, how we manage our stress and face life's challenges, how physically active we are, our sleep habits, and how we interact with each other and the larger world – has a profound effect on our health and wellness and on cancer in particular. In fact, the evidence is clear that lifestyle factors influence all the cancer hallmarks, the biological processes that are necessary to control cancer growth. We now know that most cancers are linked with our lifestyle choices,[1] empowering us to engage in lifestyle habits to lower our risk of cancer, and, for those with cancer, to improve our quality of life and clinical outcomes.

My grandmother, Vanda Scaravelli, started her yoga practice later in life. I lived with her for a year in order to learn yoga, so I felt firsthand the power of yoga. It even formed the basis of my early research, which along with research from others showed that yoga helps cancer patients sleep better, improves mood and cognitive function, reduces fatigue, improves physical functioning, and helps to regulate stress hormones and immune function, among other benefits. At a deeper level, we find that yoga can increase our ability to find meaning in the illness experience and helps to transform our lives. As Vanda wrote in her book

Awakening the Spine: Yoga for Health, Vitality, and Energy: "It [yoga] is a living process that changes moment by moment, watching when we eat, how we eat, when we walk, how we walk, what we say and how we say it. All these things must be present in us and we must be passionately interested in them all."[2] Yoga, a quintessential mind-body practice, when approached as a lifestyle, is the ideal way to prevent cancer and improve outcomes for those with cancer.

Yoga can be used throughout the cancer experience from diagnosis to survivorship as well as alongside end-of-life care. The evidence on yoga for people with cancer is so compelling that the National Comprehensive Cancer Network Clinical Practice Guidelines in Oncology now recommends yoga in managing cancer-related fatigue and treatment-related nausea/vomiting, and suggests to "consider" yoga for distress (anxiety/depression/trauma), pain, cognitive function, and menopausal symptoms. Similar recommendations are found in the joint Society for Integrative Oncology and American Society of Clinical Oncology guidelines for the use of integrative therapies during and after breast cancer treatment. Now that the evidence is in and the clinical guidelines for oncology all say that yoga is an important modality, we need to understand how to safely incorporate yoga into our healthcare system. That is where Leigh Leibel and Anne Pitman's exceptional book *Yoga Therapy Across the Cancer Care Continuum* comes in.

In *Yoga Therapy Across the Cancer Care Continuum*, we learn that a deep yoga practice can play a role at all stages of the cancer care continuum from prevention and early detection to before, during, and after treatment. We learn how yoga can help us listen to our bodies. We meet Joana (p. 83) and learn that her body awareness through yoga allowed her to feel the presence of an early stage breast cancer, even when it was barely detectable on a mammogram. Through my own yoga practice, and literally during a morning session, I noticed a strange sensation in my armpit leading

[1]Cohen L, Jefferies A. *Transform Your Life and Health with the Mix of Six*, New York, Viking (Penguin Random House), 2018.

[2]Scaravelli V. *Awakening the Spine: Yoga for Health, Vitality, and Energy*, 2nd ed. London: Pinter & Martin, 2012.

FOREWORD *continued*

to a diagnosis of melanoma. I followed the tenets of a yogic lifestyle, along with surgery and immunotherapy. It is now more than 4 years later, and I am healthier than when I was diagnosed with cancer. We know that a yogic lifestyle can reduce the incidence of most cancers and, having increased body awareness, can further allow earlier diagnosis leading to better long-term survival for those diagnosed with cancer.

Expertly written and curated with leading voices from multiple areas of yoga in oncology, *Yoga Therapy Across the Cancer Care Continuum* provides the reader with all the necessary information to understand how to safely and effectively incorporate yoga into cancer care. The combination of science alongside practical applications and the real-world examples of yoga therapists working with people across the cancer care continuum leaves the reader with an unprecedented knowledge base from which to learn. We know yoga can improve all aspects of our lives. Now it is time to incorporate yoga into all stages of the cancer continuum.

Lorenzo Cohen, PhD

Professor and Director, Integrative Medicine Program

The University of Texas MD Anderson Cancer Center

Co-author *Anticancer Living: Transform Your Life and Health with the Mix of Six*

April 20, 2022, Houston, Texas

ACKNOWLEDGMENTS *by Leigh Leibel*

As I began writing Chapter 4 of this book, my partner was diagnosed with stage II colon cancer. Through ten grueling months of treatment, Yoga helped us both find peace. I spent that difficult year at the hospital bedside, in chemotherapy and radiation suites, and when not allowed in the hospital due to Covid-19, in the back seat of my car in the parking garage. It was in these sacred spaces of healing that this book was written. With deepest respect, I acknowledge the frontline healthcare providers, including yoga therapists, who continued to provide loving, compassionate care during the Covid-19 global pandemic. Their grace imbues our pages.

This book rests on the shoulders of changemakers. I thank the National Cancer Institute (NCI) for my summer fellowship in cancer prevention and control. NCI gave me the unbelievable opportunity to join a cohort of fellows from 35 countries to study with some of the world's most prominent cancer scientists, researchers, and clinicians. It was life-changing and the genesis of this book. I am indebted to Charles and Kristin Flood and Phil and Judy DiBella for their generous philanthropy in support of my clinical work and research at Columbia University Irving Medical Center. Thanks to them, I have the privilege of working with Columbia's best: Dr Greg Mears, Dr Craig Blinderman, Dr Ian Sadler, Dr Azra Raza, Dr Siddhartha Mukherjee, Dr Gary Schwartz. I am privileged to have had extraordinary mentors at the Society for Integrative Oncology, where I serve on the Board of Trustees: Dr Lorenzo Cohen, Dr Santosh Rao, Dr Eleanor Walker, Dr Linda Carlson, Dr Eugene Ahn, Dr Ting Bao, Dr Heather Greenlee, Dr Donald Abrams, Dr Judith Lacey, Dr Gabriel Lopez, Dr Channing Paller, Dr Ana Maria Lopez, Dr Jun Mao, Dr Lynda Balneaves, Dr David Rosenthal. Their example has enriched my life. Without them, this book would not be possible. I am grateful for my beautiful co-editor Anne Pitman, our 38 contributing authors, our commissioning editor Sarena Wolfaard, and John Kepner and Alyssa Wostrel at International Association of Yoga Therapists. They helped make the dream come true. For my dear Greg and Joyce, thank you for always being there. To my beloved India; to Dr Nagendra, Dr Nagarathna, Dr Manjunath, Dr Raghavendra; to my esteemed professors, colleagues, and classmates at S-VYASA University and Ministry of AYUSH — *Dhanyavaad Bharat, mujhe itni mulyavaan shiksha dene ke liye, main aabhaari rahungi. Thank you for the gift of Yoga.* May we awaken to inequity and strive to make Yoga accessible for the well-being of all people worldwide touched by cancer.

tat tvam asi

तत् त्वम् असि

ACKNOWLEDGMENTS *by Anne Pitman*

I lay this book at the feet of those dear souls who have crossed the threshold of my yoga-office door, bless their good hearts. I pray that our book is a testimony to their endured hardship and strong spirited love. In both their living and dying, they have shown me the beauty of saying yes to it all.

I bow to my teachers, practitioners of human skillfulness and radical guides of scholarship and wonder: Stephen and Nathalie and fellow scholars at the Orphan Wisdom School, determined witnesses to the slow spin of a starry night; Sarah and Dugald and my dedicated colleagues at the Ottawa Integrative Cancer Centre, generous companions on the dream-path of equity, accessiblity and integration. To the sprightly ones who kindled my early interest in yoga: Joy, Irene and Vanda, I remember you well and fondly. To the ones who revealed the door to cancer-care; gratitude to Jane and Jennifer.

I leaned, sometimes heavily, upon many during this writing: Cassi, my dedicated and brilliant Co-Director, who lent much needed philosophy counsel and who shepherds our school so beautifully; our determined students and inspired faculty, for birthing clarity and continued wonder; Jan and Lisa, who endured numerous drafts and walking rants with heart-ears open, succinct suggestions and good humour; and Charlie who came to my rescue with her usual artistic brilliance My thanks to John for his kind invitation to present the Continuum at SYTAR; to fellow determined yoga therapists and staff at IAYT (keep going!); to Sarena and her team at Handspring for abundant patience and profound kindness; and deep gratitude also to Claire, Emma and Stephanie for adroitly picking up the reins. To Leigh, my inspired and stalwart co-editor and our accomplished contributors, I bow again and again; your determined and purposeful work enlivens this book.

To kith and kin, the seen and unseen, I offer not this book, but the rest of me. To Walter and Ida, sibs and "spice"; deepest gratitude for early attunement in beauty, kindness and care. To faithful friends, precious littles and heart-daughters: apologies for my bleary-eyed absence, may we be blessed with more days yet. For my cherished sons, Jared, Kieran and Noah and their dear partners, Emily, Charlie and Taylor, and for our beloved Elliot and Hamish, my devotion: any regret from time stolen is sweet remembrance of your enduring place in my heart and our fortunate entwined lives. For my man, Jamie, walking along the cancer continuum with rare perspective and profound strength; never so far, my love, never so far.

Introduction

Anne Pitman and Leigh Leibel

This book was born of community. What you hold in your hands is no one person's sudden flash of brilliance, or the result of any singular startling insight. Instead, it is a collective response of purpose-driven people answering the clarion call of *dharma*, yoga therapists in service to people who are, each day, facing a disease that continues to challenge and mystify us all – cancer.

In the spring of 2018, Leigh and I (Anne) were invited to facilitate a Common Interest Community (CIC) for Cancer at our annual International Association of Yoga Therapy conference (called SYTAR, Symposium on Yoga Therapy and Research). That day, as each therapist stood to speak, the hotel ballroom faded away and we were transported to the doctor's office, the infusion room, the studio, patients' homes and bedsides, as they spoke of their compassionate work with children, teens, couples and families. We listened, stilled, to tales from the shock of diagnosis to tender attendance at death. Stories were told of adaptive and accessible yoga practice, one-on-one and small group sessions, working with anxiety, lymphedema, neuropathy, fear of recurrence and all manner of client experience, in the throes of cancer. That day, we considered integrative possibilities across the globe, gleaned from those who work side by side with other oncology practitioners in psychotherapy, physiotherapy, nutrition, pain-care and more. The audience, yoga practitioners themselves, diverse in culture, lineage (or post lineage) and approach, leaned in to hear every detail, nodding with a deep acceptance, respect and shared understanding of yoga-based care; the art, science and poetry in service to the humanity and well-being of those walking with cancer.

With the last of the speakers' stories spilled, yoga therapists rose from their seats, newly determined to bring yoga therapy as a central support where they live and work. Amongst the tears and the laughter, we also considered the challenges of our profession – most notably, the need for yoga therapy, supported by research and advanced education, to be better understood by allied healthcare professionals, and more visible and available to all in oncology care.

As the session wrapped up, we just couldn't pull ourselves away from the charged atmosphere of inspiration. We lingered and shared contact information. As sometimes happens in life, "right person, right time, right place" coalesces. Sarena Wolfaard, a publisher with Handspring, and a witness to the passion and testimony of the day, introduced herself to Leigh and myself and with one simple sentence opened the door to our continuing work together: "You know", she said, "I think this could be a great book, don't you?"

Out went the call for stories from the front lines of yoga therapy. Proposals, drafts and revisions were received, until 38 contributors were chosen to offer their clients' experiences of cancer and yoga therapy. As we edited, Leigh and I, moved by each client story, began to add the context of what couldn't be expressed in a series of highlights: the role of yoga therapy in integrative care, current research and critical cancer knowledge, responsive safe practice and practical considerations, and the necessity of community self-care. As an overview, here is how we crafted the chapters.

Chapter Two – Yoga therapy in oncology: an embodied map of care
Anne Pitman

In clinical practice, I find myself regularly describing yoga therapy to both clients and colleagues in integrative cancer care. Let's just say, it is not well understood. I often have to dissuade people of the notion that it involves gymnastic poses and handstands with cancer patients. In this book we hope to reveal what oncological yoga therapy really is: therapists carrying an advanced education and knowledge of current research, married with profound and in-depth yogic and therapeutic training. All this within the possibility of compassionate integrative care.

To bring clarity, I suggested we represent yoga therapy as a seven-pointed map, something I created to use with students in our yoga therapy school, when they too, at the beginning of their studies, wonder what yoga therapy entails. It maps out the embodiment of a yoga therapist in a room with a client, the knowledge, research and wonderment required, the therapeutic skills and yogic "tools" needed and the vast humanity that is offered in each practice. While we have found it to be a useful visual to describe the complexity of yoga therapy to those outside of the profession, it is particularly useful for students in tracking their learning, enabling them to point to places on the map where they are already strong and places where they need more support.

In Chapter 2 we take some time to consider the skills of our trade, the yogic and "therapy" aspects of yoga therapy. As an overview and context for Chapter 6, we point to the diversity in yoga philosophy, lineage and/or approach and consider worldwide education, research literacy and necessary cancer-specific education. In this chapter we define, explain, and explore Sanskrit terms that are used elsewhere in the book (primarily Chapter 6), employing primary and secondary sources when possible.

Also included on the yoga therapy map is "integration," a hot topic in healthcare. There are many differing definitions. This interpretation is based on my former position as Integration Manager in an integrative cancer center in Canada, where we collaborate between the practitioners in the center (shared notes, waivers, resources and referrals between nurses, doctors, naturopaths, nutritionists, etc.) and integrate our work with our local hospital (shared medical records and client referrals/notes with oncologists). This specific form of teamwork and alliance is not easy and requires sustained effort, continuous conversations, and persistent bolstering of financial support. Critically, it requires a rare mindset in practitioners. To support best therapeutic and medical care for our

clients, and to contribute the eventual inclusion of yoga therapy as standard practice in integrated cancer care, we include this topic as worthy for your consideration.

Chapter Three – Yoga therapy in clinical practice: practicalities
Anne Pitman

In accepting each contributor's summary of session highlights (instead of formal case studies), we knew that there was a context, unwritten, supporting each story. In this chapter, we show a yoga therapist's accountability, and all the work and consideration required before, during and after the session, such as scope of practice, code of ethics, consent, assessments, notes, referrals, waivers and insurance, within local legal stipulations. As our profession evolves toward licensure, there will be more to consider, but we start here, now. We also touch briefly on resourcing ourselves in practice. Rather than only a singular focus, we view this as community self-care: how do we take care of each other (including other healthcare workers) in what can be very challenging (and ultimately fulfilling) work?

Chapter Four – Understanding cancer and its treatment
Leigh Leibel

Cancer is a fantastically complex family of diseases that affects millions of people worldwide. In 2020 alone, nearly 20 million people globally were diagnosed with cancer, and the incidence of cancer cases is projected to increase by 50% within the next two decades. Current cancer statistics suggest that two out of every three men, and one out of every three women worldwide will be diagnosed with cancer at some point in their lives. So, what *is* cancer?

In Chapter 4 we explore cancer basics including the biology of the disease, its natural history of progression, treatment and adverse events, and disparity in the access and delivery of cancer care. This chapter gives us a first glimpse into the unique challenges inherent in the safe delivery of yoga to oncology and medically fragile populations, and provides context for our contributing

Introduction

authors' patient/client stories presented in Chapter 6.

Chapter Five – The biological intersection of yoga and cancer
Leigh Leibel

For those of us who regularly practice yoga, we know that we feel pretty good after a yoga class! But *how* does yoga work impact our physiology and pathophysiology?

In Chapter 5 we'll briefly touch on DNA and gene expression, microenvironment and the immune system, inflammation, stress and the autonomic nervous system, and the evidence base for yoga's favorable effect on these various processes and its basis for cancer prevention and supportive care.

Chapter Six – Yoga in the cancer care continuum
Edited by Leigh Leibel and Anne Pitman

Cancer and its treatment are well known to cause local or systemic adverse events that can have a significant impact on the mind, body, and spirit of people with cancer, survivors, and their families at all stages of the cancer care continuum. Side effects may present during treatment or in the months or years after completion. A strong and growing evidence base shows yoga can improve quality of life and well-being for those facing cancer, mitigate many of the physical and psychological side effects of cancer and its treatment, and positively impact clinical outcomes.

In Chapter 6 we look at yoga in practice and introduce our 38 contributing authors and their patient/client stories. These stories are the *raison d'être* of the book: the *sūtra* or thread that weaves the art and science of yoga into a garland of practices across the cancer care continuum. Informed by the best empirical evidence and clinical experience, these stories show us that customized yoga therapy sessions can support mind, body, and spirit at *every* phase of the cancer care continuum – from diagnosis, treatment, post-treatment, recurrence, to

end of life. Information is presented within the context of delivering a safe, effective, accessible yoga practice to patients and survivors at all stages of care. Included throughout the chapter are editorial backgrounds on side effects and chief complaints, yoga research, information boxes, and points to remember during a yoga practice.

This section is a team effort, a collaboration with each of the 38 contributing authors. We, the editors, worked together to select each author from a pool of international candidates and edit their stories for publication. To support the stories, we adopted a cancer continuum model that Leigh designed during a fellowship at the National Cancer Institute (NCI) which was presented to and endorsed by peers at the Society for Integrative Oncology (SIO) 15th International Conference, *From Research to Practical Application*. The model is designed to be a dynamic circle of healing for yoga in oncologic care that provides continuity of patient care across the continuum and emphasizes health equity and inclusion of all people.

To provide scientific and medical context for the stories, Leigh wrote the editorial content for the chapter, including the introduction to the continuum and each of its five phases, as well as many of the backgrounds that precede each of the contributor stories (unless otherwise noted).

Chapter Seven – Yoga therapy in oncologic care: the way forward
Leigh Leibel

Chapter 7 is not the end of the story, rather, it is the beginning: a call for our global health delivery systems to prioritize the well-being of all people affected by cancer and to formally integrate yoga into standard oncologic care.

In this chapter we propose three next steps toward building a new and equitable paradigm in cancer survivorship. The goal is to positively impact health and economy at both national and global levels. Our mission aligns with and supports the World Health Organization (WHO) Sustainable Development Goal (SDG) #3 – *To ensure healthy lives and promote well-being for all at all ages.*

Editorial decisions and considerations

Use of Sanskrit (*Saṃskṛtam*)

Every book on yoga therapy must make decisions on how to respectfully communicate yoga's history, concepts, and practices to a wide audience; in this case, an audience primarily familiar with English and the language of healthcare. What is the proper etiquette, we wondered, when we are, hopefully, awake to the consequences of appropriation and commodification, and yet strive to cultivate just and inclusive approaches to the diversities embedded in culture, language, and practice? We considered deeply and consulted widely, deciding to employ the International Alphabet of Sanskrit Transliteration (IAST). Additionally, all Sanskirt (*samskṛtam*) terms are italicized. Thus, for example, breath-work is noted as *prāṇāyāma.*

Many Sanskrit words familiar to English speakers, such as *mantra*, *mudrā*, or *dharma*, are set out using diacritics (marks above or below a letter to indicate pronunciation), and italicized. The word "yoga," however, is an exception. Yoga (from the root, *yuj*) has, through a storied history, found its way into the everyday English lexicon. As such, it is generally not italicized with other Sanskrit words in yoga therapy textbooks. It is, however, sometimes capitalized. Most commonly, it is capitalized when it is a proper noun or when referring to one of the six Vedic schools (*ṣaḍdarśana*) of Indian philosophy. In the absence of any definitive guide, we have left the decision of capitalization to each author. Quotations, then, maintain each author's use of capitalization and Sanskrit (*samskṛtam*).

Considerations nothwithstanding, it is reductive to say that a word in any language means only this one particular word in another. Surely meaning is contextual, culturally embedded and nuanced. Still, we hope our choices may be received as a sign of a deep and humble respect for our authors, for the roots of Yoga (may they be watered well with our gratitude) and for the evolving practices of yoga and yoga therapy.

Use of descriptors

We live in a multicultural world and language is continually evolving. In this book we have chosen to follow the *Diversity Style Guide* (DSG) for person-centered language when using terms and phrases related to race/ethnicity, religion, sexual orientation and gender identity (see more on p. 80).

"Client" vs "patient": which term is best employed? Certified yoga therapists (C-IAYTs) utilize the term *"client"* when speaking of the person(s) they are working with. However, given that many oncological yoga therapists are imbedded in healthcare, they share the language of their colleagues, using *"patient"* more commonly. In this book we interchange the terms for inclusivity, and the contributors employ whichever term is in harmony with their workplace.

Lastly, while this book is mainly oriented toward those who are educated in and practice *yoga therapy*, we honor the *yoga teachers* who have invested considerable effort, dedication and time in advanced education in order to bring yoga to people facing cancer. We include you as respected colleagues, vital to increasing cancer care accessibility. Our future is with you, as a community of caring and engaged yoga professionals, working together to be of compassionate service to those facing cancer.

Yoga Therapy in Oncology: An Embodied Map of Care

Anne Pitman

Preface and prayer

What is yoga therapy? How does it support someone facing cancer? We come to these questions slowly, as though sitting now with a distraught client. As we breathe and offer compassion to the person in front of us, what are the many directions of engagement, care and support we might call upon? How does a therapist carry the breadth and depth of yoga, offering safe and steady accompaniment to someone enduring the steady winds of cancer, suddenly lost, blown off their well-trodden life path? Figure 2.1 is a map of yoga therapy embedded in oncology care, illustrating the landscape of intricate, intimate and intelligent work. In the nascent and growing field of yoga therapy, may it provide context, orientation and humble direction, sure footing for our personal work and our profession, beginning with a deep bow to those facing cancer.

In essence, the map:

1. **Orients a yoga therapist's knowledge, skills and devotion.** In any given session, each therapist has at their back a deep and enduring support: their own treasured understanding of yoga philosophy, current yoga and oncology research, and their vast education in yoga therapy, including a studied knowledge of cancer, its requisite treatments and its full body influence. All of this knowledge, kept alive by a dedication to wonder and curiosity, can be called upon. At their sides are the therapeutic tools of deep connection and the vast wealth of accessible yoga practices, ready and waiting, curated for each unique client. Also in the room is an often-unrecognized resource: the therapist themselves, offering a relationship of shared, equitable power. Within each therapist is a practiced and authentic presence, born in part of dedicated yoga practice, which fundamentally informs the session with a purposeful willingness to offer steady and available connection. Any of these resources

may be sensitively employed to help reduce distress and all-encompassing suffering. May this map offer the sense of safety and containment needed for such vulnerable and compassionate human work.

2. **Keeps our client in the center, encircled.** The center of a yoga therapist's devotion is the well-being of their client in the midst of the undulating and uncertain experience that ripples out from that one unforgettable moment of a cancer diagnosis. May this map highlight a depth of holistic inquiry and interconnected care, enhancing the relationship the client has with themselves, the depth of their inner resources, the engagement in their health, and all that might be brought to bear in a widening circle (including their loved ones, community resources, healthcare team, and the cultural milieu), to nourish them as they navigate the cancer continuum.

3. **Makes yoga therapy more visible in integrative cancer care, worldwide.** While many yoga therapists have already secured careers in healthcare, many more wish to join integrated teams. To be stitched into the fabric of healthcare, we must do more than simply insist upon our place at the integrative table. Instead, let us continue to craft a confident, yet humble approach, one that demonstrates a clear scope of practice, ethical guidelines, rigorous research, evidence-informed practices, client referrals, and steady professional practices, including accountability, assessments and clinical notes. In clinics, in hospitals, in infusion rooms, may we continue to offer gratitude to our oncology allies, seeing the humanity in each other and the compassion and dedication we share.

4. **Provides the context of the stories herein.** In these pages, 38 yoga professionals share the stories of their clients, a highlighted recount of their time together. These therapists are faithful witnesses to shock, fear, grief, determination and love, as they work side by

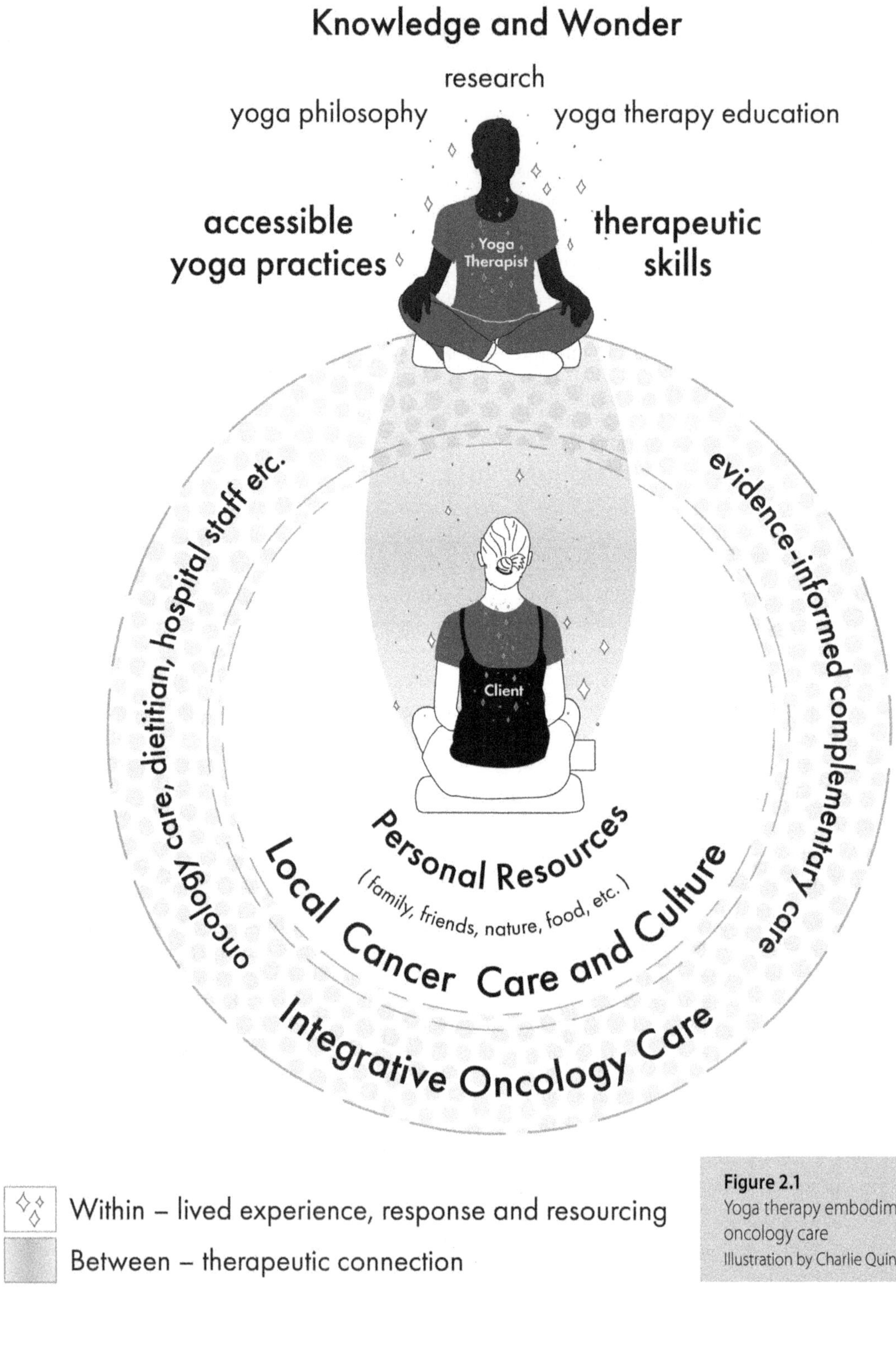

Knowledge and Wonder

research

yoga philosophy   yoga therapy education

**accessible
yoga practices**   Yoga
Therapist   **therapeutic
skills**

oncology care, dietitian, hospital staff etc.

evidence-informed complementary care

Client

Personal Resources
(family, friends, nature, food, etc.)

Local Cancer Care and Culture

Integrative Oncology Care

◇ Within – lived experience, response and resourcing

Between – therapeutic connection

Figure 2.1
Yoga therapy embodiment in
oncology care
Illustration by Charlie Quinn

side with their clients, bringing the uniquely accessible practices of yoga to lessen the suffering that often comes, gale strength, in the wake of a cancer diagnosis. Though their approaches, specific teachings and therapeutic methods may vary in kind, surely their skill born of true-hearted dedication shines. May this map lift the veil, to reveal the beauty of this practice, born of breath and wonder. And may their good work, practical, personal and professional, be truly helpful in kindling human kindness and reducing suffering, for those companionable travelers along the path of the cancer continuum.

At the yoga therapist's back: knowledge and wonder

Yoga philosophy

Cancer. Its discovery shatters normalcy and shakes us to the core. In a moment our life is wholly altered, and we're swept into a steady stream of appointments, decisions and tests. Only when there's a pause in the flood and flurry do we stop and wonder, "What just happened?"

For some, parsing existential questions is a scholarly quest. For the rest of us, our day-to-day busyness is rarely suspended long enough to wonder about the big questions in life. We don't stop until we are made to stop. But along the road of the cancer continuum, in the teeth of shock, whilst enduring seemingly endless chemo treatments, or deep in the heavy fatigue of radiation therapy, questions arise: What does this all mean, this fear, this uncertainty, this suffering? Who am I? Why am I here? What will become of me?

Surely there is good company in human wonderment. The study of philosophy brings with it a remembrance of the human heart beating through the ages: a companionship through time with those who have walked before us. Library shelves are heavy with tomes that delve into yoga's rich history, its diversity and the current scholarly wrestling with the meaning and potential steadfastness of ancient texts in modern life (Mallinson & Singleton 2017, Maas et al. 2018). Texts have been sourced across

the Indian sub-continent from the *ṛgveda*, (commonly known as the Rig Veda, said to be the earliest of the *Veda-s*), the *Upaniṣad-s* (Upanishads), the *bhagavadgītā* (Bhagavad Gītā), the *sāṁkhyakārikā* (*Sāṁkhya Kārikā*), *pātañjalayogaśāstra* (*Pātañjali's Yoga Sūtra-s*), and many more. Scholars continue rigorous discourse and study, and practitioners, turning to these texts time and again, seek guidance and search for meaning in order to navigate the challenges of life.

A cancer diagnosis can swiftly dislocate us and alter meaning. As we try to orient, we sometimes find that we've lost faith in our body, thoughts and beliefs. Perhaps akin to people that came before us who have felt similarly adrift, our uneasy questions intensify. When we find ourselves speaking to our oncologist about the disease, and the impact of its treatment upon us, we are considering *prakṛti*, or that which changes, including all the substantive aspects of this world – humans, animals, and all matter (Feuerstein 2008). But in the middle of the night, when the unwelcome question arises, "What if I die of this cancer?," we fumble towards that which is enduring, *puruṣa*, translated as witness, transcendental self, soul, or spirit (Mainkar 1972, Feuerstein 2008). In life, and when in the grip of suffering, the yogic path toward *mokṣa*, or liberation, is to contemplate, realize and come to know *puruṣa* (Mainkar 1972). These restless questions that keep us sleepless at night bring us to the heart of human wondering. A worthy companion in the wondering, come the light of day, is a yoga therapist.

So, what philosophy does a yoga therapist study? Is there one yoga philosophy that they carry, from patient to esteemed patient? On these questions, there is agreement: no. Authors and scholars, such as James Mallinson and Mark Singleton in *Roots of Yoga*, examine the possibility that there is no one singular root to what many consider "traditional yoga" (Mallinson & Singleton 2017). Yoga philosophy is rich, complex, full of contrasts and diversity and, for many of us, deep guidance. Given the cancer-focused scope of this book, please allow your wider philosophical curiosities to guide you toward the plethora of sources, primary and secondary where possible, as we have done here – breadcrumbs along the footpaths long traveled. Additionally, we suggest you rely upon extensive and well-received recent works to guide further passage along the varied pathways of modern yoga therapy (Finlayson & Hyland Robertson 2021, Majewski & Bhavanani 2020, Sullivan & Hyland Robertson 2020).

What follows, in brief, and with a deep bow to the teachers and scholars whose footprints we follow, are a few examples: a look at some of the distilled and abiding considerations and conversations that continue to arise and inform yoga therapy work in healthcare, frequently discussed at the integrative table in cancer care. When an oncologist leans in to ask, "So, how does yoga philosophy guide you when working with the fear and suffering that seems to be endemic in cancer?," what might you say, from your own studies of yoga philosophy? Arranged not by chronology, lineage or school of thought, neither fulsome nor didactic, the following are some of the philosophical threads, primarily sourced from the *Yoga Sūtra-s*, plied together from many cited sources and diverse understandings, and deftly woven by our contributors in Chapter 6.

Do no harm

In common with our medical colleagues, "do no harm" is a guiding principle in yoga. *Ahiṃsā*, translated as "non-violence," is one of the key virtues to many Indic religions, explored in many different texts, and the first stated moral restraint/rule in the *Yoga Sūtra-s*, the foundational study of ethics and part of *aṣṭāṅga* or the eightfold yogic path (Mallinson & Singleton 2017). *Ahiṃsā* is practiced at the level of body, speech and mind (Leggett 2018), and in our determination to both protect and empower our clients, we proceed with the utmost sensitivity, consciousness and conscientiousness for their well-being. Through our actions and considerations of all restraints (*yama-s*) and observances (*niyama-s*), we cultivate clarity in our relationships, and a sincere and compassionate (*karuṇa*) concern for others and their welfare (Hartranft 2003, Roy & Charlton 2019).

In practice, a therapist's attuned moral compass (with a lived practice of *yama-s* and *niyama-s* and professional accountability) is guided to speak the truth/be honest (*satya*) in communication (Mukerji 1983, Roy & Charlton 2019) and refrain from *asteya*, taking or stealing (Bryant 2009); in therapy, this may reflect a trusting and allowing of their client's experience (Roy & Charlton 2019). Also, following the *yama-s*, one is meant to consider *brahmacarya*, a wise employment of energy and attention (Roy & Charlton 2019), perhaps driving healthy boundaries, and refrainment from *aparigraha*, or acquisition, gathering only what is essential in a session (Bryant 2009, Roy & Charlton 2019). Those following a yogic path also observes *śauca*, cleanliness, *santoṣa*, contentment, and *tapas*, practice and discipline (Bryant 2009, Roy & Charlton 2019). A willingness for contemplation or self-study, *svādhyāya* (Roy & Charlton 2019) is viewed as essential, as is our willingness to yield to that which is outside of our control, *iśvāra praṇidhāna*. Some would refer to this as "trusting the process", or a devotion/surrender of all action to "Iśvara/God"/or a higher power (Bryant 2009, Mukerji 1983, Roy & Charlton 2019, Rukmani 2001).

An important aspect of "do no harm," though, is to recognize, intention aside, when harm has been done. In a Western claim on yoga, it's all there: the brutality of colonialism and commodification of spiritual teachings. Surely we must pause in the wake of our challenged awareness, reflect and be truly altered by what we have recently learned, and make amends, if at all possible. This includes the acknowledgment of abuse (Remski 2019), engagement in the work to "decolonize" Western yoga, honoring indigenous and traditional practices, and the inclusion of "post-lineage" viewpoints (Wildcroft 2020). Among us, we move toward better understandings of appropriation, differences and diversity, and work to ensure equity in our profession, a humble approach in our practice and a skillfulness in advocacy for our clients. *Ahiṃsā*, then, becomes guidance, redeemed and awakened through discourse and action, underpinning all we do.

Holistic care

Current research shows that many cancer patients are interested in holistic models of care (see Resourcing through integration of cancer care, p. 27). Rather than a (medically necessary) reductive focus on a physical diagnosis alone, yoga philosophy considers a person's experience to be complex, as represented by the many *kośa-s* (layers or sheaths), from the physical to the spiritual. Employing an historic and enduring biopsychosocial-spiritual focus, the possibilities of interrelated yoga practices explore, support and nourish the layers of the physical body/the sheath consisting of *annamaya* (food), the energetic/life-force/ the sheath consisting of *prāṇamaya* (breath), feelings, thoughts, emotions, and memory/the sheath consisting of *manomaya* (mind), discernment/the sheath consisting of *vijñānamaya* (understanding), and spirit/the sheath consisting of *ānandamaya* (bliss) (Bachman 2010, Feuerstein 2008, Müller 1897).

These are concentric layers of the human, accessed through self-inquiry (Deussen 1906), and in a modern context, through felt sense (Butera & Elgelid 2017). Getting to know and understand each *kośa*, from the *annamaya* (gross layer) to *ānandamaya* (subtle sheath), puts us in touch with *ātman* (or *puruṣa*, in this context), the self/consciousness/soul (Bachman 2010, Feuerstein 2008, Müller 1897). When a patient's presenting issue is "physical," for example, neurological pain, a yoga therapist (having read clinical notes that show the patient is well supported by pharmacological pain medication), may, with their client, consider all other influences that may be contributing to the pain. Not infrequently, a session veers toward conversations of spirituality, as a diagnosis of cancer can stimulate a fresh focus on religion or, from a secular or atheistic viewpoint, kindle a keen interest in meaning-making or life purpose.

Relationship and interconnection

Human life is interdependent and complex. *Ayurveda*, one of the indigenous medical sciences of India (Feuerstein 2008) suggests that we, like all of nature, are woven together into a symbiotic rhythm: an inherited sharing of the elements of life (air, water, earth, fire and space, or ether). *Vāta* (air and ether), *pitta* (fire and water) and *kapha* (water and earth) are "combinations of the five elements that manifest in patterns in all creation" (Lad 2002, p. 30). The *doṣa-s* (*vāta*, *pitta*,

kapha) are combinations of these elements, "the binding of the five elements into living flesh" (Lad 2002, p. 29). Much like the swaying and rebalancing inherent in tree pose (*vṛkṣāsana*), we come in and out of equilibrium throughout our days, the seasons and our life. When in a state of *vikṛti* (imbalance), through "diet, lifestyle interventions and yogic practice, one can start to come back 'home' to their *prakṛti* by honoring the elements and qualities that naturally bring about homeostasis" (Rudman in Finlayson & Hyland Robertson 2021, p. 81).

Clearly, we are deeply interconnected with nature and with each other. While the direct impact of a cancer diagnosis may rest within the patient, relationships are often impacted: the one within themselves, and with caregivers and community, including their healthcare team. While some go it alone, many cancer patients find they learn to lean into this sudden support – casseroles at the door, offers for rides to hospital treatments, walks with friends in the beauty and solace of nature.

The work of yoga therapy is relational. Especially in those difficult moments along the cancer care continuum, yoga therapy directs us to nourish and help resource our patient through caring relationships, human and beyond, building a supportive and steady kinship. More broadly, this awareness of interconnection can enhance professional integration throughout oncology. Instead of silos of care, health practitioners reach out to learn each other's practices and, with generosity of spirit, refer intelligently.

Awareness and self-knowledge

In the midst of daily cancer chaos, it can be extremely challenging to notice much at all, never mind one's unique and understandable reactions to a diagnosis, testing, treatments, and prognosis. *Avidyā*, defined broadly, is perhaps best described as not seeing things as they are, a lack of awareness, wrong cognition or ignorance (Bachman 2010, Leggett 2018, Mukerji 1983, Rukmani 2001). This lack of awareness is said to be one of five "taints" or afflictions (*kleśa-s*) (Leggett 2018, Mukerji 1983, Rukmani 2001). Much of our immediate reaction, after receiving a diagnosis, is entirely and understandably about fighting or escaping the current reality. The compassionate work of yoga therapy is to help someone, when they are ready, to see more clearly (*vidyā*). With time and accompaniment, patients begin to observe their lived experience with cancer and their *saṃskāra-s*; responses, patterns or habits (Bachman 2010), without judgment. Awareness practice, however, need not be insistent; it is more invitation than demand. The willingness to acknowledge what is happening, even for one breath, often resonates as a truthfulness, and brings with it a resultant surprising ease.

Acknowledge and reduce suffering

Cancer patients are stressed: physically (feeling weak, nauseated and in pain, for example), mentally (unable to think or focus), emotionally (feelings of anger, sadness and fear) or spiritually (loss of purpose or connection, unable to feel contented or joyful). They almost certainly will assume there is something wrong with their reactions and response. After all, everyone else seems to be "thriving."

Duḥkha is referred to throughout many yoga texts as pain, feelings of discomfort, distress, frustration, aversion and suffering (Bachman 2010, Bryant 2009, Feuerstein 2008, Rukmani 2001). Underneath much of the suffering that is sustained on the cancer continuum is *abhiniveśa*, translated as the fear of death, the will to live and the clinging to life (Bachman 2010, Bryant 2009, Leggett 2018). When we find we aren't able to be with an unarguable reality, we often stimulate *rāga*, or a clinging (Hartranft 2003, Leggett 2018) to hope or endless treatments. Or, with *dveśa*, we may attempt to avoid (Hartranft 2003) conversations that bring us closer to that inevitability.

In the *Bhagavad Gītā*, a suggested way through suffering is self-knowledge (Mitchell 2000). To work with *duḥkha* and enhance our understanding of our *kleśa-s*, a therapeutic response may be to help someone turn toward the self, especially difficult and uncomfortable emotions, when ready and with a gentle curiosity. In the shock of a diagnosis, it can feel as though a veil has been lifted, and we may suddenly be able to see more clearly. Through expression, movement, and breath, suffering

seems to soften with human accompaniment and yoga practices, from movement to meditation, become steady support, themselves promoting a shift from within. An unexpected alchemy: the willingness to be with what is, met with profound human connection, may be an integral part of suffering's relief.

Being with impermanence and uncertainty

In the days walking with cancer, we want our oncologist (or anyone) to tell us, with absolute certainty, that all will be well. We seek security and reassurance. Any change in treatment plan can topple us. Yet we know that our breathing material selves and everything around us (*prakṛti*), are subject to change. These inherent fluctuations in life, are, from a yogic point of view, a function of the *guṇa-s*, the aspects of *prakṛti* that are changing constantly. From the *Sāṃkhya Kārikā*, *guṇa-s* are attributes or qualities that are the essence of pleasure, pain and delusion, and they function to illuminate, activate and restrain (Mainkar 1972). Specifically, *rajas* is the nature of passion, stimulation and mobility, and has the capacity to activate. *Tamas* is the nature of heaviness, delusion and darkness and has the capacity to restrain. *Sattva* is goodness and pleasure; it illuminates. It is this primordial physical energy in the *guṇa-s* that is found in all of nature and the evolving cosmos (Lad 1984). Sullivan and Hyland Robertson in *Understanding Yoga Therapy* write: "The three *gunas* combine with one another to support, modify and generate all psychological and environmental content. By understanding the *gunas*, as part of *prakriti*, not *purusha*, we realize the unchanging awareness within" (2020, p. 58).

In yoga, we can accompany these fluctuations of life, and practice brief (and progressively longer) periods of sitting with the discomfort of difficult emotions, thoughts and feelings, watching sensations ebb and flow. We can be a witness to change when relationships shift, seasons progress, and our bodies age. We realize, in small moments, that all that we are experiencing is impermanent, even our suffering. Nothing of this world lasts forever; that's also the sorrow of it. Yet our willingness to see this clearly, returning to a state of *sattva* even when it's hard (and it is), can reaffirm our contract with life.

Returning to the present moment

A cancer patient commonly finds themselves looking in two directions at once: the past, trying to figure out why they have cancer in the first place, and the future, worrying about how serious their prognosis may be. Even at the end of treatment, when we might, in relief, put it all behind us, the fear of recurrence can be intense and enduring. While there is, of course, a need to plan for the future and make decisions at all points on the cancer continuum, sometimes we need help finding our way back to the present, and the shelter of this moment.

Stilling the fluctuations of the mind and coming, now, to yoga practice, is how the *Yoga Sūtra-s* begin (Bachman 2010). For someone suffering the more impactful side effects of cancer treatment, it can be hard to make a case for "present moment awareness": now hurts too. And yet, there can be a full-body softness in acknowledging this human experience, small moments of noticing the impermanent fluctuations, and practices selected to ease the pain. In times of trouble, there can be an uncanny spaciousness and momentary rest in the present moment. We often only need a gentle reminder.

Practice and engagement

In cultures where people are taught to be independent and self-reliant, a cancer patient is often surprised at how much practical and emotional help they may need. It then becomes a time of unlearning, accepting the support and blessings from those around them. Beyond and including medical care, many wonderful therapies in integrative oncology (massage, acupuncture, reflexology) allow a patient to receive much-needed human comfort. While yoga practices are well known for teaching us to "let go" and relax, each uniquely begins with client engagement. Even the most simple meditations and/or restorative practices require us to pause and respond, rather than only react, to rely on agency rather than grasping for control. Yoga practice intentionally leads you back to your own embodiment, breath by breath. Not perfect practice, or practice to make perfect. Practice. In this way engagement can be a stepping-stone to further healthful action, developing solid habits in good nutrition, exercise, and stress relief, and an enduring commitment to lifelong well-being.

Purposeful life

Not uncommonly in the early stages of cancer, a patient can feel as though the wind has been utterly taken out of their sails. Their life trajectory, as they see it, has taken an unexpected and unwelcome turn. They may feel that they have lost their identity and direction. *Dharma* can be translated as "one's own nature" or "that which upholds" (Bachman 2010, Bryant 2009), a poetic understanding of life purpose. For many, their temporary purpose becomes a matter of getting themselves to cancer treatment – no small feat. Some people change radically in the course of their cancer experience, shifting their perspective, relationships and life goals. Yoga encourages pause, contemplation and compassionate study to know the self. For those who find themselves facing the ending of their days, purpose asks more of them still, possibly deepening the meaning of their remaining time.

Yoga therapists, guided by their own call of *dharma*, help their clients to face all that arrives in life (including death), with practiced equanimity. For some, the study of yoga philosophy reflects to them their own ancestral history, remembered deep in their bones. Some may apply yoga philosophy directly, in practical and esoteric conversations with interested patients struggling to piece together rhyme or reason in their days met with cancer. For others, these and many other strands of philosophy are quietly embedded in their approach to their work and embodied in their manner with patients and colleagues. In remembrance of humankind over time, the study of yoga philosophy can inform and provide guidance to our days, sustain human wonderment in difficult times, and heighten our capacity to see the beauty of our work in yoga therapy and that which shines from our oncology colleagues.

Chapter two

Access to scientific research

Supporting a therapist's daily work are the ongoing efforts and stalwart labors of the worldwide scientific community, studying the efficacy of yoga across the spectrum of healthcare (Balaji, Varne & Ali 2012, Jeter et al. 2015, Mohammad et al. 2019). Yoga therapists already working in healthcare depend on continually updated research to guide their practice and inform lively integration discussions with colleagues. Yoga therapists, when trained well, raise themselves up to a standard of academic rigor, research literacy and evidence-informed practice. In this way, they participate in ongoing debate and discourse, more easily recognize misinformation, and stand up amongst those calling for validated and reliable research to temper unsubstantiated claims ("Yoga can cure your cancer!") in mainstream media. We, as a profession, rely on research.

From *prāṇāyāma* (breath) to *āsana* (movement), from *dhyāna* (meditation) to *vidyā* (mindfulness or awareness), many yoga practices have been studied in clinical trials (see Chapters 4–6). Over the last ten years, there has been a steady increase in peer-reviewed research, much of it published in integrative health and medical journals, such as the *Journal for Integrative Oncology*, and many meet the gold standard of randomized controlled trial (RCT) design (Cramer et al. 2014).

On the heels of so much growth, there is a continued profession-wide determination to improve and refine ongoing research. In 2021, Delphi-based guidelines were published to enhance the transparency of reporting yoga interventions (Moonaz et al. 2021). Gathering 128 global researchers, and with a consensus-based methodology, they developed CLARIFY, a 21-item checklist outlining "details considered necessary for high quality reporting of yoga research." This work spearheads the persistent call for increased clarity and research detail to inform in-person clinical application. When we understand what works, we can customize it for individual needs: most appropriate practices and optimal "dose."

Research, when relevant and rigorous, in combination with in-clinic experience, informs adaptive practice and helps to define future research directions and policy decisions. Rather than dampening inquisitiveness, good research fosters curiosity and wonder. The therapist's daily work, then, is to burnish critical thinking and weave the depth of their knowledge, bolstered by scientific inquiry, with companionable human caring, in real time.

Yoga therapy education

Worldwide, yoga therapy education takes an experienced yoga teacher on the purposeful path to becoming a yoga therapist. Some programs, particularly in India, are long established (many at a post-graduate degree level at universities), with the majority, now in more than 50 countries, founded as independent schools. Through the years, the International Association of Yoga Therapists (IAYT) has created an accreditation process for yoga therapy schools (with accompanying competencies) and a certification for credentialing individual yoga therapists (C-IAYT), including a detailed code of ethics (COE) and a clarifying professional scope of practice (SOP). Recently, IAYT has supported the study of the cultural and social determinants of health, and collaborative measures taken within the membership to ensure diversity, equity and inclusion (www.iayt.org/dei) in yoga therapy schools and professional yoga therapy practice.

Revised in 2020, the definition for general practice remains:

Yoga therapy is the professional application of the principles and practices of yoga to promote health and well-being within a therapeutic relationship that includes personalized assessment, goal setting, lifestyle management, and yoga practices for individuals or small groups.

www.iayt.org

Each IAYT accredited school, while maintaining their unique approach or deference to lineage, directs the education of experienced yoga teachers (entering with a teacher's certification of at least 200 hours) with an additional 800+ hours of advanced training. Studies include advanced safety-oriented training in applied anatomy, neurophysiology, and biomechanics, as well as a focus on yogic lifestyle: a holistic combination of healthful diet, exercise, restful sleep and resourceful social connection. Their studies are broad and encompass traditional yoga philosophy and the depth, beauty and intelligence found in the enduring practices of yoga (see Yoga practices, p. 21). Foundational are the necessary practical and therapeutic skills to individualize yoga practices for complex conditions and medically diverse populations, all supported by unwavering compassionate care. Guided by IAYT competencies, each accredited school brings holistic inquiry, peer-reviewed research, and compassionate evidence-informed yoga practice in service to human suffering: conditions, injuries, disease, mental health, pain, trauma, all that might befall fellow humans throughout their lifetime. At a therapist's back on this "map" is the enduring support of their yogic scholarship, augmented continually and deepened with time and face-to-face clinical experience with individuals and small groups (see Chapter 3).

Towards the end of their yoga therapy training, many yoga therapy students define a clinical focus, such as oncology. As part of their clinical training (or "mentored practicum"), yoga therapists begin, under supervision, to see clients, employing an expanded biopsychosocial-spiritual framework (see Chapter 3). More and more, doctors, nurses and psychotherapists, recognizing the need for expanding holistic care, are embarking on yoga therapy training themselves. In this way, through their devotion to yoga and health, they see clients in compliance with their prevailing colleges and licensure.

Specialization in yoga therapy: education in cancer

Yoga therapists, working in oncology care, must have knowledge and skills beyond general practice, both in patient care and in integrative practice (see Chapter 3). Through extensive and ongoing clinical education (see Advanced Professional Development courses at www.iayt.org and Crucial education, below) many yoga therapy students focus their studies toward understanding a cancer patient's experience, from diagnosis to remission, and for some patients, from recurrence to their dying days. Yoga teachers, while not having a yoga therapy credential, may learn the skills of teaching oncology-based yoga classes by taking advanced teacher training (see YACEP certification at www.yogaalliance.org), thus becoming "advanced-practice yoga teachers" (see Chapter 6 for their work). Yoga professionals find their work with people facing cancer, who are often in distress and sometimes medically fragile, both profoundly rewarding and requiring more of them: amplifying a need for cancer-specific knowledge applied clinically, a fulsome understanding of the therapeutic relationship, and their own resilience-enhancing yoga practice. They recognize the reality that each cancer patient is unique in the lived experience of their cancer diagnosis, and often presents with concomitant health issues prior to, or running alongside their cancer experience (such as a psychological response, physical injury, or medical comorbidities). A yoga therapist, attending to the complexity of each person, and seeing through a wide *kośa* lens, brings care and practice to their client's lived and present moment experience, regarding them as a whole person, not only the sum of their disease.

Working knowledge of cancer

A yoga therapist will want to have a working understanding of cancer and the many conditions that influence its growth. They should understand cancer typing, staging and the many and varied treatments (see Chapter 4). While cancer treatments and medications are complex and evolving, a yoga therapist's understanding must support due diligence in offering safe, evidence-informed therapeutic work, within their scope of practice (see below and Chapters 3 and 6). In curating yoga practices, therapists will be aware of red flags and contraindications based on current best practices for particular cancer conditions and/or side effects of treatment (see Chapters 3, 4 and 6). This understanding is imperative, especially when side effects influence range of movement or physical safety (lymphedema, neuropathy, osteoporosis, etc.).

A clear understanding of oncological services, both medical and complementary (such as psychotherapy, physiotherapy, massage, and lymphedema therapy), is also mandatory, including a solid integrative referral network, to ensure each client's safe and timely support. Carrying cancer-specific knowledge and informed by integrative clinical notes and reports, they effectively remove the heavy burden of repeated clinical explanations from their client. They listen and nod as their client speaks, understanding both the medical terminology and the mosaic of challenges at every stage of the continuum. Normalizing any confusion and fear, they offer steady accompaniment with germane, safe, individualized practice (see Chapter 6) for one-on-one or small group sessions.

A focus on lifestyle and social connection

Yoga, in-clinic and beyond, is understood as a philosophy, a practice, and a lifestyle. Each session offers the client an opportunity to reflect upon their choices beyond the mat, and the lifestyle variables that influence their health. Lee Majewski and Ananda Balayogi Bhavanani, in their well-received book, *Yoga Therapy as a Whole-Person Approach to Health* (2020), extol the importance of a "yogic lifestyle" (*yogacāra*). The components discussed are, in brief: *ācāra* (healthy activities), *vicāra* (healthy thoughts and attitudes), *āhāra* (healthy diet), *vihāra* (relaxation and connection with others), and *vyavahāra* (healthy interpersonal relationships) (2020, p. 35).

What might a healthy lifestyle look like in the throes of cancer-care and beyond? Lorenzo Cohen and Alison Jefferies make a strong case in *Anti-Cancer Living* (2018) for "a mix of six". This prescient book, backed by rigorous research, presents six areas of lifestyle focus, many shared with yoga therapy: the importance of social connection, stress relief, quality sleep, joyful movement, healthy diet, and an increased awareness of environmental toxins. A comprehensive lifestyle randomized control trial offered diet, exercise, mind/body practices (including yoga therapy) and behavioral counseling to radiation therapy patients (Arun et al. 2017). They reported both on the important

comprehensive nature of the program and, through testimonials, stressed the significance of the mind/body components, lifestyle transformations and meaningful social support offered to the participants.

A yoga therapist, emanating an authentic availability for social connection themselves, will help a client identify and nurture meaningful social support, between them in a one-on-one session, in the refuge of a yoga class, and when engaged with family, friends, community and local cancer networks within the vast embrace of the culture of cancer.

Crucial education alongside oncological yoga therapy: five vital topics

Cancer patients often feel broken apart by their diagnosis. They spend the next many months, or in some cases, their lifetime, parsing the impact. Most immediately they will be contending with the cancer itself: the ongoing treatments, medications and side effects (see Chapters 4 and 6). Yoga therapists must be aware of cancer's complexity and be well educated to provide nuanced evidenced-informed care. But there is often more in the room. Even as they step onto the cancer continuum, a patient may already be struggling with their mental health or have a lived experience of trauma. They may present with comorbidities, such as diabetes or a heart condition, or have prior physical injuries, perhaps already having borne a lifetime of chronic pain. They may also, life being life, have an uneasy acquaintance with grief and death. Add to that, cancer.

In oncology we regularly meet with patients carrying a heavy load. Fortunately, the science, research, and best practice experience of clinical yoga is ever evolving. To stay current and to build adaptive and accessible skills, yoga therapists must participate in ongoing and additional specialized training through certified yoga therapy schools, take Advanced Professional Development courses (www.iayt.com) or learn with local oncology colleagues at cancer hospitals and clinics. In addition to furthering their education and enhancing hard-won knowledge, a yoga therapist must continue to do their

(continued)

own work (*svādhyāya*), otherwise their habits, judgments and attitudes (*saṃskāra-s*), may surface involuntarily, impacting needed therapeutic connection. Clear on their scope of practice, a yoga therapist proceeds with sensitivity, places trust in professional partnerships, engages in supervision and peer support, and refers out to licensed oncological practitioners.

Note: evidence for the efficacy of yoga in cancer care is referred to in Chapter 6. Here we focus on what appears in the room alongside cancer and make a call for advanced education in these five areas of concern.

1. Mental health

Some would say that yoga is a state of mind. Pointing to **Yoga Sutra 1.2**, "*yogaś citta-vṛtti-nirodhaḥ*," translated as "yoga is directing and containing the activities of the mind," Roy and Charlton, in *Embodying the Yoga Sūtra* (2019, p.14), explore the nature of the mind and *duḥkha*, the mental or emotional suffering that arises from a real or imagined situation. Ultimately, they suggest that "exerting effort to 'stop the mind' will not stop the suffering. Instead, the route to quieting the mind is to focus it, not suppress it" (2019, p. 14). In a well-researched and supportive response to the breadth (some might say an epidemic) of societal mental health struggles, Mason and Birch, in *Yoga for Mental Health* (2018), reveal the deep compassion and broad efficacy of yoga practice in the face of anxiety, depression, schizophrenia, and more. As evidenced in Chapter 6, it's fair to say that every yoga therapist in cancer care will meet regularly with clients exhibiting heightened distress, anxiety, depression (Cramer et al. 2017, Carreira et al. 2018, Pham et al. 2019), and overwhelming fears about specific treatments, tests and recurrence, and an underlying indefatigable fear of death (Butow et al. 2018, Sharpe et al. 2018).

In light of evolving research and clinical knowledge, **yoga professionals are wise to undertake specialized training in mental health and to consider referrals to:** *yoga therapists and meditation/mindfulness teachers with specialization in mental health and integrative oncology colleagues: mental health nurses, psychotherapists, psychologists, psychiatrists, social workers, somatic practitioners.*

2. Pain

The experience of pain, acute or persistent, can be confounding, exasperating and isolating; all possibly contributing to *duḥkha,* a sense of suffering. Patients experiencing pain can sometimes conflate discomfort entirely with tissue damage. Research (and clinical experience) tells a different story; pain is remarkably complex. Colleagues in yoga therapy, incorporating their training in physiotherapy, have revealed the need for evidenced-based and creative approaches in meeting with each individual's unique experience of pain (Pearson et al. 2019, Taylor 2018). When facing cancer, pain can reside in every moment, from the aggravating tingling of neuropathy (Yoon & Oh 2018) to the many discomforts associated with dying (Renz et al. 2018). "Total pain" is a term used in medical settings, where pharmaceutical pain management meets expertise that respects whole-person complexity (Fink & Gallagher 2019). And yet, while cancer-related pain is reported by more than 70% of patients, it may be inadequately managed in up to 50% of patients (Neufeld et al. 2017). Says Neil Pearson, physiotherapist, yoga therapist, and co-author of *Yoga and Science in Pain Care* (personal contact, July 2021): "Every aspect of a person's existence, every *kośa*, all the *kleśa-s*, the proximal environment, current life history, genetics, relationships, culture and our society (everything actually), influences pain." In addition to the variety of accessible yoga practices in pain-care, the compassion offered by a therapist, that begets the client's own self-compassion, can profoundly impact recovery and well-being (Prosko, 2019).

In light of evolving research and clinical knowledge, **yoga professionals are wise to undertake specialized training in pain-care and to consider referrals to:** *yoga therapists with a specialization in pain care, pain care physiotherapists and integrative oncology colleagues: acute and chronic pain physicians, palliative care physicians, acupuncturists.*

3. Trauma

Yoga's enduring and compassionate response to trauma is well documented in many seminal works (Emerson 2015, NurrieStearns & NurrieStearns 2013, Hopper

(continued)

et al. 2011, Turner 2020). Recent trailblazing books shed light on ethnic/race-based trauma (Parker 2020), sexual trauma (Rousseau 2020) and care for survivors of severe abuse (Byron 2021) with resonant practices employed in support for those carrying these often-invisible burdens. In their chapter in *Yoga for Mental Health* (Mason and Birch 2018), Moore and Libby point to the need for a supplementary training and a deepened human sensitivity in order to be of sound service, including wise use of assists and trauma-sensitive language. As yoga is becoming widely known as useful support (Cramer et al. 2018, Taylor et al. 2020, Van der Kolk et al. 2014), Erin Byron, yoga therapist and psychotherapist, suggests that: "Yoga provides the tools required to accept and move through hardships, including unwanted happenings and difficult emotions. By allowing 'what is to just be', we steadily increase resilience" (personal contact, August 2021). A cancer diagnosis and its treatment are recognized as potentially traumatic and persistently so throughout the continuum, leading to current research in cancer-related PTSD (Brown et al. 2020, Cordova et al. 2017, Yang et al. 2017).

In light of evolving research and clinical knowledge, **yoga professionals are wise to undertake specialized training in trauma-care and to consider referrals to:** *yoga therapists with a specialization in trauma care, trauma-focused psychotherapists, psychologists and psychiatrists, somatic practitioners.*

4. Grief

A familiar companion on the cancer continuum, grief may be the most mysterious and unrecognized emotion that arrives in a yoga therapist's office. Such is the profound cultural disavowal of grieving, that patients don't initially see what they are carrying. No matter the issue – injury, disease, pain, trauma – there is often a deep sense of loss. After a cancer diagnosis, it can feel as though the rug has been pulled out from underneath us. Losses abound: loss of a job, loss of identity, surgical loss of an organ or limb, loss of naivete and innocence, perhaps even the anticipated loss of a future self. Sadly, many cultures remain grief illiterate and the pressure to "get over it, and on with it" is immense. Add to that an insistent "toxic positivity"

(see p. 29), and it becomes more and more difficult to recognize and tend to grief.

Greatly misunderstood, grief is a natural and intelligent response to life and love. Stephen Jenkinson, author of *Die Wise* (2015), suggests that grief is better understood as a skill, a human-making possibility, and deeply worthy of respect and practice. Seen as necessary and vital to human life, grief's inward spiraling, discomforts, and unraveling can be beautifully sustained and supported by awareness, compassion and community support (Weller 2015). Gathered in, enduring sources of deep connection binds people with affirming conversations, shared mourning and remembered ritual. Yoga therapists are well suited to sit with grief, not to banish it, but to listen well and provide nourishing practice. While the spirit mourns, the body bears an obvious burden: tight throat, taut stomach, and gripped heart, riding the inevitable waves of despair. We can start our practice here (Sausys 2014).

In light of evolving research and clinical knowledge, **yoga professionals are wise to undertake specialized training in remembering and honoring grief and to consider referrals to:** *yoga therapists with a specialization in grief, grief therapists, spiritual health practitioners, clergy and integrative oncology colleagues: nurses, psycho-oncology practitioners, palliative care team.*

5. Dying

A cancer diagnosis can unearth long-buried fears of death. Even if the diagnosis is hopeful, it can be enough to revitalize *abhiniveśa*, a suffering kindled by our fear of death or "ending of Me" (Stone 2008). These fears are difficult to voice in a death-phobic culture and can further contribute to isolation and loneliness when cancer patients turn away from the rumor of their own death or are unable to find any kind of shared acceptance with family (Taylor 2008). Yoga therapists, through their understanding of yoga philosophy and their practice of "sitting with," absent of judgment or advice, are well positioned to be of help to their palliative colleagues. Yet without self-reflection on their culturally embedded death phobia, a yoga therapist, naïve to the labors of dying, can inadvertently forestall the dawning of awareness (*vidyā*) in

(continued)

their clients and in so doing, unintentionally steal (*asteya*) the opportunity for people to speak candidly, wrestle openly with their dying, make decisions (if there are any to make), or place flowers on the altar of regrets. Tragically, when death is kept out of the conversation so determinedly it often is too late to receive the depth of palliative care that may otherwise be afforded.

The way we come to our dying time surely informs those who come after us (Jenkinson 2015), yet most of us don't grow up in a culture that reveres aging or honors death. When someone dies of cancer, obituaries speak of "losing the battle" or "failing in their fight"; they are evermore portrayed as the victim of death. While some prepare for a peaceful transcendent "yogic" dying (Foos-Graber 1989), death, like birth, is often unpredictable; perhaps rightfully so. It is both devastating and catastrophic, and yet stitched lovingly into the fabric of life. Perhaps *Pātañjali* has been preparing us for death all along. Perhaps the practice of yoga is, by design, bereavement sensitive, relying on the foundational practice of *śavāsana* or "corpse pose" in every practice. More than a practice of relaxation, *śavāsana* can, by befriending death, turn us toward a refreshed love of life. Yoga therapists may have their greatest influence on a culture by offering death a radical hospitality and heartful presence, demonstrating a willingness to accompany uncertainty, honor endings and befriend death. A yoga therapist working at the bedside with others in palliative care can offer easeful breath and subtle practice to relieve the aching body and the fearful mind. In service to the soul, with philosophical and ethical wonderings embodied, the yoga therapist witnesses, supports, and yields gracefully to the client's most faithful and loving community, the old ones who have come before them, and those to whom they offer their life and legacy.

*In light of evolving research and clinical knowledge, **yoga professionals are wise to undertake specialized training, to remember the importance of family/community knowledge and ritual, and to consider referrals to:** yoga therapists with a specialization in death care, community death care practitioners, family therapists, spiritual health practitioners and integrative oncology colleagues: psycho-oncology practitioners and palliative care teams.*

Therapeutic principles: education to enhance presence, safety, and connection

When considering the unique approach of yoga therapy in oncological care, we could say that yoga philosophy differentiates us, and the diverse practices of yoga define us. True, and there's more. Embedded in the name and definition of yoga therapy is "therapy" itself. "Therapeutic relationship" (see Between the therapist and client, below) is central in yoga therapy and is a principal competency in our training as defined by IAYT. As such, each accredited school must provide relevant education. Authentic presence is key, emerging, in part, from devoted and dedicated practice (see Within the therapist, below). It is this embodied presence, offering genuine human connection and steady engagement in safe clinical experience, that fosters authentic therapeutic relationship.

Here, yoga therapy (one of many body-centered therapies) finds kinship with body-centered psychotherapy (Ogden & Fisher 2015, Caplan 2018, Lutz 2021, Winhall 2021) and shares a focus of "present moment" experience with a host of somatic therapies, from Focusing to Somatic Experiencing (Gendlin 1982, Cornell 2013, Levine 2010). Yoga therapy, as a holistic body, mind, and spirit practice, similarly views the body as intelligent, responsive, and conversant. By bringing awareness through the body, we can, through practice, become present to our multilayered experience (*kośa-s*), and ultimately come to understand our "true self" (Bryant 2009). Our approach, then, becomes one of expanding our capacity to turn inward and listen.

Therapeutic relationship, in yoga therapy, is an attuned and shared responsibility, the safe-making intention that allows for entrusted collaborative work, one-to-one, or with small groups (see Chapter 3). Studied in the realm of psychotherapy, therapeutic alliance alone predicts a reduction in psychological distress (Baier et al. 2020, Bisseling et al. 2019) and this alliance, and a therapist's empathy and genuineness, are all integral parts of the therapeutic relationship

(Nienhuis et al. 2018). Navigating the path of cancer, the therapist/client relationship provides social connection, offers compassionate co-regulation or attunement, and brings the vast neuro-immuno-biological benefits that accrue when a client can rest in a secure sense of belonging. Emanating from the clarity and good will of the therapist, it includes a well-defined scope of practice and healthy boundaries, patient autonomy, safe containment of practice, and compassionate and authentic communication with a depth of embodied listening (See Body-centered therapuetic skills, p. 24).

Scope of practice

Important for establishing a firm foundation for orientation, safety and professional conduct, a C-IAYT accredited yoga therapist must learn and be conversant on the IAYT's detailed Scope of Practice, Code of Ethics and Professional Responsibilities (www.iayt.org). This is always foremost, but especially so when working with the complexity of cancer. Not diagnostic, oncology-educated yoga therapists see through a holistic *kośa* lens and help each client regain agency, awareness, and self-compassion by offering evidence-informed, philosophy-inspired, individualized practices to find refuge in the present moment and reduce suffering. Their work is relational (see Chapter 3), with therapists better described as willing witnesses, co-regulators, and safe-making practice guides, walking peaceably with each client on their winding cancer path, offering kindness and compassion at every turn.

From the earliest conversations with a client, clarity of work establishes a strong sense of professional and embodied boundaries (*brahmacarya*), and a reciprocal understanding of what may be expected in any given session (see Chapter 3). It is sagacious, as part of informed consent, to point out differences between yoga therapy (see current definition, p. 12) and diagnostic/licensed/regulated oncology practices, which offer support for body (such as physiotherapy), mind (such as psychotherapy) and spirit (such as spiritual health practices or palliative care). For example, Tracey Meyers, who penned "Relationships in yoga therapy: developing collaboration within a healing presence" (2021) discusses how yoga therapy and psychotherapy, though occasionally overlapping, differ in terms of fundamental models of practice, procedures in session and the role of the therapist (Meyers 2021, p. 265). Yoga therapists must be oncology-educated (within their scope of practice) and know their role, both with their client and within their workplace (see Chapter 3 for waivers, confidentiality, and health records), and regularly refer to their many

---

Cancer diagnosis through the lens of Polyvagal Theory and the *Guṇa-s*

"You have cancer." Instantly, before we can steady ourselves, before we can rationalize or strategize, we react. In a swift instant, the autonomic nervous system (ANS) rises up as our quick-acting protector, our wise (but fast!) arbiter of safety and the unconscious modulator of our biological response for ongoing survival. The capacity to sense into safety, danger and threat is called "neuroception," a term coined by Stephen Porges, creator of Polyvagal Theory (Porges 2011). Porges's theory (PVT) is a working hypothesis that explores how the mammalian nervous system has adapted to react in the moment and pattern through experience. To deepen our understanding of our patient's lived experience of facing cancer, and discern how best to help, we can view the experience of facing cancer through an overlapping polyvagal and yogic lens.

Typically, upon hearing "bad news," patients feel their heart hammering in panic, or a numbed sense of having left their bodies behind. According to PVT, sensing an immediate danger or possible life-threat (for some, a cancer diagnosis) immediately stimulates a defensive mobilization (sympathetic arousal) or precipitates a defensive immobilization (in theory, a stimulation of the dorsal vagal complex, or DVC). Depending on many factors, such as how and where the cancer diagnosis is delivered (Figg et al. 2010), and past experiences with disease or complex trauma, we respond in what may be the height of neurobiological brilliance.

(continued)

Fight/flight, freeze or shutdown are intelligent reactions, immediately resourceful and protective.

Cascading neurohormonal responses further our defense: "fight and flight" (sympathetic response), governed by the limbic system ("emotional brain"), releases epinephrine (adrenalin) which mobilizes the body for quick action with a rapid rise in breathing, heart rate, and blood pressure (Chu et al. 2021). In rapid choreography, the hypothalamic–pituitary–adrenal (HPA) axis mobilizes, releasing a flush of cortisol for sustained energy. All the better to fight or flee. If "freeze or shutdown" dominates, a withdrawing or numbing can result in a heightened physiological response, such as a possible lowering of heart and breathing rates (Roelofs 2017). In this state, a patient can feel utterly immobilized, unable to move at all. Heart rate variability (HRV), currently considered a reliable indicator of resonant emotions and the responsivity of our ANS (Ernst 2017, Rainville et al. 2006, Thayer et al. 2012), suggests that our health and well-being depend on this body intelligence: our ability to act defensively when necessary, and in contrast, to relax when no danger is perceived. Being scared when something is scary is intelligent. Also, understandably unpleasant and difficult. And hopefully temporary.

This complex and highly nuanced dance of the nervous system is witnessed every day in a doctor's office. People arrive vulnerable, anxious and largely unprepared to hear their doctor's words, even if anticipated. Should they also live in an achievement-oriented culture, or a situation where they live in a state of perceived constant threat (including racial persecution, and health or financial inequities), they may already be living a chronic sympathetic pattern. Adding to this is the challenge of the hospital environment. Geared toward a sanitary efficiency, it can be perceived as cold, clinical, and for some patients, dangerous. Best of intentions aside, the conditions don't always allow for deep human comfort and support.

In this understandable state of shock (referred to clinically, depending on many factors, as "acute stress disorder," or "adjustment disorder" in the *DSM-5-TR* (*American Psychiatric Association, 2022*), patients often find it immediately difficult to be present, hear clearly (Porges 2011), or make decisions (Yu 2016, Mazzocco et al. 2019). With the accompanying neurological changes in executive functioning (Shansky & Lipps 2013, Arnsten 2015) it may be nigh on impossible to understand and retain anything said after "you have cancer." Inevitably, all of these reactions, when not fully understood, can themselves create feelings of confusion, frustration, isolation and fear. Patients, lonely in their heightened state of distress, often say they fear they are doing cancer "wrong."

And there is more. ANS "dysregulation" can become habitual, as patients continue down the cancer continuum. In the first many months after a diagnosis, the continuing stress can be relentless, a shock-upon-shock, with increased testing, endless waiting and difficult treatment conversations. Reports of cognitive dysfunction are common, perhaps contributing to the baffling and frustrating experience of "brain fog" (Hermelink et al. 2017, Kaiser et al. 2019). Chronic patterns of sleeplessness, heightened anxiety, and preoccupied worry can continue (Trill 2013). Equally likely, a patient may swing toward a depressive state; not able to get out of bed, or to convince themselves to exercise, or, in some cases, unable to muster the momentum to pursue further tests and/or treatment. Continuing research focuses on how these patterns of dysregulation may contribute to long term "cancer-related PTSD" (Cordova et al. 2017).

From a yogic point of view, we see the remarkable intercommunication (through the *kośa-s*) demonstrated in the "stress response"; emotions (*manomaya*) can affect the body (*annamaya*), and the body can influence the mind. Even in the absence of immediate danger, "top-down" information (Taylor et al. 2010) flowing from brain to body (through efferent neural pathways), such as perseverating "negative" thoughts, attitudes, and emotions, can re-stimulate physical patterns of defense. Anecdotally, both "upregulated" and "numbed" responses share an increased physical tension in the central body (eyes, jaw, shoulders, spine, and hip flexors), theoretically in preparation to fight, run or draw away from the situation. Physical symp-

(continued)

toms of defense, like a bracing tension in the center of the body (O'Clair 2021), can likewise inform our brain (through "bottom-up" afferent pathways) that we are under threat, even when we are not. Without help in regulating these patterns, a patient can stay in chronic distress, well past their cancer treatment, possibly promoting cancer development (Dai et al. 2020).

Our compassionate capacity to acknowledge and help mindfully mediate these stress responses, in the moment and over time, may well be the "superpower" of yoga therapy (Matthew Taylor, PT, C-IAYT, Integrating Yoga Therapy and Health Care, Global Yoga Therapy Day, Aug 13, 2021). "Nervous system dysregulation," common parlance in healthcare, sends consistent referrals to yoga therapy, identifies patients who are anxious or panicking, or conversely displaying signs of depression and "dissociation," or both. While a steady yogic intention is to help someone, over time, learn to self-regulate, it may be immediately impossible. What might be of assistance, in addition to emergency yogic support (see Chapter 3) is to help patients "normalize" and understand the brilliance of this protective neurobiological reaction. A therapist, offering compassionate acknowledgment and calming practices, can help de-escalate the response, possibly activating the ventral vagal parasympathetic complex (VVC), or the "social engagement" aspect of the ANS (Porges 2011). When "regulated," our heart rate and blood pressure return to homeostasis, and systemic inflammation decreases (Chovatiya & Medzhitov 2014). The body softens, calms and feels more relaxed. We think more clearly, and, with oxytocin released (Kemp et al. 2012), we may enjoy a strong feeling of belonging. "*Sattva*" a yogic term for the *guṇa* that reflects balance or ease, "goodness and pleasure" (Mainkar 1972), shares many of the attributes ascribed to the VVC.

Indeed, much of the language and philosophy of yoga may run in parallel to the understanding of this neurology, offering a new validity to the integration of ancient knowledge in modern times. Take the current explanation of "hybrid states" (Porges 2011). These occur when we perceive safety and are, theoretically, a neural co-activation of the sympathetic nervous system and ventral vagal complex. In *Understanding Yoga Therapy* (2020), Sullivan and Hyland Robertson show us how a convergence of the neural platforms identified by polyvagal theory can mirror the yogic concepts of the *guṇa-s*, qualities or attributes that make up *prakṛti* (see Yoga Philosophy, pp. 7–12). Someone, for example, playing a friendly game of tag with their kids, may be in the neural state of "safe mobilization" (a co-activation of ventral vagal complex and sympathetic nervous system). Understood from a yogic point of view, co-activation represents a balance of the essence of *sattva and rajas*, the substrate of energy, turbulence and activity (Sullivan & Hyland Robertson 2020). When we sit peacefully, enjoying a beautiful sunset, the neural state of "safe immobilization" (a co-activation of dorsal vagal complex and ventral vagal complex) may be active. Understood from a yogic point of view, this represents a co-mingling of *sattva and tamas*, the substrate of restraint, mass and form (Sullivan & Hyland Robertson 2020). Yoga wisely meets distress when we can offer a range of yoga practices to enhance safe mobilization (playful movement, "joint loosening/*pavanamuktāsana*, flowing postures/*āsana* etc.) and safe immobilization (loving kindness meditation/*maitrī*, visualization/*bhāvanā* etc.). In fact, all yoga practices, including lifestyle and ethical guidance (see Chapters 3 and 6) can be skillfully curated to enhance calm and the return to the resilient state of *sattva* (see Yoga practices, below): "the substrate of calm, light, buoyancy and illumination...from which tranquility, harmony, equanimity, patience, joy, forgiveness, truth, contentment, humility and compassion emerge" (Sullivan & Hyland Robertson 2020, p. 58).

Co-regulation

An indispensable "neural tool" for compassionate support is based on the concept of co-regulation. Polyvagal theory, inspired by studies of mothers and newborns, shows us how humans are wired for connection to facilitate survival (Porges 2011). This nurturance goes beyond basic survival. Co-regulation refers to the beauty of a reciprocal caring relationship: a profound and nuanced connection married with a sense of assured safety resourced from an

(continued)

authentic regulated presence. According to psychotherapist Deb Dana (2020), the ability to self-regulate is built on ongoing experiences of co-regulation. Through establishment of therapeutic trust, the therapist becomes the "reliable, regulating other" (Dana 2020, p. 3).

Understanding the need for social connection after a shocking diagnosis of cancer, a yoga therapist can create the many conditions necessary to enhance a trustworthy sense of safety, modulate their own nervous system and broadcast a compassionate accessibility (see Chapter 3). It is in the palm of this kinship that we can decrease a desperate loneliness, and help clients to develop a resilient inner and outer resourcing, on the mat and beyond. With enduring compassion, we can offer cancer patients ethically enhanced, evidence-informed, personalized nervous-system-friendly practices in the intimacy of a resonant one-on-one meeting, and also in the sweet embrace of a caring yoga class (see Chapter 6). With our good colleagues in oncology care, we can encircle patients with professional experience, life-honed expertise and steady human warmth – necessary accompaniments on their travels and travails along the cancer continuum.

A caveat: yoga therapists are experts in helping someone become calmer, true. However, patients sometimes get the idea (see "Toxic" positivity, p. 29) that they should be calm all the time. This is near impossible and, one could argue, not entirely functional on the cancer roller coaster, when there is near constant stress and protective reactivation of fight/ flight/freeze or collapse/shut down. There is intelligence here. Maybe anger is occasionally necessary to propel us to action; in this case, testing and treatment. Maybe "collapse" stimulates a surrounding community to "show up" and offer more nourishment and care. Perhaps anxiety brings a distressed patient to many doors, ready to receive help. Welcomed, "dysregulation" is not wrong. Instead, with genuine connection and yoga practice, the patient's return to their true nature can begin with self-compassion, no matter what. This, perhaps, is the heart of yoga therapy work.

Author's note: in a balanced and cautious academic approach, a yoga therapist looks for counterarguments to any research, including PVT, such as those proposed by Grossman and Taylor (2007) and added to more recently (such as Gourine et al. 2016). The PV theory does not purport to tell the whole neurophysiological story of distress, and therapists, utilizing it in their practice, should first educate themselves on the theory, consider the validity of counterarguments for themselves, and additionally caution themselves in simplifying or overstating. More broadly, however, we might ask why PVT (or any theory) captures the imagination of therapists of all stripes. In this case it seems to offer a common language that emphasizes the importance of a therapist's self-regulated embodiment. Additionally, PV theory, in normalizing involuntary responses, may help a patient find self-compassion and motivate them to consider practices and resources to balance their fight and flight responses. It may additionally provide insight for yoga therapists on how yoga philosophy reflects current real-world practice. The benefits of tethering yoga therapy to science fosters sound and reliable knowledge when married to an openness to change our approach in response to further discoveries. In this way, we make room for both science and wonder, and keep our keen eyes open for continuing research.

oncology colleagues when outside their scope of practice (see Crucial education box, above).

At the yoga therapist's side: yoga practices and therapeutic skills

Yoga practices

Here sits beside us our gold, our revered, honed "tools of the trade", offering a time-honored doorway to engaged and contemplative well-being, and an interconnected, interdependent health-filled life. These practices, imbued with philosophy and carried by time, speak of accrued wisdom and discernment born of diverse cultures (a deep bow) and now brought to bear in service to those facing cancer. Steady practice in turbulent times – some might call it embodied prayer. While there are innumerable tomes penned that open the gates to the many streams of yoga philosophy, books written about the day-to-day, on-the-mat practices of yoga would measure in the tons. Important works speak of these practices, endlessly adaptable, answering a vital call for equity, diversity, shared humanity and accessibility (Heyman 2019). Many have been written specifically to offer adaptive practice for those living with cancer and are excellent references (Carlson & Speca 2011, Mills 2021, Neargardner 2019, Prinster 2014).

As a framework for Chapter 6, we present an adapted list of yoga practices. It is a menu that denotes but does not detail the vast richness of varied cross-cultural yoga practices and traditions, ancient and modern. Yoga therapists, depending on their lineage or education, may carry additional understandings and practices or may teach customary practices differently. Each heading epitomizes a deep well of lived knowledge. For example, open the door of *āsana* to appreciate the vast variety of purposeful and responsive shapes, planes of movement, gravitational choices, approaches of noticing (for example, interoception or proprioception) and the creative and intentional adaptability that arises, including the use of supportive walls, floors, blocks, and bolsters. Practices may be chosen and refined to build *brāhmaṇa* (strength), *laṅghana* (calm) or *samana* (balance) (Desikachar 1998). Various poses and shapes may connect you with a kinship to nature (e.g., tree pose/*vṛkṣāsana* or crow pose/*bakāsana*) or remind you of the wisdom born of humanity and strength (e.g., sage pose/*marīcyāsana* or warrior pose/*vīrabhadrāsana*). What follows is an adapted list (description is ours) from the Scope of Practice Guidelines and Yoga Therapy Tools (www.iayt.org). Additions reflect practices from various yoga traditions (see Chapter 6) for which the therapist has received guidance and training. They are treasured jewels carried by each therapist in responsible and accountable stewardship.

In Chapter 6 experienced yoga professionals invite us into hospitals, clinics, and homes, to see these practices beyond theory, in service to those making their way through the cancer continuum, breath by anxious breath. We leave the details of their work, choices made, and the lineage-based or personalized practices they have offered, to them. Many of our contributors also use the modalities of restorative yoga, *yoganidrā*, and iRest, and are inspired to adapt poses through the work of Accessible Yoga (see Boxes 2.1–2.4).

- Lifestyle inquiry (*vihāra*): includes consideration of lifestyle factors, such as sleep, relationships, and daily patterns.

- Breath-work (*prāṇāyāma*): breathing patterns that inform the energetic body.

- Postures and movement (*āsana*): physical shapes, some historic, some modern.

- Meditation (*dhyāna*), mindfulness, and relaxation: various focused and non-cognitive awareness practices for the mind (*citta*) and body.

- Energetic gestures and seals (*nyāsa and mudrā*): symbolic hand and body gestures.

- Energetic locks (*bandha*): the use of diaphragms to contain or encourage the flow of *prāṇa* (life-force).

- Sacred sounds and chant (*mantra*): word or phrase, sometimes with accompanied melody.

- Visualization (*bhāvanā*): imagined object, response or resourceful situation.

- Affirmation and intention (*saṅkalpa*): positive words informing an aim or plan of action.

BOX 2.1 Accessible Yoga

Accessible Yoga is about unearthing our essential self, or spirit. This same spirit exists in all of us, regardless of the diversity of our experiences, our bodies, or our minds. All of the tools of yoga can be adapted in a multitude of ways when the therapist is sensitive to each person's unique and remarkable capabilities. In a chair, a bed, or even just in the mind, yoga can be made accessible to all people facing cancer. Whether it's breathing or movement practices, meditation, or ethical guidance, no one is left out.

Jivana Heyman, C-IAYT, founder of Accessible Yoga

BOX 2.2 iRest

iRest is a form of *yoga nidrā*, a guided meditative practice that can create a feeling of deep rest, and restore a sense of well-being. It is an effective tool to relieve pain, improve sleep and increase immune functioning and resiliency. A sense of safety and security is cultivated, coupled with guidance to meet sensations, emotions and beliefs. Through a process of dis-identification with various states of body, mind and thought, we come to rest in our essential wholeness. In this way, iRest helps cancer patients befriend the range of experiences that accompany their cancer experience.

Karen Soltes, LCSW, C-IAYT, certified iRest® Meditation teacher, senior iRest Trainer

BOX 2.3 *Yoga nidrā*

Yoga nidrā ("yoga sleep") is an effortless, lying-down, listening meditation which welcomes conscious rest at the threshold of sleep. It usually includes settling, intentions, breath and body scans, witnessing paradox and externalizing attention to finish. In co-creative *yoga nidrā*, client and facilitator collaborate to create unique *yoga nidrā* for specific purposes, such as reframing chemotherapy to transform the infusion into liquid golden light, or the elixir of life. *Yoga nidrā* recordings can be very comforting for people living and dying with cancer, helping to relieve pain and fear.

Uma Dinsmore-Tuli, PhD, C-IAYT

BOX 2.4 Restorative yoga

Restorative yoga is the use of props, like bolsters and blankets, to support the body in adaptable positions of ease and comfort to facilitate relaxation and health. Cancer is one of the most stressful things to live through, as the patient, and as the family of the patient. Restorative yoga is a proven and easy way to reduce stress and allow the body to martial its resources for healing. Restorative yoga can be done on the floor, on your couch, or in a hospital bed, all in silence.

Judith Hanson Lasater, PhD, PT, C-IAYT, E-RYT-500

Two words on breath: light and low

Those who suffer from lung disease, long COVID, or lung cancer can experience a pervasive sense of breath deprivation. They often appear in-clinic believing that they are supposed to be taking "deep breaths," though they often can't. Understandably, this causes increased worry, anxiety and distress, and can begin a vicious circle. In addition to needed pharmacological and respiratory care, diaphragmatic breath is often suggested (Yates et al. 2013). But is a diaphragmatic breath what we understand as a "deep breath"? Robin Rothenberg, C-IAYT, author of *Restoring Prana: A Guide to Pranayama and Healing through Breath for Yoga Therapists, Yoga Teachers and Healthcare Practitioners* (2020), offers further explanation:

The insistence on deep breathing is less than helpful for people suffering with lung disease and especially for those with lung cancer. Unfortunately, forced inhale or exhale will trigger the accessory muscles of the chest, often increasing mouth-breathing and making the whole act of taking a single breath more effortful and exhausting. Compounding this experience, chest-breathing triggers the sympathetic nervous system, which will increase tension in the body, elevate respiratory rate, and cause the airways to constrict, thus making it even harder to breathe. The focus on volume of air is ultimately unhelpful, in terms of increasing perfusion in the lungs, in fact if anything, it does the opposite.

It is far better to coach our clients to breathe lightly, to sip the breath in – as much as possible through the nose – and either exhale gently through nasal breathing or soft, pursed lips. Light, nasal breathing increases diaphragmatic action while inducing a relaxed, parasympathetic response in the body and mind. The activation of the diaphragm low in the ribcage, rather than up in the chest, increases perfusion (gas exchange) in the lungs with far less effort. Engaging the abdominals lightly inward on the exhale furthers both this relaxation response and optimal movement of the diaphragm.

In addition, nasal breathing helps regulate the velocity of the air stream as we breathe and prepare the air to land softly on the lungs through thin networks of bone, vessels,

(continued)

and soft tissue called turbinates. Within the sinus cavity, nitric oxide is produced. NO has been shown to increase oxygen uptake in the upper airways, thereby increasing ventilation into the lungs with far less effort than mouth and chest inhalation [Lundberg et al. 1996, Taneja 2020]. For maximum health, all breathing instruction needs to emphasize subtle, nasal breathing, and proceed with gentleness – low and light. Teaching yoga therapists to "befriend the breath" in this way, rather than fight or force it, will help them assist their clients to experience greater ease and calm.

Integrative oncology referrals: thoracic physicians, respiratory therapists.

Body-centered therapeutic skills

Yoga therapists develop various therapeutic skills in their accredited training in accordance with their lineage, school or approach to yoga therapy. The following terms are offered as examples of how therapists offer their skillfulness and equanimity in yoga therapeutics (while these definitions are ours, for more on somatic terms like these, check Ogden & Fisher 2015, Caplan 2018, Levine 2010 and Lutz 2021).

- Authentic presence: truthful, presence as a non-judgmental witness.

- Compassionate communication: employing invitational, non-declarative, trauma-sensitive language, expressions, gestures, and behavior.

- Embodied listening: generous, full-bodied listening with an in-the-moment presence.

- Compassionate embodied inquiry: guided awareness, call and response; employing curiosity and wonder, moment-by-moment practice exploration, following emergent directions and co-creating a therapeutic plan. A continued non-insistent interoceptive return to body, breath, and present moment, noticing holistic response.

- Attunement, modulation, and resonance: a therapist's capacity to attune and resonate with their client, modulate their nervous system and embodiment and provide a willing co-regulation or connection.

- Acknowledgment and accompaniment: an assurance of understanding and compassion, a "walking alongside."

- Co-assessment: client-centered interoceptive-based observing, noticing, sensing. Tracking response and refining of practices.

- Titration: providing small doses (*krama*) of practice with deep respect for a client's level of tolerance, preferences, allostatic load and lived experience.

- Pause and silence: allowing space for both client and therapist to reflect, sense, feel, collect thoughts, and wonder.

- Resourcing: identifying inner full-body nourishment that can be supported and enhanced through practices that lead to a sense of balance, ease and authenticity (*sattva*). Recognizing internal and external resources (in the environment and community) to enhance connection and healthful lifestyle.

- Yielding and letting go: a practiced capacity to soften and be supported, by the earth, community, perhaps even by medical treatments. The rare practice of letting go of an attachment to outcome.

Within the therapist

Being human, a yoga therapist carries their own lived experience and will, more than likely, be well acquainted with life's unpredictable shatterings, uncontrollable events and deeply uncertain times. While this is true for all therapists, a yoga therapist's path includes turning toward these lived experiences and through yoga practice, cultivating an increased awareness and skillfulness such that they are uniquely available and present to others.

Through philosophic study (see Yoga philosphy, above) and requisite *svādhyāya* (self-study), a yoga therapist will have delved deeply into their own *saṃskāra-s* (patterns), know their personal *doṣa* (constitutional type), regularly explore their *kośa-s* (layers or sheaths of self/experience), the ongoing changes of the *guṇa-s* (attributes or qualities) throughout the seasons, and the signature of their own *kleśa-s* (afflictions) and *duḥkha* (suffering). Cultivating self-knowledge, they continually examine the way they move in the world, know their own personal and community resources, surface their own beliefs, and regularly tend to the ethics (*yama-s* and *niyama-s*) that keep them on their path personally, and in their work. In assessing their own assumptions and biases, "triggers" and "projections," they labor to build integrity and honesty, and call on collegial community support to help them see clearly (see Chapter 3). Their maturing experience, personal or professional, develop in them a steadiness, a willingness, a learned capacity, and a honed intention (*saṅkalpa*) to accompany suffering – their own and others'. As they have long "sat on the mat," they have companianble relationship with stillness and silence. Informed thus, and working in the area of cancer, a therapist practices a counter-cultural willingness to simply "be" with illness. To resist turning their client's suffering into a problem to solve; instead offering the refuge of compassion and practice, where they can work together, helping to reduce suffering where they can.

Practiced over time, a therapist holds a steady, regulated and willing availability, a fluency and resilience useful to their clients and for themselves. The work of a yoga therapist is to show up, skills and knowledge honed and in hand, responsible and accountable, as an available, professional, imperfect human, acutely aware that they could just as easily be in that client's place, just as shocked, facing the precarious road of cancer. Through their embodiment, boundaries, behavior, and bottomless compassion they work to become a trustworthy presence in the eyes of the client. In this way, kindness, intention and expertise are kindled, and service meets life purpose (*dharma*).

Between the therapist and client: the meeting ground of therapeutic relationship and practice

Here in the infusion room, in the clinic, in the studio, in our client's living room, we come together, therapist and client. With an approach akin to entering Rumi's field (Rumi & Barks 2005), we meet in non-judgmental and welcoming space. In the beginnings of compassionate inquiry, a gossamer trust is stitched, guided not by scrutiny, but by wonder. In a slow and imperfect sidestep off the fast-moving path of tests and treatment, here is time and space, a resonant receptive calm, a warm presence, a skillful containment and a slow reach for gentle understanding. Together we pick up each trouble tenderly and hold it up to the light. With generous listening and attuned heart-led dialogue, we sift last night's sleeplessness, tomorrow's fears, this moment's thoughts and feelings through open hands. Nourished and unearthed by soft movement, breath and companionable silence, feelings and long-held beliefs find their way to the surface, and we listen anew. Here is a place to doubt, to cry, to unveil a hidden anger or surprising joy; all are welcomed by genuine care and non-judgmental presence.

Side-by-side now, in an affinity of connection, we hold possibilities for yogic practice in wide consideration, weighing all preferences, assessments, and evidence: reports, side effects, contraindications, lived experience, patterning, and lingering worries. Attuned to their role, the therapist looks beyond themselves, calling in treasured colleagues, stitching a wide net of care. A practiced therapist will draw on the knowledge needed to respond to each unique client – sometimes reaching back for supportive philosophy or a specific aspect of current research – all informing accessible yoga practice. This is steadying practice within the wider circle of uncertainty and life's mysteries.

A yoga therapist creates an atmosphere of deep respect for how things are, at present. Returning again and again to the body, the breath, with a fresh curiosity and in some rare moments, a sense of awe and wonder. Over time, a slow and steady alliance is knit, a devotion and emerging trust, a professional collaborative kinship that is tethered to a deep humanity. (See Chapter 3 for clinical practicalities, such as detailed descriptions of yoga therapy sessions).

Within the client

In front of us sits our client. Here is someone, undoubtedly with a life lived before cancer, full of busyness, relationships, accomplishments, disappointments, and pleasures. They have their unique constitution, personality, patterns, and habits, and their own stories of loneliness and love. Perhaps they've weathered previous illness or injury, and carry a lived experience with trauma or mental/emotional health conditions. They may be lucky with privilege, or be struggling with social, racial, or financial inequities. What might become new resources, through explorations of breath, movement, meditation, and self-compassion?

What is their story of cancer? Perhaps this is all new to them or maybe this is not their first time with cancer. What tests and treatments have they already undergone and what lies before them on the continuum? What is the impact of cancer upon them, including symptoms and side effects and all that is experienced beyond the physical? Slowly, their experience is remembered, felt, and collected. In all likelihood, they are anxious. And, if still in treatment, utterly exhausted. Here in front of us now, bedraggled by overwhelm or driven by hope, is a complex person living with cancer, requesting help and human care. (See Chapter 3 for clinical practicalities, such as oncology assessments and yoga therapy co-assessments).

Encircling the client

Personal resourcing

Fanning out behind each client are, ideally, many potential resources, unique to each person: kith and kin, home and the wider natural world; all that matters to them. In their days of trouble and treatment, where can they source security, easefulness, remembrance, and even a for a moment, joy? As they sense into what could be most helpful to navigate the continuum, are they able to access any lifestyle resources deemed useful, whether this be yoga, walks in nature, deep connection with family, or good nutritious food?

Who are their people? Is there nourishment in their relationships or are their most intimate relations, post-diagnosis, quite challenged? Caregivers, family and friends may need help, understanding and referrals too (see Chapters 3 and 6). In deep respect to differing religious and spiritual beliefs, are there cherished churches, or a grand temple of trees, that would be of solace and inspiration? Any return to a sense of safety and nourishment, any breath of ease in meditation can bolster *sattva*, a place of calm equanimity.

Perhaps most vital, do they have the financial and practical accessibility to enable needed cancer therapies, both medical and complementary? Are they able to afford transport, childcare, and fees of services required? If receiving care online, do they have fair and affordable access to computers and internet? Established systems of care can tragically and unfairly welcome some and exclude others. There is an unsettling and frustrating futility in recommending healthy lifestyle changes or referring to enhanced integrative care, if, for all intents and purposes, it is not possible. As such, yoga therapists, beyond time in a session, often lead the charge, becoming fierce advocates for equitable and compassionate care (see Chapter 6).

Impact of personal beliefs about cancer

"But why did I get cancer?" While understandable in the human-scale search for meaning, this line of questioning often results in exhausting spells of late-night research displacing all self-care. While there is mounting evidence of environmental and lifestyle correlation (see Chapter 6), it's difficult for any particular individual to pinpoint one source; a genetic link may be the exception.

(continued)

Some beliefs, however, seem to contribute to a patient's suffering, rather than assuage it, such as the idea that the appearance of cancer is entirely due to an inadequate diet or evidence of a punishment from God. (See Global culture and the culture of cancer, p. 28). Resulting shame and self-blame can promote isolation and adversely affect a client's mental health and their willingness to care for themselves. As yoga therapists, we meet this question with curiosity and non-judgment. The therapist's role is not to insist on a particular viewpoint, but to slowly foster an awareness of beliefs, and any suffering or barriers to care they may create. Given cancer's complexity, a simple offering of compassion and welcoming a modicum of mystery, may suffice to soften the mental grip and allow movement toward growth, care, and self-compassion.

Resourcing through local cancer groups

One of the beautiful surprises of this work is the upswell of tender support given by people and organizations, who educate, fund research, and connect people living with cancer. Think dragon boats and lemonade stands. Drives to appointments and lending of wigs. Community fundraisers and Gofundme websites. When our clients "join the club they never wanted to be a part of," what peer support networks and local programs are available? How might social engagement, if desired, be sought out and enhanced? In addition to one-to-one and group yoga therapy classes (see Chapter 3), many yoga therapists help to facilitate cancer support groups; rare and vital opportunities to sit with others who truly understand.

Resourcing through integration of cancer care

Encircled, a patient is potentially supported by a host of oncology practitioners, from medical to "complementary," including yoga therapy. Patients, worldwide, are leading the growing call for such encircled integration, during and after their conventional medical care (Buckner et al. 2018, Posadzki et al. 2013, Zuniga et al. 2019), with some reporting that more than half of all participating cancer patients use complementary services (Weeks et al. 2013). Studies are beginning to explore the efficacy of CAM therapies alongside medical oncology care (Seely et al. 2019), and the Society for Integrative Oncology was founded in 2003 to ensure that: "evidenced-based complementary care is accessible and part of standard cancer care for all patients across the cancer continuum" (www.integrativeonc.org).

One definition of integrative oncology care is as follows:

Integrative oncology is a patient-centered, evidence-informed field of cancer care that utilizes mind and body practices, natural products, and/or lifestyle modifications from different traditions alongside conventional cancer treatments. Integrative oncology aims to optimize health, quality of life, and clinical outcomes across the cancer care continuum and to empower people to prevent cancer and become active participants before, during, and beyond cancer treatment.

Witt et al. (2017)

Many models of oncological integration have been studied. Seely, Weeks and Young (2012) focused on integrative oncology (primarily in the US and England) and found that half of the programs existed in hospitals with most patients self-referred. Lopez, Mao and Cohen (2017) point toward the benefits of integrative communication, stating that: "efforts at enhancing communication between patients and healthcare providers, as well as between integrative practitioners and conventional healthcare teams, are critical to achieving optimal health and healing for patients with cancer." When working at an integrative clinic or hospital, records are often shared between practitioners, with client permission (see Chapter 3). Funding and provision of affordable services was a common barrier in programs studied across three continents (Grant et al. 2019). Financing for integrative programs and clinics varies by country and region and currently includes direct patient billing, third party billing, public or hospital funds, research grants, and charitable donations, with some dependence on volunteer support (Seely et al. 2012).

While so much collaborative progress has been made over the years, yoga therapists rally with their medical and complementary colleagues to further equity, inclusion and belonging in healthcare, supporting diverse needs and embracing local, traditional and indigenous medical/healthcare systems. Clearly, there is much work ahead of us to seek licensure, enhance integration, and secure a sustainable financial path for yoga therapy.

The "othering" language of cancer

There are aspects of facing cancer, well known by those who have lived it, that rankle. These are ways of speaking, in a well-meaning culture, that result in cancer patients feeling misunderstood or "othered."

Personal choices

As soon as they enter their doctor's office, each patient realizes that there is a new language to learn. Names of the many varieties of cancer, ways of staging, specific treatments and possible side effects; all of this is initially baffling, but by necessity, quickly adopted. Beyond the medical terminology is the language of personal impact and response. Some people call themselves a "victim" of cancer and speak of the need to "be brave," "fight," or "battle" the cancer, while others find a gentler language more resonant. Some bristle at the term "patient" and prefer "client" or the other way around. Some identify as "having" cancer, others see themselves as a person who is "facing" cancer. "Survivor" is another possibly contentious label; some love the empowerment it speaks of, and others feel the term doesn't meet their experience, preferring "recovering from cancer treatment" or "living with cancer" (which includes the truthful possibility of its return). Here, we take our lead from the client, with the language that speaks to their current lived experience, without judgment. Language often evolves through time and the experience of cancer, and may change to reflect a shift in therapeutic direction or change in a sense of personal agency.

"Toxic" positivity

Of course, everyone wants to feel "positive." But the insistence that a cancer patient is 100% positive, 100% of the time, is asking a lot from someone who may be understandably shocked and afraid. When riding the cancer roller coaster, a full range of human emotion is responsive and natural, including culturally defined "negative" emotions, such as fear, anger and sadness. Cajoled and "cheerleaded" to "put on a happy face" by well-meaning friends and family, this false positivity may instead increase feelings of "otherness," guilt and shame; hence the term "toxic." Surely therapy sessions are meant to be a safe place to speak of difficult things. Turning toward difficult emotions, in a titrated and trauma-sensitive way, helps clients feel seen and met, when they are often simply trying to stay afloat. Kindness, and the stabilizing effects of yoga practice, can shift attitude (*bhāvanā*), modulate "visiting" emotions and allow a genuine positivity to surface. One might proffer that a state of equanimity or *sattva* could be understood not as positivity, but as authentic presence.

Global culture and the culture of cancer

Behind each patient, beyond their personal resources and community connections, is something less visible, but equally potent. Born of a culture, each person carries beliefs informed over time by their heritage, their shared struggles, the society they engage in, perhaps even influenced by the land they live upon. Through family, relations, and local education (and somewhat mysteriously), we come to our beliefs, in part, through lived collective experience. Worldwide, cultures differ in their beliefs about cancer, some ascribing to fatalism (Sawadogo et al. 2014, Lee & Lee 2018), "unhealthy" lifestyle, or a punishment from God (Hamilton 2017). Most certainly, views of grief and dying are not universally shared (Bhuvaneswar & Stern 2013, Braun et al. 2014, Gupta 2011, Jenkinson 2015).

So invisible is this pull of cultural communion that we are fish in the ocean, utterly unable to see the water we swim in. Until we are met with crisis, a persistent cough or a discovered lump, our beliefs may not surface. A therapist and client sitting together, both citizens of a country that encompasses a multitude of cultures, can easily find themselves with vastly different understandings of cancer and cancer treatment. A continued call for increased diversity across yoga therapists is relevant here, a determined intention for a felt safety in commonality. In the absence of a shared identity or understanding, we center on the work and our client's viewpoint. We pause, wonder together and make room for a client's self-inquiry, with a practiced and collaborative cultural sensitivity (Orest Weber et al. 2016).

Globally, there are vast cultural differences in understandings of illness, aging, grief, and death. Some cultures, many indigenous, seem to engage differently in the ending of days. Rather than interpreting death as a sign of personal failure, these days are more akin to a summons sent out to the wider community. In these places, they heed a silent call; first, to attend the ailing person, then in their willingness to gather around them, to nourish an interconnected life (Jenkinson 2015).

Perhaps, at the end of the day, when a therapist pauses to wonder more widely about cancer, culture, and yoga, the lingering question becomes, "So, what does cancer ask of us?" as patients, as therapists, as a community in relationship with our natural world. How would we come to a cancer diagnosis differently if we saw our role, even when we are sick, beyond our individuality? Might we weigh the complexity of illness and suffering, of health and healing, and begin to see the need to nourish the interconnected health of all sentient beings? Does cancer ask us to wonder about other manifestations of unstoppable growth, in consideration of consumerism, commodification, and eco-politics?

Perhaps this is where cancer becomes metaphor, and philosophical wonderings from long ago circle back, offering needed human companionship in times of trouble. It's a big wondering, returning us to the question of *puruṣa and prakṛti*, the life entrusted to us and the great mysteries. We remember, as we pause, that a yoga therapy map is not the terrain and there is so much more to learn about cancer and well-being in the midst of it all. So, we do what we can to help each other? We listen, we offer prayers and we practice. We seek an abiding awareness and gratitude for our compassion-soaked interdependent time together, where our suffering and resilience can be shared, gathered as we are now, breathing together, in the shelter of this present moment.

A meditation to embody the map: awaiting your client

Stand, honoring the presence of all those who have walked the earth before you, breathing the nourishment of interrelationship: you with all of humanity and this beautiful world. Feel, at your back, the treasure of yoga philosophy and the support of your studies, informed by research and human skillfulness. Knowledge and wonder, in wait. At your sides, acknowledge the breadth of steadying yoga practices and your availability in therapeutic relationship. Skillfulness in wait.

Notice the fullness of your lived experience and your own resources, as you embody the present moment. Imagine, with breath, attuning your eyes, your ears, and your heart to your client, coming toward you. Imagine all that is within them (their lived experience and inner resources) and all that fans out behind them (their life, friends and family, home place and resources of deep nourishment). Visualize sitting with them, fully present, encircled by the compassionate integrated care of their oncology team, the wider companionship of a caring cancer community and kinship of culture.

Feel yourself grounded, willing and spacious, as you imagine holding their story, offering equanimity, positive regard and responsive, accessible whole-person practice. Breathe.

References

American Psychiatric Association, 2022. *Diagnostic and Statistical Manual of Mental Disorders: DSM-5-TR.* 5th ed. Text revision. American Psychiatric Association Publishing; Washington, D.C.

Arnsten, A.F., 2015. Stress weakens prefrontal networks: molecular insults to higher cognition. *Nature Neuroscience.* 18(10):1376–1385.

Arun, B., Austin, T., Babiera, G.V., et al., 2017. A comprehensive lifestyle randomized clinical trial: design and initial patient experience. *Integrative Cancer Therapies.* 16(1):3–20.

Bachman, N., 2010. *The Yoga Sutras.* Sounds True; Louisville, CO.

Baier, A.L., Kline, A.C., Feeny, N.C., 2020. Therapeutic alliance as a mediator of change: a systematic review and evaluation of research. *Clinical Psychology Review.* 82:101921.

Balaji, P.A., Varne, S.R., Ali, S.S., 2012. Physiological effects of yogic practices and transcendental meditation in health and disease. *North American Journal of Medical Sciences.* 4(10):442.

Bhuvaneswar, C.G., Stern, T.A., 2013. Teaching cross-cultural aspects of mourning: a Hindu perspective on death and dying. *Palliative & Supportive Care.* 11(1):79–84.

Bisseling, E.M., Schellekens, M.P., Spinhoven, P., et al., 2019. Therapeutic alliance—not therapist competence or group cohesion—contributes to reduction of psychological distress in group-based mindfulness-based cognitive therapy for cancer patients. *Clinical Psychology & Psychotherapy.* 26(3):309–318.

Braun, M., Hasson-Ohayon, I., Hales, S., et al., 2014. Quality of dying and death with cancer in Israel. *Supportive Care in Cancer.* 22(7):1973–1980.

Brown, L.C., Murphy, A.R., Lalonde, C.S., Subhedar, P.D., Miller, A.H, Stevens, J.S., 2020. Posttraumatic stress disorder and breast cancer: risk factors and the role of inflammation and endocrine function. *Cancer.* 126(14):3181–3191.

Bryant, E.F., 2009. *The Yoga Sūtras of Patañjali.* North Point Press; Berkeley, CA.

Buckner, C.A., Lafrenie, R.M., Dénommée, J.A., et al., 2018. Complementary and alternative medicine use in patients before and after a cancer diagnosis. *Current Oncology.* 25(4):275–281.

Butera, K., Elgelid, S., 2017. *Yoga Therapy: A Personalized Approach for Your Active Lifestyle.* Human Kinetics; UK.

Butow, P., Sharpe, L., Thewes, B., et al., 2018. Fear of cancer recurrence: a practical guide for clinicians. *Oncology (Williston Park).* 32(1):32–38.

Byron, E., 2021. Survivors of severe abuse. In: Finlayson, D., Hyland Robertson, L. (eds). *Yoga Therapy Foundations, Tools and Practice.* Jessica Kingsley Publishers; London, UK: 484–485.

Caplan, M., 2018. *Yoga & Psyche: Integrating the Paths of Yoga and Psychology for Healing, Transformation, and Joy.* Sounds True; Louisville, CO.

Carlson, L., Speca, M., 2011. *Mindfulness-Based Cancer Recovery: A Step-by-Step MBSR Approach to Help You Cope With Treatment and Reclaim Your Life.* New Harbinger Publications; Oakland, CA.

Carreira, H., Williams, R., Müller, M., et al., 2018. Associations between breast cancer survivorship and adverse mental health outcomes: a systematic review. *Journal of the National Cancer Institute.* 110(12):1311–1327.

Chovatiya, R., Medzhitov, R., 2014. Stress, inflammation, and defense of homeostasis. *Molecular Cell.* 54(2):281–288.

Chu, B., Marwaha, K., Sanvictores, T., Ayers, D., 2021. Physiology, stress reaction. *StatPearls.* Available from: https://www.ncbi.nlm.nih.gov/books/NBK541120/.

Cohen, L., Jefferies, A., 2018. *Anti-Cancer Living.* Penguin Books; America.

Cordova, M.J., Riba, M.B., Spiegel, D., 2017. Post-traumatic stress disorder and cancer. *The Lancet Psychiatry.* 4(4):330–338.

Cornell, A.W., 2013. *Focusing in Clinical Practice: The Essence of Change.* WW Norton & Company; New York.

Cramer, H., Lauche, R., Dobos, G., 2014. Characteristics of randomized controlled trials of yoga: a bibliometric analysis. *BMC Complementary and Alternative Medicine.* 14(1):1–20.

Cramer, H., Lauche, R., Klose, P., et al., 2017. Yoga for improving health-related quality of life, mental health and cancer-related symptoms in women diagnosed with breast cancer. *Cochrane Database of Systematic Reviews.* 1(1):CD010802.

Cramer, H., Anheyer, D., Saha, FJ., Dobos, G., 2018. Yoga for posttraumatic stress disorder – a systematic review and meta-analysis. *BMC Psychiatry.* 22(18/1):72.

Dai, S., Mo, Y., Wang, Y., et al., 2020. Chronic stress promotes cancer development. *Frontiers in Oncology.* 10:1492.

Dana, D., 2020. *Polyvagal Exercises for Safety and Connection: 50 Client-Centered Practices* (Norton Series on Interpersonal Neurobiology). WW Norton & Company; Manhattan, NY.

Danhauer S.C., Addington E.L., Sohl S.J., et al., 2017. Review of yoga therapy during cancer treatment. *Supportive Care in Cancer.* 25(4):1357–1372.

Desikachar, T.K.V., Cravens, R.H., 1998. *Health, Healing and Beyond: Yoga and the Living Tradition of Krishnamacharya.* C&C Offset Printing Co. Ltd; New Jersey.

Deussen, P., 1906. *The Philosophy of the Upanishads* (Vol. 1). Dover Publications; New York.

Emerson, D., 2015. *Trauma-Sensitive Yoga in Therapy: Bringing the Body into Treatment.* WW Norton & Company; Manhattan, NY.

Ernst, G., 2017. Heart-rate variability—more than heart beats? *Frontiers in Public Health.* 5:240.

Feuerstein, G., 2008. *The Yoga Tradition: Its History, Literature, Philosophy and Practice.* Hohm Press; Arizona.

Figg, W.D., Smith, E.K., Price, D.K., et al., 2010. Disclosing a diagnosis of cancer: where and how does it occur? *Journal of Clinical Oncology.* 28(22):3630.

Finlayson, D., Hyland Robertson, L., 2021. *Yoga Therapy Foundations, Tools and Practice.* Jessica Kingsley Publishers; London, UK.

Fink, R.M., Gallagher, E., 2019. Cancer pain assessment and measurement. *Seminars in Oncology Nursing.* 35(3):229–234.

Foos-Graber, A., 1989. *Deathing: An Intelligent Alternative for the Final Moments of Life.* Nicolas-Hays, Inc.; Florida.

Gendlin, E., 1982. *Focusing.* Random House Publishing Group; Manhattan, NY.

Grant, S.J., Hunter, J., Seely, D., et al., 2019. Integrative oncology: international perspectives. *Integrative Cancer Therapies.* 18:1534735418823266.

Grossman, P., Taylor, E., 2007. Toward understanding respiratory sinus arrhythmia: relations to cardiac vagal tone, evolution and biobehavioral functions. *Biological Psychology.* 74(2):263–285.

Gourine, A., Machhada, A., Trapp, S., Spyer, K., 2016. Cardiac vagal preganglionic neurones: an update. *Autonomic Neuroscience.* 199:24–28.

Gupta, R., 2011. Death beliefs and practices from an Asian Indian American Hindu perspective. *Death Studies.* 35(3):244–266.

Hamilton, J., 2017. Cultural beliefs and cancer care: are we doing everything we can? *Cancer Nursing.* 40(1):84–85.

Hartranft, C., 2003. *The Yoga-Sutra of Patanjali: A New Translation with Commentary.* Shambhala Publications; Boulder, CO.

Hermelink, K., Bühner, M., Sckopke, P., et al., 2017. Chemotherapy and post-traumatic stress in the causation of cognitive dysfunction in breast cancer patients. *Journal of the National Cancer Institute.* 109(10):djx057.

Heyman, J., 2019. *Accessible Yoga: Poses and Practices for Every Body.* Shambhala Publications; Boulder, CO.

Hopper, E., Emerson, D., Levine, P.A., et al. 2011, *Overcoming Trauma Through Yoga: Reclaiming Your Body.* North Atlantic Books; Berkeley, CA.

Jenkinson, S., 2015. *Die Wise: A Manifesto for Sanity and Soul.* North Atlantic Books; Berkeley, CA.

Jeter, P.E., Slutsky, J., Singh, N., Khalsa, S.B.S., 2015. Yoga as a therapeutic intervention: a bibliometric analysis of published research studies from 1967 to 2013. *Journal of Alternative and Complementary Medicine.* 21(10):586–592.

Kaiser, J., Dietrich, J., Amiri, M., et al., 2019. Cognitive performance and psychological distress in breast cancer patients at disease onset. *Frontiers in Psychology.* 10:2584.

Kemp, A.H., Quintana, D.S., Kuhnert, R.L., et al., 2012. Oxytocin increases heart rate variability in humans at rest: implications for social approach-related motivation and capacity for social engagement. *PLoS One.* 7(8):e44014.

Lad, V., 1984. *Ayurveda: The Science of Self-Healing: A Practical Guide.* Lotus Press; Twin Lakes, WI.

Lad, V., 2002. *Textbook of Ayurveda.* Ayurvedic Press; Albuquerque, NM.

Lee, S.Y., Lee, E.E., 2018. Access to health care, beliefs, and behaviors about colorectal cancer screening among Korean Americans. *Asian Pacific Journal of Cancer Prevention.* 19(7):2021.

Leggett, T., 2018. *The Complete Commentary by Śaṅkara on the Yoga Sūtra-s.* Trevor Leggett Adhyatma Yoga Trust; UK.

Levine, P.A., 2010. *In an Unspoken Voice: How the Body Releases Trauma and Restores Goodness.* North Atlantic Books; Berkeley, CA.

Lopez, G., Mao, J.J., Cohen, L., 2017. Integrative oncology. *Medical Clinics of North America.* 101(5):977–985.

Lundberg, J.O.N., Settergren, G., Gelinder, S., et al., 1996. Inhalation of nasally derived nitric oxide modulates pulmonary function in humans. *Acta Physiologica Scandinavica.* 158(4):343–347.

Lutz, J., 2021. *Trauma Healing in the Yoga Zone.* Handspring Publishing Limited; Edinburgh, UK.

Maas, P., Baier, K., Preisendanz, K., 2018. *Yoga in Transformation.* Vienna University Press; Vienna.

Mainkar, T.G., 1972. *Sāṃkhya-Kārikā of Iśvarakṛṣṇa.* Chaukhamba Sanskrit Pratishthan; Delhi.

Majewski, L., Bhavanani, A.B., 2020. *Yoga Therapy as a Whole-Person Approach to Health.* Singing Dragon; London & Philadelphia.

Mallinson, J., Singleton, M., 2017. *Roots of Yoga.* Penguin Books, UK.

Mason, H., Birch, K., 2018. *Yoga for Mental Health.* Handspring Publishing Limited; Edinburgh, UK.

Mazzocco, K., Masiero, M., Carriero, M.C., Pravettoni, G., 2019. The role of emotions in cancer patients' decision-making. *Ecancermedicalscience.* 13:914.

Meyers, T., 2021. Relationships in yoga therapy: developing collaboration within a healing presence. In: Finlayson, D., Hyland Robertson, L. (eds). *Yoga Therapy Foundations, Tools and Practice.* Jessica Kingsley Publishers; London, UK: 263–281.

Mills, J., 2021. *Adapting Yoga for People Living with Cancer.* Singing Dragon; London, UK.

Mitchell, S., 2000. *Bhagavad-Gita: A New Translation.* Three Rivers Press; New York.

Mohammad, A., Thakur, P., Kumar, R., et al., 2019. Biological markers for the effects of yoga as a complementary and alternative medicine. *Journal of Complementary and Integrative Medicine.* 16(1).

Moonaz, S., Nault, D., Cramer, H., Ward, L., 2021. CLARIFY 2021: Explanation and elaboration of the Delphi-based guidelines for the reporting of yoga research. *BMJ Open.* 11(8):e045812.

Moore, D., Libby, D.J., 2018. Trauma. In: Mason, H., Birch, K. (eds). *Yoga for Mental Health.* Handspring Publishing Limited; Edinburgh, UK: 105–130.

Mukerji, P.N., 1983. *Yoga Philosophy of Patanjali.* State University of New York Press, Albany, NY.

Müller, F.M., 1897. *The Upanishads.* Christian Literature; Sheffield, UK.

Neargardner, L., 2019. *Cancer + Yoga: For People Living with Cancer and Their Yoga Teachers.* Lulu Publishing Services; Morrisville, NC.

Neufeld, N.J., Elnahal, S.M., Alvarez, R.H., 2017. Cancer pain: a review of epidemiology, clinical quality and value impact. *Future Oncology.* 13(9):833–841.

Nienhuis, J.B., Owen, J., Valentine, J.C., et al., 2018. Therapeutic alliance, empathy and genuineness in individual adult psychotherapy. *Psychother Res.* 28(4):593–605.

NurrieStearns, M., NurrieStearns, R., 2013. *Yoga for Emotional Trauma.* New Harbinger Publications; Oakland, CA.

O'Clair, P.G., 2021. Movement therapy for breast cancer survivors. In: Schleip, R., Wilke J. (eds). *Fascia in Sport and Movement.* Handspring Publishing; Edinburgh, UK: 552–567.

Ogden, P., Fisher, J., 2015. *Sensorimotor Psychotherapy.* W.W. Norton & Company, New York, NY.

Orest Weber, M.A., Sulstarova, B., Pascal Singy, M.A., 2016. Cross-cultural communication in oncology: challenges and training interests. *Oncology Nursing Forum.* 43(1):e24.

Parker, G., 2020. *Restorative Yoga for Ethnic and Race-Based Stress and Trauma:* Singing Dragon; London, UK.

Pearson, N., Prosko, S., Sullivan, M., 2019. *Yoga and Science in Pain Care.* Singing Dragon; London, UK.

Pham, H., Torres, H., Sharma, P., 2019. Mental health implications in bladder cancer patients: a review. *Urologic Oncology: Seminars and Original Investigations.* 37(2):97–107.

Porges, P.G., 2011. *The Polyvagal Theory: Neurophysiological Foundations of Emotions, Attachment,*

Communication, Self Regulation. W.W. Norton & Company; New York, NY.

Posadzki, P., Watson, L., Alotaibi, A., Ernst, E., 2013. Prevalence of complementary and alternative medicine (CAM)-use in UK paediatric patients: a systematic review of surveys. *Complementary Therapies in Medicine.* 21(3):224–231.

Prinster, T., 2014. *Yoga for Cancer: A Guide to Managing Side Effects, Boosting Immunity, and Improving Recovery for Cancer Survivors.* Simon and Schuster.

Prosko, S., 2019. Compassion in Pain Care. In: Pearson, N., Prosko, S., Sullivan, M., 2019. *Yoga and Science in Pain Care.* Singing Dragon; London, UK: 235–256.

Rainville, P., Bechara, A., Naqvi, N., Damasio, A.R., 2006. Basic emotions are associated with distinct patterns of cardiorespiratory activity. *International Journal Of Psychophysiology.* 61(1):5–18.

Remski, M.D., 2019. *Practice and All is Coming: Abuse, Cult Dynamics, and Healing in Yoga and Beyond.* Embodied Wisdom Publishing; New Zealand.

Renz, M., Reichmuth, O., Bueche, D., et al., 2018. Fear, pain, denial, and spiritual experiences in dying processes. *American Journal of Hospice and Palliative Medicine.* 35(3):478–491.

Roelofs, K., 2017. Freeze for action: neurobiological mechanisms in animal and human freezing. *Philosophical Transactions of the Royal Society B: Biological Sciences.* 372(1718):20160206.

Rousseau, D. (ed.), 2020. *Yoga and Resilience.* Handspring Publishing Limited; Edinburgh, UK.

Rothenberg, R., 2020. *Restoring Prana: A Guide to Pranayama and Healing through Breath for Yoga Therapists, Yoga Teachers and Healthcare Practitioners.* Singing Dragon; London, UK.

Roy R., Charlton, D., 2019. *Embodying the Yoga Sutra: Support, Direction, Space.* Yogawords Limited; UK.

Rudman, S., 2021. Ayurveda for the yoga therapist. In: Finlayson, D., Hyland Robertson, L. (eds). *Yoga Therapy Foundations, Tools and Practice.* Jessica Kingsley Publishers; London, UK: 78–87.

Rukmani, T.S., 2001. *Yogasutrabhasyavivarana of Sankar.* Munshiram Manoharial Publishers Pvt, Ltd.; New Delhi, India.

Rumi, J.A.D., Barks, C., 2005. A Great Wagon. In: *Rumi: The Book of Love: Poems of Ecstasy and Longing.* Harper and Collins; Toronto.

Sausys, A., 2014. *Yoga for Grief Relief: Simple Practices for Transforming Your Grieving Mind and Body.* New Harbinger Publications; Oakland, CA.

Sawadogo, B., Gitta, S.N., Rutebemberwa, E., et al., 2014. Knowledge and beliefs on cervical cancer and practices on cervical cancer screening among women aged 20 to 50 years in Ouagadougou, Burkina Faso, 2012: a cross-sectional study. *Pan African Medical Journal.* 18:175.

Seely, D., Ennis, J.E., McDonell, E., et al., 2019. Intervention development process for a pragmatic randomized controlled trial: the thoracic peri-operative integrative surgical care evaluation trial. *Journal of Alternative and Complementary Medicine.* 25(S1): S112–S123.

Seely, D.M., Weeks, L.C., Young, S., 2012. A systematic review of integrative oncology programs. *Current Oncology.* 19(6):436–461.

Shansky, R.M., Lipps, J., 2013. Stress-induced cognitive dysfunction: hormone-neurotransmitter interactions in the prefrontal cortex. *Frontiers in Human Neuroscience.* 7:123.

Sharpe, L., Curran, L., Butow, P., Thewes, B., 2018. Fear of cancer recurrence and death anxiety. *Psycho-oncology.* 27(11):2559–2565.

Stone, M., 2008. *The Inner Tradition of Yoga: A Guide to Yoga Philosophy for the Contemporary Practitioner.* Shambhala Publications; Boulder, CO.

Sullivan, M., Hyland Robertson, L.C., 2020. *Understanding Yoga Therapy.* Routledge; New York.

Taneja, M.K., 2020. Modified bhramari pranayama in COVID infection. *Indian J Otolaryngol Head Neck Surg.* 72:395–397.

Taylor, A.G., Goehler L.E., Galper,D.I., et al., 2010. Top-down and bottom-up mechanisms in mind-body medicine: development of an integrative framework for psychophysiological research. *Explore.* 6(1):29–41.

Taylor, J., 2008. End-of-life yoga therapy: exploring life and death. *International Journal of Yoga Therapy.* 18(1):97–103.

Taylor, J., McLean, L., Korner, A., et al., 2020. Mindfulness and yoga for psychological trauma: systematic review and meta-analysis. *Journal of Trauma & Dissociation.* 21(5):536–573.

Taylor, M., 2018. *Yoga Therapy as a Creative Response to Pain.* Singing Dragon; London, UK.

Thayer, J.F., Åhs, F., Fredrikson, M., et al., 2012. A meta-analysis of heart rate variability and neuroimaging studies: implications for heart rate variability as a marker of stress and health. *Neuroscience & Biobehavioral Reviews.* 36(2):747–756.

Trill, M.D., 2013. Anxiety and sleep disorders in cancer patients. *EJC Supplements.* 11(2):216.

Turner, J., 2020. *Embodied Healing.* North Atlantic Books; Berkeley, CA.

Van der Kolk, B.A., Stone, L., West, J., et al., 2014. Yoga as an adjunctive treatment for posttraumatic stress disorder: a randomized controlled trial. *Journal of Clinical Psychiatry.* 75(6):1–1.

Weeks, L.C., Seely, D., Balneaves, L.G., et al., 2013. Canadian integrative oncology research priorities: results of a consensus-building process. *Current Oncology.* 20(4):289–299.

Weller, F., 2015. *The Wild Edge of Sorrow.* North Atlantic Books; Berkeley, CA.

Wildcroft, T., 2020. *Post-Lineage Yoga.* Equinox Publishing Limited; Sheffield, UK.

Winhall, J., 2021. *Treating Trauma and Addiction with the Felt Sense Polyvagal Model: A Bottom-Up Approach.* Routledge; UK.

Witt, C.M., Balneaves, L.G., Cardoso, M.J., et al., 2017. A comprehensive definition for integrative oncology. *JNCI Monographs.* 2017(52).

Yang, J., Guo, J., Jiang, X., 2017. Executive function in cancer patients with posttraumatic stress disorder. *International Journal of Psychiatry in Medicine.* 52(2):137–146.

Yates, P., Schofield, P., Zhao, I., Currow, D., 2013. Supportive and palliative care for lung cancer patients. *Journal of Thoracic Disease.* 5(Suppl 5):S623.

Yoon, S.Y., Oh, J., 2018. Neuropathic cancer pain: prevalence, pathophysiology, and management. *Korean Journal of Internal Medicine.* 33(6):1058.

Yu, R., 2016. Stress potentiates decision biases: a stress induced deliberation-to-intuition (SIDI) model. *Neurobiology of Stress.* 3:83–95.

Zuniga, K.B., Zhao, S., Kenfield, S.A., et al., 2019. Trends in complementary and alternative medicine use among patients with prostate cancer. *Journal of Urology.* 202(4):689–695.

Yoga Therapy in Clinical Practice: Practicalities 3

Anne Pitman

Cancer patients, riding on the continuum roller coaster, often come to yoga therapy anxious and in a state of distress. They are best met with consistent calm and kindness, and an intention of creating a safe place to breathe, reflect, and explore: a strong yet flexible containment of practice where human work can be undertaken. There is no one breath, no particular posture, that all cancer patients must do. There is no unwavering protocol that is necessary or curative. There is no rigid systematization; this is human work. Tender, weepy, sometimes bursting with laughter, real.

Yoga therapists[1] welcome patients in one-on-one sessions or small-group work, sometimes both (see client stories in Chapter 6). There are notable differences between the two, and one arrangement often works better for some patients than the other. Both share a distinct advantage in oncological care, and serve each patient's neurobiological need for connection: one with the co-regulating therapist alone, the other in a group of students who share in the cancer experience. As such, a therapist's capacity to establish trust and an authentic alliance is a heart-centered imperative (see Chapter 2). An in-depth and advanced knowledge of evidence-informed oncology yoga practice, from movement to meditation, in service to a person's unique needs, is essential (see Chapters 2 and 6). The safety and integrity of each and every practice, breath and beyond, are the foundation of yoga therapy education and continuing oncology care.

"First aid" for distressed clients

While many yoga therapists arrange sessions with their clients (one-on-one or in a small-group), others are on call, in hospital or clinic, available when a need arises. In one moment, they may be summoned to the infusion center to help a client who is panicking prior to treatment, the next waved into an office by the doctor, to be at hand when "bad news" is delivered. As part of a palliative team, they may be called to assist a bed-ridden patient with gentle movement and easeful breath practice. All yoga therapists, using their steadying voice and presence, carry a plethora of immediate "emergency" practices (see Chapter 6) which tend toward calming: a slow exhaled breath, a seated, subtle cat/cow-like movement (*mārjaryāsana*) of the spine, an easy forward bend with elbows on knees and hands on forehead, a whispered *mantra* (sacred sound), a steadying *mudrā* (hand gesture), a grounded feeling of weight in the chair. Immediate care when most needed.

Yoga therapy in clinical practice: scheduled sessions

Yoga therapists carry diverse philosophies and lineage are educated in different cultures and may vary somewhat in therapeutic approach, but all C-IAYT therapists share a scope of practice, as outlined by the International Association of Yoga Therapists (www.iayt.org) (see Yoga teacher education in Chapter 2). They come to a session, well-skilled in both the art and science of yoga therapy, practice a sensitivity in their embodied presence, and are best supported with additional training in mental health, pain, trauma, grief and dying (see Crucial education in Chapter 2). The following format for a scheduled non-emergency session is offered as an example, to make visible a strong container for safe, steady, reliable, and negotiable therapeutic practice. The order and focus of sessions may vary by school, lineage, and approach or differ by location. Appointments last anywhere from 45 to 90 minutes, in person, or online via a secure telehealth platform.

One-on-one yoga therapy sessions

Individual sessions are the pinnacle of creative evidence-informed curation. Yoga therapists draw on the many threads of what has been learned about a person though referrals, chart notes, integrative conversations, co-assessments,

---

[1] We recognize that some yoga teachers, while not having yoga therapy certification, have extended oncology education (see Chapter 2, Specialization in yoga therapy: education in cancer). We include them here, with welcome (see Chapter 1).

and in compassionate embodied inquiry with each client. Co-assessments gather lived experience and current expressions of their client's biopsychosocial-emotional and spiritual state. Informed further by current research and clinical collaboration in cancer care, they incorporate each client's evolving clinical picture, curating and adapting the practice to ease symptomatology (see Chapters 5 and 6). They bring multidimensional support with a vast array of yoga practices as neural exercises to relieve distress and promote self-regulation. Yoga therapists are, additionally, lifestyle guides, exploring any barriers to practice and well-being, practical or otherwise, while cultivating client autonomy, intention and motivation. With an embodied understanding of adaptive practice, yoga therapists are champions of support, using blocks, ties, blankets, pillows, walls, floors, chairs, and beds, when necessary, for individualized optimal experience. Listening well and sensing into lived and responsive experience in the moment, they envision a therapeutic plan, weaving all of these threads into a relevant, safe, evolving, and nourishing practice.

Before the session – integration of referrals, charts and lab results: A yoga therapist, depending on place of work, accesses medical charts, records and referrals prior to the first appointment. They make note of cancer type and stage, embark on necessary research, study pre-morbidities, comorbidities and contraindications to yoga practice, read about cancer treatments considered, or if already started, consider any side effects currently experienced (see Inclusion of clinical oncology assessments, p. 46). Referral notes from doctors or other therapists may provide initial direction on their "presenting condition" (see Records etc. p. 48). Some clients are self-referred; their self-advocacy (or that of their family and friends) prompts first contact. In either case, all clients must be medically cleared for yoga practice. Waiver forms with secured informed consent may be included in hospital/clinic forms sent out separately by the therapist before the session, or discussed and signed in the initial appointment (see The forms, p. 48). Like any other professional therapy, confidentiality (within legal limits) is assured. At some places of work, there may be the option for a short phone call before the meeting, to hear more about a client's intentions and goals. In practical terms, a yoga therapist will want to be sure that emergency procedures are intact, and that the space, if at all possible, is accessible, quiet, clean, comfortable, and scent free. To begin, the yoga therapist breathes, regulates, and resources themselves to be warm-heartedly available to their client.

Introduction to the yoga therapist and scope of practice: A personal introduction ensues if they are newly met, and an introduction to the work of yoga therapy provides the framework – its scope and what can be expected in the session (see Yoga therapy co-assessment, p. 46). It is not the goal of a yoga therapist to "fix" a client, but to instead assist them in developing awareness and to healthfully mediate the impact of cancer and its treatment, in their body and in their life. Although waivers may already be signed, a verbal discussion of scope of practice is useful and necessary for informed consent.

Compassionate embodied inquiry – the meeting ground: The yoga therapist is guided by studies in yoga philosophy, informed by current research and additional studies in cancer care. They carry a depth of adaptive yoga practice and body-centered therapeutic skills. All of this quiets into the background, ready when and if needed. So begins a back and forth, a deep listening, an easy silence, a slow wondering, and a resulting softness around the eyes. Here is a willingness to be a trusted witness, to join the patient in engaged and relevant yoga practice to reduce suffering. Professional and human-making accompaniment in hard times.

Listening and observing, witnessing, sensing and co-assessment: Many patients come to a session with a "presenting condition." Perhaps something is troubling them physically (difficulty breathing, fatigue, lymphedema, etc.) or they are struggling with shifting a perspective (in beliefs, motivation, fear of death, etc.). A yoga therapist attends with deep listening and gentle observation, enhancing their client's capacity to notice their own body's lived experience, including breath, movement, sensations, thoughts, beliefs, and emotions. This requires a deliberate slowing down, a mindful approach, and the learned skill of interoception (see p. 89). One might observe a sense of "freeze" after a diagnosis (eyes staring, tension and breath mostly held, thoughts stalled) while others may display a "fight or flight" response (agitated, breath rapid, thoughts racing). The yoga therapist will slowly explore the impact of their experience of cancer upon the broader biopsychosocial-spiritual aspects (*kośa-s*) of each unique person. Several yoga therapy assessment tools have been developed, based on ancient texts and current research (see p. 46). Throughout, a yoga therapist hopes to learn, as best they can, the many answers to the questions: What is your inner experience? What would you like a yoga therapist to know? All red flags, previous injuries, contraindications, comorbidities, and modifications needed to address any devices (such as PICCs and ports; see box on General instructions for yoga practice in oncology, p. 43 and Chapters 4 and 6), specific to each cancer client, will be noted and discussed.

Client education: In the midst of listening and noticing, "misapprehensions" may emerge from conversation or from an interoception of sensation. The yoga therapist may choose to titrate some knowledge, either coming from yoga philosophy or recent research that allows the client to "normalize" their reaction or better understand their experience; perhaps with regard to a profound existential questioning, the complexity of pain, the benefit of particular breath practices during medical treatment, or a current understanding of how the nervous system works. For example, learning that a flight/fight response is protective and normal after a diagnosis can be immediately reassuring, even withstanding the continued worrying, sleeplessness, and ongoing vigilance. These moments can bring a sense of relief and have the felt quality of two humans, sitting together, however briefly, in wonder about the vast intelligence of the body and the grand, if troubling, mysteries of life.

Curation of yoga practice: A seasoned yoga therapist will curate possibilities of practice in response to what they have heard, observed, sensed, and learned, creating a therapeutic plan, and individualized practice, in concert with their client, with a beginning gentle dose. This requires a depth of yoga knowledge and of cancer itself, as well as mental agility and discernment on the part of the therapist. The practices offered may be subtle or strong, physical or visualized, with each practice attuned to the needs presented by the client, depending on where they find themselves on the continuum of cancer care, and any side effects of treatment they may be experiencing (see Chapter 6). Based on a *kośa* assessment, yoga practices may be sampled to support the layers of each person: physical (*annamayakośa*, e.g., a restorative bolstered pose to support healing after surgery), energetic (*prāṇamayakośa*, e.g., alternate nostril breath to regulate), emotional/mental (*manomayakośa*, e.g., a warrior pose to remember grounded steadiness), wider witnessing/wisdom (*vijñānamayakośa*, e.g., a loving kindness meditation) or spiritual/connection (*ānandamayakośa*, e.g., chanting a *mantra*).

Co-assessment and refinement: Responses to conversation and practices offered (changes in breath, voice, behavior, tension, pain, affect, etc.) are discussed. The yoga therapist will be curious about what is developing in their client's awareness: what is the lived experience of this moment, their response to connection, acknowledgment, and practice? Thankfully, assumptions are unnecessary. Instead, a therapist may ask: How did this breath feel? What did you sense when you held this *mudrā*? What is the felt response to this guided meditation? How comfortable was this movement? Did the feeling of discomfort change in this posture? How could the practice be easier, softer, more grounded? If other formal assessments are employed, there may be a specific interest in the before and after measurements (see Inclusion of oncology assessments and Yoga therapy co-assessments, p. 46). A shared wondering and curiosity can elicit a heightened interest in the client toward their body and its changeable nature, adding to a sense of embodied agency.

Home practice and lifestyle recommendations: Any small shifts in initial practice can be enhanced through further practice, on and off the mat, beyond the session. What elements of the session's practice would be useful to continue? What might be added? When and where, and for how long is a home practice do-able and enjoyable? What lifestyle shifts would allow a yoga practice to be possible? Say, for example, if the presenting issue is insomnia, what sleep hygiene and calming practices could be included before bed, or when awakened with troubling thoughts? The therapist, if informed by "neural platforms" (see Cancer diagnosis through the lens of Polyvagal Theory and the *Guṇa-s*, Chapter 2), may have a conversation with their client about resourcing themselves with and beyond their yoga practice: for example, with suggestions for "safe mobilized movement" (such as curated *āsana* practice, playing active games with friends or walking in the woods), and safe immobilized practices (such as mindful meditation or sitting by their favorite stream and listening to the music of moving water). Depending on the interest of each patient, and what may be most supportive to encourage practice outside of the therapy session, written yoga practice notes, recordings of the session, or relevant meditations may be offered to assist in home practice.

Healthcare referrals: As part of integrated healthcare, a yoga therapist, in conversation with their client, will make recommendations and referrals to other oncology focused practitioners, such as a psychotherapist, nutritionist, or physiotherapist (see Records etc., p. 48). Referrals can be made to complement yoga therapy (for example, for increased relaxation through oncological massage), to recommend a yoga therapist with a specialization (such as pain or lymphedema), or to defer in consideration of complex need (for example, long term psychological support). An agreement is made between the pair with regard to best next steps and the timing and frequency of yoga therapy sessions that is easeful for the patient.

After the session – yoga therapy charting and notes: The yoga therapist will keep professional clinical notes, including assessments, as required by their workplace. Hospital and medical clinics may require charting in electronic medical records. SOAP (Subjective, Objective, Assessment, and Plan) notes are also common, and *kośa* notes are often written for a yoga therapist's own purposes (see Records etc., p. 48).

Returning clients: Although yoga therapists may see a client once, they primarily work with people over many sessions throughout the continuum. As such, they re-assess and gather information on each client's changing clinical picture from their client and/or medical charts as they proceed. Therapeutic trust deepens as the yoga therapist learns about their continued experience, yoga practice and their life beyond the mat. Response to

any specific homework practices or lifestyle changes are noted and discussed, and new practices are layered in, when needed and desired.

Reasons for practitioner referrals or self-referral to one-on-one therapy

One-on-one sessions can be very personal, quiet and (professionally) intimate. Here are some reasons, among many, that a client might prefer a one-on-one session, over or in addition to a small-group practice.

To feel a calm and practiced presence: The cancer world can feel chaotic at the best of times; tests, appointments, waiting (and more waiting), and feeling continually in the throes of swirling thoughts and fears. While the medical system is chock full of good and caring people, its immediate function is efficiency. It can be a (necessarily) sterile situation that doesn't always lend itself to an intimate, unhurried conversation. Friends and family, should one be lucky enough to have them, can be even more anxious than the patients themselves. When nervous systems are "upregulated," we tend to gravitate to people who are genuinely calm, if only to "borrow their nervous system" until we can modulate our own. While yoga therapists are practitioners of a wide range of skills, the foremost is a practiced and authentic calm.

To examine beliefs: Not only can the diagnosis of cancer be a shock, but it often deeply confusing, especially for people who take the utmost care of their bodies, their minds and their souls. To these "health-conscious" folks, a cancer diagnosis can feel like a betrayal. Some come to a yoga therapist to parse out beliefs laid bare by the diagnosis. Whether it is to contend with beliefs that can no longer hold water ("if you eat enough broccoli, all will be well" or "bad things don't happen to 'good' people"), or to open a door to renewed religious or spiritual wonderings, a yoga therapy session can hold a space for a person to reflect and contemplate in good company.

For help in listening to the body: A cancer diagnosis can be an "out-of-body experience" and it can be helpful to have a willing guide to embodiment. Sometimes people realize, post-diagnosis, that they have not been truly connected to their bodies in a very long time. They may, by extension, also be disconnected from their daily life (and often, from their loved ones) and the present moment. It can be difficult to know where to start. A yoga therapist can offer a variety of practices to help someone find the bread crumb trail back to a friendly, listening relationship with their body.

To establish agency: Many of us think, pre-cancer, that we are masterfully "running the show" and in control of present and future plans. A cancer diagnosis can shatter this illusion very quickly. Through practice, we can become aware of what is truly in our purview by practicing skillful response (with compassion for our autonomic reactions) to life's happenings. No one and no cancer can take away our inner experience, our capacity to choose breath and movement, when possible, and our learned capacity to soften our heart in uncertain times.

To satisfy complex needs: Each cancer is unique, true. And each person will be impacted in unique ways, will have specific acute or lingering side effects (or no side effects at all!), differing available social support, and particular needs for connection. Additionally, each client carries their lived embodied experience before cancer, which can include significant trauma, injury, or comorbidities, all met with individualized practices. Sometimes it isn't the cancer that has someone worried, but something that is, for them, even more stressful, such as severe financial difficulties, lack of housing, or having to care for an incapacitated family member or friend. Life is complex, more so with cancer. A yoga therapist will want to understand these complexities, learn how cancer is specifically affecting the individual, their family, and their life and advocate for their best care.

To express difficult feelings: A diagnosis of cancer may be a shock, no matter how anticipated. Then comes a rush of unwelcome and more challenging feelings, such as sadness, grief, and anger. While completely normal, these feelings are classified as "negative" in many cultures. Unfortunately, in a positive-only cancer culture, it can be hard to admit that you are sad, angry, frustrated, fearful, and in despair (see "Toxic positivity," p. 29). Feelings may remain unexpressed or "unmoved," yet embodied, causing undue tension and stress. Conversely, emotions, well met, often are restored to their impermanent "visiting" nature. In this way, yoga therapy allows authenticity to reign. A one-on-one session creates space for feelings to be fully heard and well met with compassion and practice.

To work with specific fears and traumas: As people progress down the path of cancer treatment, they may find themselves up against some very specific fears, such as a fear of enclosed places (like an MRI machine), fear of needles, or "scanxiety," an anticipation of testing and the following anxiety-filled wait for results. Fear of recurrence, when finished with medical treatment, can be uniquely incapacitating. Very consistently, running underneath every worry, concern and anxiety, is the fear of death. Yoga therapists, trained in trauma, work sensitively and slowly with a range of trauma-informed yoga practices and can bring awareness and human companionship to fears that can otherwise become a barrier to treatment and holistic health.

To protect a compromised immune system: Cancer patients may be more susceptible to higher risk of infections due to systemic immunodeficiency, depending on their treatment (see Chapter 4). They may feel more safe and secure meeting with just one other person, who is vigilant with distancing and sanitizing. This protective need may also be met with virtual session on a secure telehealth or HIPPA-compliant Zoom platform.

To maintain sense of privacy: People can understandably feel emotionally vulnerable when they have cancer, their boundaries regularly breached by (necessary) questioning, poking and prodding. When their bald head, even when covered, broadcasts their state of health to the world, they often wish their cancer was less public. The confidentiality and privacy of a one-on-one appointment can often better meet these needs.

To feel "safe-enough": Emotional safety is foremost, offered by a trustworthy depth of human understanding, compassionate negotiation, and attunement to more subtle emotional needs. For someone with significant trauma, an individual session (supported by their mental health team) allows for slow and titrated practice, interoceptively negotiated. Comfort-making props, such as a weighted or warmed blanket, may be very welcome.

To avoid emotional flooding: Although most people want supportive human connection as they move through cancer treatment, they sometimes can't bear to hear other people's cancer stories. They can be profoundly impacted by the suffering of others, easily flooded by their own empathy for others, and may not be able to bring their own self-care to the fore when faced with difficult and possibly "triggering" stories. In addition, some patients prefer to proceed one day at a time, shielding themselves from treatment stories offered by others further down the cancer road.

To create individualized, "cancer-informed" practice: A cancer diagnosis can stop us. Specifically, it can stop us from moving at all, even for some people with established fitness and yoga practices. For other patients, a cancer diagnosis can be the motivating factor to begin moving more regularly (or for the first time), but they don't know where to start. It is critical to work with a therapist well-versed in physical safety (see General considerations, p. 43), with knowledge of breath and movement modifications for particular cancers (such as modifications in movement after a mastectomy). If particular conditions (see Chapter 6) arise during or after treatment, such as lymphedema, osteoporosis, or complex pain, expertise (and possible referral) is required.

Physical safety can also be met in wise use of props, such as bolsters to support or modify position, or a chair or wall to aid in balance. In treatment, the practice is often subtle, gentle, and includes the necessity of rest. After treatments end, while rest is always important, the focus may be more on strengthening. A compassionate conversation about each individual's unique abilities and barriers is helpful, whether it is finding a suitable practice space, the best timing of practice around a myriad of appointments, or the consideration of each client's immediate limits (fatigue, pain, surgical sites, safe range of motion, other injuries or comorbidities). Working with each person to create a doable and satisfying practice is key to ongoing engagement.

To expand and connect with an integrated healthcare team: A yoga therapist can be the missing piece of the integrated healthcare puzzle. Clients are sometimes looking for a particular balance between top-down practices (such as meditation or visualization), and bottom-up practices, initiated in the body (such as *āsana* or free-movement). Sometimes this balance is found within yoga therapy, sometimes it is shared between therapies. For example, a patient who already has a movement plan suggested by a physiotherapist, seeks guidance from a yoga therapist to add a contemplative meditation practice. Or the yoga therapist, having established an accessible *āsana*/movement practice for a client, may refer them to a psychotherapist, for expanded psychological care. When a yoga therapist finds themselves outside of their scope of practice or knowledge, they will happily refer onward. If they work at a hospital or clinic, these colleagues may be right down the hall, available for a personal introduction.

To have a constant companion on the continuum: As a patient moves through the cancer continuum it can be helpful to have constant practitioners, perhaps one person who knows them well and has worked with them from diagnosis to remission, throughout their survivorship, "chronic" disease or recurrence, or continuing to practice with them through palliative care and dying, offering responsive practice to changing treatments and experiences. It can be a great relief to know you don't have to tell your story to one more person. Integrated, yet set apart from their medical treatments, a one-on-one session can be a time together of calm reflection, and steadying practice throughout undulating waves of life with cancer.

Small-group yoga therapy sessions

A person living with cancer can sometimes feel as though they can't "do" yoga – they aren't flexible enough or aren't strong enough for those vigorous practices seen in magazines, ads, and books. This is a tragic misunderstanding of the variety, breadth, and accommodation of yoga practice (which includes non-physically demanding options, such as subtle movement, meditation and breath-work), and a teacher's learned capacity to alter and modify all practices for the ease and benefit of the student. Yoga is meant to fit the person, not the other way around.

Yoga therapists have extensive experience in the skill of practice modification, originally from their teacher training, and deepened throughout their training and experience as a yoga therapist. Keeping their potential clients in mind, their capacity and limitations, a therapist will create a supportive and inclusive class, with a sequence of relevant, accessible, and trauma-sensitive breath and movement practices, possibly including meditation, visualization, *mudrā*, chanting, and relaxation (and more), all in an atmosphere of responsive compassion. It will take into account the attending population: their lived experience (injuries, trauma, and shocks), how they may be feeling (possibly anxious, depressed, etc.) and any typical needs of people during and after cancer care (see Chapter 6). Once they know more about individual preference and needs, they modify accordingly. As such, small-group practice is complex, requiring both intake and assessments, and the discernment, acuity, and flexibility of the therapist.

The yoga therapist is a virtuoso, orchestrating adaptable sequencing and necessary modifications to ensure a safe and engaging class for people with different needs, sometimes with opposite capabilities. For example, in one class they must be able to include someone who can't sit (perhaps as a result of pelvic floor radiation), someone who can't easily stand (perhaps they are dizzy from chemo), and someone who can't lie down perhaps (they are not yet comfortable with their head touching the mat after a long recovery from brain surgery). This is the nimble work of an experienced and knowledgeable teacher.

Group classes for those facing cancer are popular and take place in clinics, hospitals, recreation centers and private studios, and may be privately run or linked with cancer associations. Sometimes these classes are designated by cancer type (breast or prostate etc.), and some are open to people with all types of cancer. Some are married to specific times on the continuum,

for example, welcoming patients during treatment, or a class specifically for "survivors." Many offer a particular kind of yoga (such as "chair" or "restorative"), adapted for accessibility. Classes provide both a strong container for accountability in practice and a shared social connection (in community/*saṅgha)*, so important to many patients. Similar to one-on-one sessions, these can be in-person or online via a secure platform.

Before the class – integration of referrals, records, and lab results: In some locations, yoga therapists have access to records for each member of their group. All students of the class must have medical clearance for yoga practice, and waivers/informed consent discussed and signed (see The forms, p. 48). In many cases yoga therapists connect with clients before class with a phone call, or they meet for an intake as the client enters the class. They ask about current treatments, making notes of red flags (see box on General considerations for yoga practice in oncology, p. 45, and Chapters 4 and 6), side effects of treatment, or contraindications to yoga practice, so they can incorporate this information in their ever-changing class plan (see Assessment in oncological yoga therapy, p. 45). Some worthy questions might include: Do you have any discomfort or pain? Can you describe it? What makes it feel better? What positions do you find to be most comfortable? Can you tell right away that a movement or position is bothering you, or do you feel the discomfort the next day? Have you checked with your healthcare team on this? The answers to these questions can direct the yoga therapist toward particular adaptive modifications and allow a conversation about how to ensure safe practice. If a teacher suspects that their class wouldn't be suitable or safe for any given individual, suggestions can be offered for one-on-one yoga therapy or an alternative modality (physiotherapy or oncological massage, for example), or the yoga therapist might ask to be in contact with their healthcare provider to receive further guidance on their condition. Before a group arrives, a yoga therapist will want to be sure that the space, if at all possible, is accessible, warm, quiet, comfortable, and scent free. There may be a moment to breathe and to embody their compassionate heart before students trickle in.

Compassionate embodied inquiry, group style: The yoga therapist, who teaches group classes, has cultivated a "wide-lens" capacity to enable them to notice many people at the same time, and an ability to respond to many differing physical capacities, change direction depending on client response, and tend to the emotional temperature of the room. An embodied, welcoming presence is key to ensuring clients, new and long-standing, feel seen and included.

Introduction to the yoga therapist and scope of practice: An introduction to yoga and the intention of the practice helps everyone settle. This is a meeting place of a different kind, a place where, even given the difference in cancer experiences, there can be a deep acceptance and rare understanding between students. It can help to suggest the following agreement: the therapist, observing and assisting if desired, will offer a variable practice based on education in oncological yoga, with a variety of adaptations and options for what they know about each individual present. The student is welcome to pause, rest, breathe differently, choose a different movement or more comfortable position (sit, stand, lie down), ask questions or wave the therapist over for individual assistance. Important here, is to plant the hardy seeds of self-awareness or interoception, so the client can learn to sense into an inner "yes" or "no", and to see themselves as "response-able," the architects of their own practice.

Check-in (optional) and group witnessing: Beyond a private check-in with the yoga therapist (see Yoga therapy co-assessment, p. 46), a group check-in allows everyone to witness and benefit from the experience of the collective: sometimes a report on side effects they are noticing, or emotions that are surfacing, such as a sadness they feel in leaving a job or the fear of recurrence that is growing stronger as they end treatment. This heart-felt sharing can help people feel less alone. Clients can also learn from each other's practical cancer experience: the best hospital parking spaces, what recommendations they found helpful for mouth sores, and what prosthesis shop has the best quality goods. However, some people may be understandably overwhelmed, shy or have previous social trauma, and may want to pass

on a check-in or choose classes that don't include this aspect. Invitation and sensitive care are the focus.

Client education: There is so much to know about the human body and the challenges when facing cancer. For the newly diagnosed, it is a whole new world with a whole new language. In order to broach cancer-related knowledge and evolving research, some teachers speak to a different theme each week, including: Your Brilliant Nervous System, Little Known Facts about Lymphedema, Authenticity is the New Positivity. Information that speaks to the experience of all students, such as Working with Anxiety, can also be sprinkled through the yoga practice. Shared experience can foster a feeling of connection.

Yoga practice with modifications and co-assessments: People come to class with a wide variety of physical abilities; add to this the impact of cancer. Yoga therapists must have well-honed skills in assessing postural needs and offering a variety of modifications, such as changing the intensity of a movement (a smaller, more comfortable range of movement), changing the postural plane of movement (instead of cat/cow or *mārjaryāsana* on hands and knees, replicating this movement sitting on a chair or standing against a wall), selecting a similar but easier direction of movement (instead of a seated forward fold, achieving the desired flexion by lying down and drawing knees to chest), or adding props for support (under knees, lower back, cervical spine, wherever needed). Therapists must cultivate well-tuned ears and eyes, in addition to a caring heart.

Check out (optional) and group witnessing: Here is a time for each client to track, for themselves, any shift in thoughts, feelings or sensations as they finish their practice. Noticing any change in experience, such as a calming of anxiety or a softening of discomfort, can give people great hope and motivation for sustained practice. Again, the shared experience can be the antidote to loneliness. After-class "good vibes" can foster personal contacts outside of class, further enhancing a sense of community connection.

After the class – notes and referrals: Any needed referrals can be given to clients as they leave or written in charts, if applicable. Yoga therapy notes, assessments and anything that stood out in class, along with referral records, may be kept by the yoga therapist or by the clinic/hospital, and can augment an understanding of the benefits of yoga therapy in colleagues (see Records etc., p. 48). Many therapists also call or send emails to receive patient feedback and response.

Reasons for practitioner referral or self-referral to small-group yoga therapy

Group sessions can provide both knowledgeable guidance and group support. Here are some reasons, among many, that a client might prefer group classes, over or in addition to, one-on-one yoga therapy sessions.

Shared companionship: There is nothing like the feeling when you are amidst people who appreciate what you are going through. When we suffer, we make up a story that we are the only ones troubled, and thus, we must be doing cancer "all wrong." In a class, you can let down your guard, speak your fears without worry for/of others, take off your wig, and feel less alone. The lived experience is a rare co-regulation with people who understand the depth of your experience and fears. An enduring sense of belonging can be cultivated in such a class. Suffering shared can be suffering lifted. Acceptance from others is gold.

Discomfort in being the center of attention: Some folks prefer being one amongst many, not singled out, even in a compassionate way. They relax into the general chatter, moving, chanting and meditating with others, and would rather avoid a spotlight or focus that can come with one-on-one sessions. It is important that their preferences are respected, without judgment. As such, the "check in" should be optional, as it may provoke anxiety for some. Advertisements for classes could be clear on whether this is included, to allow for comfort.

To ensure safety: There may be contraindications and safety concerns (see General considerations, p 43), even when a client is far beyond their active medical treatment (such as persistent lymphedema or osteoporosis). Having a yoga therapist who is well versed and experienced with oncological yoga, both in- and post-treatment, can

feel more supportive, and can provide a wider range of research-informed modifications than can be given in a (non-cancer focused) community yoga class.

To learn from others farther down the path: Some people like to know what may be upcoming in their treatment and recovery. In class, patients share practical tips, learned from their oncology team (a local place to buy great wigs, a great cancer website for nutritious recipes) and emotional support ("Oh, I cried a lot at first too," "Walking every day really helped me feel more grounded"). Experienced patients often reach out to those newly diagnosed, perhaps offering the former a fresh sense of purpose.

To find one's voice: Sometimes after discovering cancer, clients feel depleted, diminished, small and, all of a sudden, without a strong voice in order to direct their care. In the rush of tests and treatments, they can feel as though they have become invisible. Chanting in a group class has no equal for slowly building confidence, and a willingness to stand firmly and speak. Voice married to compassion can help enormously in continuing communication with family, therapists, and doctors.

Less expensive option: Group classes are usually a low-cost option (compared to individual sessions), but sometimes both can be found free of charge, if associated with a hospital or cancer foundation. Financial equity in cancer care has a long way to go (see Cancer health disparity, p. 66) and it must be remembered that for some people, cancer is disproportionally financially burdensome.

General considerations for yoga practice in oncology

Yoga therapy specializes in research-informed individualized practice. Nevertheless, it's useful to keep some general safety considerations in mind when working with people in cancer treatment. See Chapters 4 and 6 for more detailed information on treatment side-effects and modifications for specific conditions.

- **Medical clearance:** All clients should have medical clearance for yoga therapy. Yoga therapists may want to provide a pamphlet that

(continued)

cites yoga research and explains the vast range of yoga therapy approaches (including the benefits of a subtle in-treatment approach and safe and progressive strengthening/restorative practices, post-treatment) so that the oncology team can make effective and knowledgeable referrals.

- **Side effect care:** Inquire with regard to common side effects of treatment in every session and understand contraindications to practice. Yoga therapy is not diagnostic. Refer clients back to their oncology team and work collaboratively with any symptomology that suggests lymphedema, neuropathy, anemia, or if they experience discomfort/pain or shortness of breath.

- **Pain:** Never work through pain. Instead insist that your client check with their oncology team to rule out, or better understand progression or metastasis (see Table 4.2 in Chapter 4). If the client is cleared, provide safe and relevant accommodation for any discomfort or condition, such as changing positions, adding supports or including non-movement practices. Be sure your patient refers back to their oncological team with any symptoms of swelling.

- **Compromised immunity:** Make sure your space is clean, props are regularly cleaned and/or have clients bring a towel from home to lay over any props. Be sure your conduct (mask wearing and hand washing) is in keeping with your clients' needs and comfort. Patients and therapists with active infections should postpone their sessions.

- **Hydration:** Be sure your client stays hydrated during practice, as many people find cancer treatments drying. Drinking water more frequently can reduce the intensity of some side effects, such as nausea. See that everyone has a water bottle.

- **Room and body temperature:** Practice in comfortable room temperatures; now is not the time for hot yoga. Some patients, especially in the midst of treatment, can sometimes feel chilly, so have clean blankets available. Those with a fever should immediately consult medical care.

- **Cognitive issues:** Many patients and their caregivers experience "brain fog" or cognitive overwhelm, in and beyond treatment. Keep conversations simple and clear, if needed, and always compassionate.

- **Devices:** Make proper accommodations for devices such as PICCs and ports. Review each client's current status at every appointment and know any contraindications (for example, avoiding movement in the days after a port surgery) or necessary comfort measures for all devices (such as placing bolsters under the hands in table position or under the arms in reclining postures for PICC lines).

- **Dizziness/weakness/numbness/tingling:** Have props available, including chairs and wall space or shift practices on the floor to support clients who feel weak or are prone to dizziness. Similarly, modify practice for those with neuropathy (numbness/tingling) who find it hard to practice standing or on hands and knees.

- **Skin health:** Note location of any radiation treatments, as the skin in that area may be compromised. For example, if your patient has received pelvic region radiation, they may want to avoid long sitting practices or may need strategic bolstering.

- **Compressive garments:** Be sure your client is using (if needed) a compressive garment fitted specifically for them (not store bought), and is following the recommendations of its use in yoga practice from their lymphedema/oncology team.

- **Steroid alert:** Watch for an uptick in energy. Patients taking chemo may be given steroids prior to their treatment. In these days they may find stillness and meditation more challenging. A focus on gentle movement can be helpful.

- **Frailty:** Depending on the treatment, your client may experience extreme fatigue or have lost significant weight and muscle tone (cachexia). Turn instead toward the wide range of subtle bed-yoga practices (for example, breath awareness, visualization, meditation, or gentle joint movements).

Where are sessions held?

Yoga therapy sessions are held in various locations: yoga studios, complementary healthcare clinics, hospital outpatient centers and infusion rooms, or a client's home, to name a few (see Chapter 6). Each place of work has its own idiosyncrasies, such as the need for therapist flexibility in starting and stopping yoga practices to allow for necessary medical interruptions, if in hospital. Online work in yoga therapy is not new, but the COVID-19 pandemic demanded that yoga therapists pivot quickly, creating what is now considered an important option for many. Secure telehealth platforms and HIPPA-compliant sessions are now popular places of virtual gathering for both small-groups and individuals. While there are some downsides, such as a possible decrease in social cues for nervous system regulation, or a reduced ability for teachers to clearly assess physical poses (depending on the client's computer set-up), time, research, and increased online experience will help therapists refine best practices for future work.

Advantages to yoga therapy on medical virtual platforms or Zoom

Anecdotally, the advantages of telehealth for cancer populations have become quickly apparent. For those in treatment, practicing at home may simply be less hassle, more accessible, and more convenient. Cancer patients who are medically fragile or immunocompromised may reasonably feel safer at home in front of their computers. In group classes, students can sometimes feel less intimidated or self-conscious when practicing together online – they enjoy the freedom and privacy to move differently, or more easily take self-directed breaks. While for some, virtual practice can feel disconnecting, others appreciate the sense of distance and space to self-regulate their nervous system.

Interestingly, groups can continue to feel socially supported, especially with a yoga therapist who has a strong capacity to cultivate online relationships with, and between participants. Rural patients, formerly at a disadvantage for attending in-person cancer-based classes, may find increased availability of online programs, depending on their internet connection. Appropriate technology, though, is certainly not available to all patients, so effort must be taken to ensure equity for marginalized populations, and democratize accessibility to best care. On a practical note, online classes underline the need for individualized detailed intakes and waivers that include both emergency contacts and immediate addresses for all participants, should an in-session emergency arise.

Whom do we serve?

Yoga therapists, in collaboration with colleagues in oncology, work with people at any stage of the cancer care continuum. Their clients include children, teens, and adults facing cancer, and they refine their practices for each unique population. In addition to working directly with diagnosed clients, yoga therapists offer care to families of patients, and couples, recognizing that the shock and burden of cancer ripple out beyond the patient. Over the past decade, emphasis and education has been purposefully oriented toward diversity, equity and inclusion in both medical and yoga-based care (www.iayt.org/dei). We are sadly mistaken if we presume all patients can easily access holistic and integrative care (see Chapter 4 on Cancer health disparity). The ethics of human compassion demand that we keep these inequities in our sight, work to attune ourselves to the suffering of all, and find creative ways to bring care, compassionate practice, and kinship to all communities.

Assessment in oncological yoga therapy

The yoga therapist seeks to understand the experience of their client and to discern whether the therapy employed is relevant and helpful as they continue down the cancer continuum. Inspired by *Patañjali-s Yoga Sūtra-s* (Bryant 2009), a yoga therapist looks for as complete and comprehensive an understanding of the problem (*heyam*) as possible. Together with their client, they try to understand the cause (*hetu*) of the suffering, as best they can. They then proceed with the negotiated goals of healing (*hanam*), and the selection and utilization of therapeutic tools (*upayam*). Assessment refers to the formal means of recognizing the ways in which the client is suffering, tracking any changes, and appraising how therapeutic practices are being received. "Co-assessments," a term used by many in yoga therapy, points to a collaborative process. Simply said, it is an assessment that includes the client's willingness to engage and explore, and their capacity to notice, sense, track, and report from their interior present moment experience.

Inclusion of clinical oncology assessments

In integrative oncology care, referrals, containing diagnostics, are often made available to yoga therapists, with physical and/or psychological assessments prepared by licensed practitioners. A familiarity with these can help a yoga therapist understand more about their client's "presenting condition" (from a colleague's vantage point and expertise), and the assessed impact of said diagnosis. Yoga therapists may receive information with regard to psychological state (anxiety or depression, for example), or cancer side effects or progression (lymphedema, bone metastasis), and/or non-cancer related diagnostics (injuries, such as knee or shoulder pain, or comorbidities such as diabetes, or heart conditions).

It is incumbent on the yoga therapist, while not interpreting medical or psychological tests, nor providing diagnostics, to understand the vetted testing supplied by other professions and to safely dovetail their therapy practice, in accordance with their scope of practice. For example, a shared client chart may include scores for a host of inventories, such as the Edmonton Symptom Assessment Scale (ESAS), the Eastern Cooperative Oncology Group Performance Scale (ECOG) or the Functional Assessment of Cancer Therapy Fatigue Scale (FACT-F). Many patients fill in the NCCN "Distress Thermom-

eter" each time they go to a medical appointment. While these are not specifically yoga therapy assessments, they can provide pertinent foundational information.

In integrated practice, yoga therapists can be agile when working with colleagues, while always remaining in their scope. For example, a psychologist, while providing care for a client exhibiting depression, may ask a yoga therapist for help in establishing a movement practice. The yoga therapist, through compassionate embodied inquiry, then provides a range of interrelated practices (see Chapters 2 and 6) that support and complement the client's work with the psychologist. Ongoing communication between psychologist and yoga therapist ensues (after obtaining written permission from the client). In the case of more severe and complex psychological or physical issues, this close collaborative approach with other practitioners in oncology is mandatory, and reciprocal referrals are necessary.

Yoga therapy co-assessments

The yoga therapy profession is young and is currently devising formal assessment tools (too many to detail here) to better understand their clients through their breath, movement, behavior, thoughts, emotions, and nervous system regulation through the lens of yoga philosophy (Butera & Elgelid 2017, Garner 2016, Wheeler 2021, Sullivan & Hyland Robertson 2020, Rothenberg 2019, Majewski & Bhavanani 2020, Krentzman & Sullivan 2021). In yogic terms, therapists would be listening for evidence of suffering, signs of distress, and disharmonies or imbalances in the *kośa-s, doṣa-s, kleśa-s,* and *guṇa-s* (and more, see Chapter 2); These co-assessments both reveal our client's inner experience and direct the selection of relevant resourcing yoga practices, including philosophical discussion and possible lifestyle changes.

As an example, a common yoga therapy co-assessment is one that considers all five *kośa-s* (see Yoga Philosophy in Chapter 2). In a collection of notes, referrals, and clinical assessments, in consideration of the evolving clinical picture of any given patient in what emerges throughout compassionate inquiry, a therapist will consider the obstacles to vitality of each sheath. They detail what a client is experiencing on each layer of their experience, at each stage of the cancer continuum. As an example, here are some common areas of concern during cancer treatment seen through a *kośa* lens (see Chapter 4 for side effects of treatment and Chapter 6 for expansive and personalized *kośa* approaches):

- *annamaya* – the physical/body systems sheath. All physical impacts of treatment are considered, such as effects on systems (circulatory, digestive, respiratory, muscular, endocrine, reproductive, etc.), including nausea, burns, hair loss, pain, etc. (see Chapter 4 for each treatment's possible side effects).

- *prāṇamaya* – the energy/vital air/life-force sheath. Yoga therapists will want to understand a client's level of energy or vitality. Many clients in treatment endure long periods of fatigue or weakness, and many struggle with insomnia. Some struggle with shallow breath or shortness of breath that may be part of the disease (e.g., lung cancer) or a symptom of anxiety.

- *manomaya* – the emotional/mental/thoughts sheath. Many clients are very mentally active, researching their own cancer. Conversely, "brain fog" affects many. Beliefs about cancer are very personal. Common emotions include shock, fear, anger, frustration, loneliness, and despair. Anxiety and depression may be constant companions.

- *vijñānamaya* – the wisdom/witness/knowledge/personality/metacognition sheath. Bringing awareness to the many impacts of cancer and cultivating discernment in this sheath can inform the many decisions facing someone in treatment. Many clients speak of looking at their life differently after a diagnosis and experience significant growth in knowledge and wisdom.

- *ānandamaya* – the bliss/connection/meaning/spiritual development/life purpose sheath. The meaning of suffering, and life-purpose itself, can change radically during cancer treatment. Yoga therapy inquiries regarding connection, joy, "bliss," and for some, spiritual faith, are warranted.

(Using the combined definitions of *kośa-s* from: Wheeler 2021, Rudman 2021, Pearson et al. 2019.)

Many clients report enjoying the process of yoga therapy assessments and see them as invaluable for self-reflection and inner awareness. Yet therapists must be sensitive to the everyday medical experience of their client. Cancer patients are regularly inundated with physical and psychological testing as part of their medical care, filling in surveys each time they enter a hospital or clinic. They may, at least initially, be coming to yoga therapy to move, breathe, and express, not to spend inordinate amounts of time in formal assessments.

Ultimately, a yoga therapist is interested in inner state of their client and their changing capacity for awareness. To this end, yoga therapists employ non-intrusive observation skills to help a client co-assess and track change objectively (for example, breath pace and depth) and subjectively (such as changes in pain, sensation, and emotional intensity). For example, it isn't until our client mentions the strange tightness in their throat and is asked to pause, that they realize they are carrying a much deeper grief than they had thought. Or when they are asked to become more aware of their clenched stomach and restricted breath, their apprehension for an upcoming test is revealed to them. This kind of sensing requires a change of tempo, a slowing down.

Yoga practices, from *āsana* to *mudrā*, are themselves reflective and offer ongoing possibility for co-assessment throughout the session. Breath can be a good place to start. While a slow breath may reveal an inner calm, it may also mask a frozen response to trauma (see Cancer diagnosis through the lens of Polyvagal Theory and the *Guṇa-s*, Chapter 2). Therapists have the advantage of not having to rely on assumption. They can, instead, offer a short practice, say a bee breath (*bhramarī*), and take time to observe and listen to the client's experience and response during and after the practice, what they noticed and how they feel. They can similarly observe how a client moves through *āsana* practice, the general tension displayed, and their sense of embodiment, offering practices to enhance stability or grounding, or mobility and fluidity, depending on what is needed.

Perhaps the most informal co-assessment, and arguably the most important, is in a continued curiosity-based conversation with the client. We are, with their permission, holding up a mirror, helping them to see themselves and their situation more clearly. This compassionate inquiry, back and forth: How does this feel for you? Do you notice any changes in your breathing? How would you describe the sensation of discomfort now? How could it be more

"Spiritual bypass"

Related to "toxic positivity" (see p. 29) is a similar insistence on good-feelings-only, but from a spiritual point of view. Coined by John Wellwood, spiritual bypass can be defined as:

a defensive psychological posture cultivated by a tendency to privilege or exaggerate spiritual beliefs, emotions or experiences over and against psychological needs creating a means of avoiding or bypassing difficult emotions or experiences.

Picciotto et al. (2018)

Although this term has seen limited systematic study, it has anecdotal prevalence in spiritual communities, including yoga. In cancer-land it can sound simplistic: "people with cancer have created their own reality," and "if you were purer and more enlightened, you wouldn't need the lesson of cancer," and now that you've "made yourself sick, you can manifest your way to health," and other such statements devoid of empathy. Unfortunately, these declarations can suggest to people facing cancer that they aren't good enough or trying hard enough, which can be both devastating as well as silencing. Yoga therapists, themselves misjudged or tragically held up as "enlightened beings", can rein this in, and bring a more compassionate, equitable, and grounded humanity to the room.

easeful or effortless? All of this affirms the therapist's interest and their companionable presence, and helps them to select practices, to try now and practice at home, in waiting rooms, in MRI machines, while infusions drip, or when nervous, speaking to doctors, family, and friends.

Records, referrals, notes, clinical integration and insurance coverage

Depending on their workplace, yoga therapists keep their own notes (often from a *kośa* perspective) and/or enter notes into appropriate integrative records (hospital charts or clinical SOAP notes – Subjective, Objective, Assessment and Plan). Secure record keeping (destruction of personal information and legal access to records) must be in compliance with local laws and governance. Referrals are made to other healthcare practitioners when the work needed is outside of their scope of practice, or if diagnostic information is required to proceed.

Referrals to yoga therapy are received from a wide variety of healthcare and oncological practitioners. Integrative teams (see Resourcing through integration of cancer care in Chapter 2), working together in-hospital or in-clinic, may, with written permission, share clinical notes, minimizing overlapping care and relieving the burden on the patient to tirelessly repeat their story/or health information. If working in-clinic or in a hospital, the institution's waivers and insurance may cover all oncology practitioners, but they may not. Be sure to check. Best practice would suggest that yoga therapists working in or adjacent to a healthcare setting procure their own liability insurance, including insurance for online work, if needed. Not all "yoga insurance" covers yoga therapy, so buyer beware!

The forms: waivers, informed consent, and disciplinary action

If a yoga therapist is working under the auspices of a hospital or medical clinic, they will follow their procedures for waivers, intake forms, informed consent, insurance, reporting of adverse effects/breach of conduct, and disciplinary actions. If a therapist is dual-credentialed (for example, they are also a nurse or psychotherapist), they will follow the guidelines of their licensing board.

Yoga therapists with a C-IAYT credential are beholden to the requirements of IAYT. As such, they must follow IAYT's Code of Ethics (COE) and Scope of Practice (SOP) and share these with their client. Before a session, intakes and waivers, including informed consent, must be completed by the client for either one-on-one or group sessions. All forms should be discussed to be sure all is understood, and any questions fully answered.

Yoga therapists (C-IAYT) creating their own waiver forms, may consider including the following. Legal requirements may vary from jurisdiction to jurisdiction.

1. Scope of practice: A clear description of yoga therapy practice should be included: what the therapy entails; what to expect with regard to cost; timing and cancellation policies; risks, benefits, and contraindications for practice; and details of how referrals are made to licensed practitioners. See IAYT's Scope of Practice for Yoga Therapists document for details (www.iayt.org).

2. Code of ethics: The IAYT's Code of Ethics (www.iayt.org) is best included in waivers and discussed. Accountability is key, and clear details for reporting of adverse experiences to an accrediting body or workplace should also be included.

3. Informed consent: Therapists must provide full disclosure of SOP, COE, and the specific yoga therapy and practices that will be used, including if the therapist regularly employs physical contact or touch. The patient must agree to what has been described and understand that consent can be withdrawn at any time in the session. If gentle touch, clearly defined, is within a particular therapist's practice (check local jurisdictions for "hands-on" stipulations), consent must be received before touch is therapeutically employed. (For more on the scope of practice with regard to touch, see addendum to SOP at www.iayt.org). Disclaimers should be included, as much to guide clients as to protect yoga therapists, such as: "Yoga therapy is not a substitute for medical care. Full medical clearance must be attained before your yoga therapy session."

4. Client details: Name, address, phone number and urgent emergency contact are requested and kept confidential. If practicing on a secure, HIPPA-compliant virtual platform, it is recommended, in case of emergency, to double-check the client's current location and immediate emergency contact. Email address and/or mobile number should be verified in case there are technical difficulties that interrupt a session. Sharing of client information and record keeping (destruction of personal information, legal access to records) must be in compliance with local laws and governance.

5. Confidentiality agreement: The yoga therapist must maintain the client's privacy and the confidentiality of their personal information, including health records. Depending on jurisdiction, a client's records could be required by law, and a yoga therapist may be required to report if the client is in a life-threatening emergency, or is likely to harm themselves or others.

6. Grounds and procedures for disciplinary action: IAYT has a policy setting out procedures that apply in the event of an alleged breach of the conduct for those credentialed as C-IAYT. A clear process to file a complaint should be included in the waiver, whether that be IAYT or the hospital/clinic/institution a therapist is working for. IAYT policy describes the disciplinary process which, in some cases, could result in the involvement of the Ethics and Disciplinary Review Panel (EDRP) for those with C-IAYT status.

Community self-care for therapists: staying resourced and connected

"Isn't it hard to work with people who have cancer? It must be so dismal, sad and exhausting?"

Ask an oncological yoga therapist and you'll likely hear more about witnessing love, joy, and a deep humanity. Truthfully, it is both fulfilling and intensely challenging. There is daily shock, sadness, heartbreak, and despair amongst the sweetness of working with good humans. "Burnout," "compassion fatigue" and what Joan Halifax might call "pathological empathy" are common in healthcare (West et al. 2018, Halifax 2018). Doctors, nurses, and now therapists are beginning to see the need to regularly bolster their boundaries of care and turn toward themselves and their communities with yoga-focused practices. A sense of connection within healthcare teams is vital and has been shown to enhance, in house, a profound culture of caring (Wei et al. 2020). In *Yoga as Self-Care for Healthcare Professionals* (2019), Aggie Stewart brings much needed philosophical and practical foundations to support well-being in our valued and often overwhelmed and overworked healthcare practitioners, setting out yoga practices to cultivate resilience and self-compassion in their practices and in their communities.

Working in cancer care can bring unique challenges. While a clear sense of embodied boundaries (Ogden & Fisher 2015) and a well-defined and professional scope of practice can create a strong container, even therapists who have this clarity can experience burnout. A yoga therapist may have their own cancer history, or remembered experience with a loved one. All this can come roaring back when faced with a client who has a similar diagnosis, treatment and/or side effect. This is difficult territory and requires pause and discernment. Some yoga therapists refer these clients to other therapists or choose to work in cancers beyond what they have personally experienced. Even so, we may, at times, continue to feel reactive. This may not be a problem to solve, but simply a surge of empathy to notice. Awareness, self-regulation and compassion, resourcing (before, during, and after sessions), and reaching out to colleagues can be of great help. Find a yoga therapy supervisor, a peer, or a group of therapists to connect with regularly. Cultivate co-regulated collegiality and be both accountable and well appreciated.

While oncological yoga therapists will celebrate moments of healing and witness resilience, remissions and "cure" with their clients, they will endure as many losses. For some, it's too much, a too-heavy weight on their shoulders and heart. Some therapists seem mysteriously wired for an enduring empathy or have cultivated sustaining practices to fill their cup, over and over. Many in the field of oncology simply find a way to walk with a "brokenheartedness" that doesn't weary them, but makes inarguable room for life as it is, suffering included. In avoiding the crush of burnout, it is

Yoga therapy for the oncologist: a personalized approach to reducing burnout and compassion fatigue

Lois Ramondetta MD, 500 RYT, C-IAYT, Gynecological Surgeon

The pressures of working as a gynecologic oncologist in an academic medical center are intense. Days are spent with patients discussing treatment deci-sions, performing difficult surgeries, and attending to those facing their death. End-of-life discussions, especially the ones early in my career, sat heavily on my heart. So much stress can lead to burnout, shortened reaction time, compassion fatigue, as well as difficulties identifying self-worth outside of a medical professional identity. Working with advanced cancer patients, my thoughts, not infrequently, landed here: I'm never doing enough, I'm never good enough, and

(continued)

I need to accomplish more. Sometimes at night, when work responsibilities quieted down, these thoughts become insidious ruminations. Although I had committed to "do no harm," I was clearly harming myself. Many symptoms of burnout eventually forced me into an intense period of self-reflection and a needed change in self-care. Eleven years of medical training had focused me almost entirely on the physical aspects of disease (*annamayakośa*, see Chapter 2). I came to realize that suffering and resilience are much more complex.

Using my yoga mat as the training ground, I slowly learned to release and self-regulate. I more purposefully engaged in *svādhyāya* (self-study) by first enrolling in a 200hr, then a 300hr teacher training and finally Yoga Therapist certification. Being part of a supportive community of yogis reminds me of the benefits of stilling the mind through meditation, breath, and movement. When faced with difficult interactions (and the stressors of academic oncology), I address *iśvāra praṇidhāna*, a personal humbling or surrendering, by silently reciting the "Teacher's Mantra" (*Sahanā Vavatu*) specifically noting the words: "May we work together with great energy, may our intellect be sharpened, may our study be effective and let there be no animosity amongst us." I quiet my mind, reconnect with "my true self," and remember that my relationships with others (patients, colleagues, family) matter more than my academic accomplishments.

My yoga practice (and study) remains vital to my inner peace. At the hospital, I give myself more time to pause when dealing with a disappointed or angry patient, to feel compassion instead of defensiveness; more time to pause when a colleague is successful, to feel delight instead of competition. In these pauses, I take a few slow extended exhalations, stand in mountain (*tāḍāsana*) and watch the veil of smoke clear around my own inner light. In doing so, I become more loving and accepting of myself and as a result, have more compassion to give to others. Through these ever-so-subtle actions, I am able to feel lighter at the scrub sink, before entering the next exam room, and before entering my home and greeting my family. Instead of a *rajasic* achiever, I become a contented healer.

important to know who we are, our personal needs and available resources, and to regularly turn toward our sustaining yoga practice and the support of our community for ample servings of compassion and care. Surely our capacity to be with others is also sourced from within, enhanced by cultivating an enduring relationship with self, nature and life, through to and including our dying time. So, a hearty recommendation for more yoga practice for the yoga therapist! Meditation, *mantra*, movement…all of it. For you, for others, for the health of our planet and the breath that is shared.

References

Bryant, E.F., 2009. *The Yoga Sūtras of Patañjali*. North Point Press; Berkeley, CA.

Butera, K., Elgelid, S., 2017. *Yoga Therapy: A Personalized Approach for Your Active Lifestyle*. Human Kinetics; UK.

Garner, G., 2016. *Medical Therapeutic Yoga: Biopsychosocial Rehabilitation and Wellness Care*. Handspring Publishing; Edinburgh, UK.

Halifax, J., 2018. *Standing at the Edge: Finding Freedom Where Fear and Courage Meet*. Flatiron Books, New York, NY.

Krentzman, R., Sullivan, M., 2021. Assessing musculoskeletal balance in yoga therapy. In: Finlayson, D., Hyland Robertson, L. (eds). *Yoga Therapy Foundations, Tools and Practice*. Jessica Kingsley Publishers; London, UK: 175–196.

Majewski, L., Bhavanani, A.B., 2020. *Yoga Therapy as a Whole-Person Approach to Health*. Singing Dragon; London & Philadelphia.

Ogden, P., Fisher, J., 2015. *Sensorimotor Psychotherapy*. W.W. Norton & Company; New York, NY.

Pearson, N., Prosko, S., Sullivan, M., 2019. *Yoga and Science in Pain Care*. Singing Dragon; London, UK.

Picciotto, G., Fox, J., Neto, F., 2018. A phenomenology of spiritual bypass: causes, consequences, and implications. *Journal of Spirituality in Mental Health*. 20;4:333–354.

Rothenberg, R.L., 2019. *Restoring Prana: A Therapeutic Guide to Pranayama and Healing Through the Breath for Yoga Therapists, Yoga Teachers, and Healthcare Practitioners*. Singing Dragon; London & Philadelphia.

Rudman, S., 2021. Ayurveda for the yoga therapist. In: Finlayson, D., Hyland Robertson, L. (eds). *Yoga Therapy Foundations, Tools and Practice*. Jessica Kingsley Publishers; London, UK: 78–87.

Stewart, A., 2019. *Yoga as Self-care for Healthcare Practitioners: Cultivating Resilience, Compassion, and Empathy*. Singing Dragon; London & Philadelphia.

Sullivan, M., Hyland Robertson, L.C., 2020. *Understanding Yoga Therapy*. Routledge; New York, NY.

Wei, H., Corbett, R.W., Ray, J., Wei, T.L., 2020. A culture of caring: the essence of healthcare interprofessional collaboration. *Journal of Interprofessional Care*. 34(3): 324–331.

West, C.P., Dyrbye, L.N., Shanafelt, T.D., 2018. Physician burnout: contributors, consequences and solutions. *Journal of Internal Medicine*. 283(6): 516–529.

Wheeler, A., 2021. Foundations of yoga as therapy: assessments and healing approach. In: Finlayson, D., Hyland Robertson, L. (eds). *Yoga Therapy Foundations, Tools and Practice*. Jessica Kingsley Publishers; London, UK: 60–77.

Understanding Cancer and its Treatment

Leigh Leibel

Cancer is an expansionist disease; it invades through tissues, sets up colonies in hostile landscapes, seeking "sanctuary" in one organ and then immigrating to another. It lives desperately, inventively, fiercely, territorially, cannily, and defensively – at times, as if teaching us how to survive. To confront cancer is to encounter a parallel species, one perhaps more adapted to survival than even we are.

Siddhartha Mukherjee, MD
The Emperor of All Maladies: A Biography of Cancer

Cancer is a fantastically complex family of diseases, as Dr. Mukherjee lyrically posits in his Pulitzer Prize-winning book *The Emperor of All Maladies*. In 2020 alone, nearly 20 million people globally were diagnosed with cancer, and the incidence of cancer cases is projected to increase by 50% within the next two decades (Sung et al. 2021). Current cancer statistics suggest that two out of every three men, and one out of every three women worldwide will be diagnosed with cancer at some point in their lives (Ferlay et al. 2020).

So, what *is* cancer? Throughout this chapter we'll explore the basics of this complex disease, including its biology; natural history of progression (diagnosis, staging, grading, recurrence, metastasis); treatment side effects and adverse events; and disparity in access and delivery of cancer care. This information gives us a first glimpse into the unique challenges inherent in the safe delivery of yoga and yoga therapy to people with cancer and survivors, and provides the foundation and context for our contributing authors' patient/client stories presented in Chapter 6.

Cancer as a collection of related diseases

Cancer is a collection of more than 100 related diseases. It begins as a cellular disease, where normal cells are trans-

formed into cancer cells.

While there are many different kinds of cancers, they all fall into two basic categories, blood and solid:

- Blood (hematologic) cancers, which include malignancies such as acute and chronic leukemias, lymphoma (Hodgkin lymphoma and non-Hodgkin lymphoma), and multiple myeloma.

- Solid tumors or cancers, which include malignancies in any of the other body organs or tissues. The most common solid cancers in the United States are breast, lung, colorectal, and prostate.

Characteristics of cancer cells[1]

Cancer cells are different from normal cells in many ways that allow them to grow out of control and become invasive, as described in the six bullets below:

- **Cancer cells lose specific cellular functions:** One important difference is that cancer cells are less "specialized" than normal cells. That is, whereas normal cells mature into very distinct cell types with specific functions, cancer cells do not.

- **Cancer cells evade growth suppressors:** Normally, human cells grow, divide, and form new cells as the body needs them. Tumor suppressor genes regulate normal cell growth and facilitate senescence (cellular aging) and apoptosis (programmed cell death, where the body gets rid of old or damaged cells). Normal cell growth is limited by contact inhibition, which causes cells to stop growing upon physical contact with other cells.

- **Cancer cells divide uncontrollably:** When a malignancy develops, the controlled and orderly process of growth and division breaks down. Cancer cells evade the tumor growth suppressors and continue to divide and grow, even though they are not needed in the body. Cancer cells also ignore signals that normally tell cells to stop dividing, such as apoptosis. Some cancer cells have mutations that disable gatekeeper proteins that control mitosis and inactivate contact inhibition.

- **Cancer cells evade immune destruction:** The immune system is a network of organs, tissues, and specialized cells. Normally, the immune system identifies and eradicates foreign microbes (including cancer cells), repairs tissue damage, and defends the host through the ability to distinguish self from non-self and prevent malignant proliferation. Although the immune system normally removes damaged or abnormal cells from the body, some cancer cells are able to "hide" from the immune system so they can survive and grow. For example, cancer cells can suppress components of the immune system (e.g., natural killer cells) that would normally kill cancer cells. Evidence indicates that deficiencies in T-lymphocytes, T helper cells, and natural killer cells increase the risk of cancer development.

- **Cancer cells induce angiogenesis:** In the process of angiogenesis, new blood vessels are created from existing ones to provide nutrients and remove waste products. In normal tissues, angiogenesis takes place during embryogenesis with tissue and organ development. In adults, this process is usually dormant, except during wound healing and during the female reproductive cycle. However, cancer cells can also induce the angiogenesis process, so that nearby blood vessels in the microenvironment will form additional blood vessels. These newly created blood vessels will supply tumors with oxygen and nutrients to assist in their growth, and will remove waste products from the tumors (see Chapter 5 for more on the microenvironment).

- **Cancer cells activate invasion and metastasis:** Cancer cells have invasive properties and can invade the blood and lymphatic system. As these tumors grow, some cancerous cells can break off and travel via blood or the lymphatic system to distant places in the body to form new tumors far from the original tumor. This process is "metastasis", described more fully later in this chapter.

Cancer arises from the acquisition of gene changes[2]

Cancer arises from the acquisition of gene changes (see Chapter 5). That is, cancer is caused by changes to our genes, which are the basic physical units of inheritance that control the way our cells develop and function. Genetic changes that can drive cancer can occur:

- Through inheritance from our parents.

- During a person's lifetime as a result of errors that occur as cells divide.

- From damage to DNA caused by certain environmental exposures (e.g., chemicals in tobacco smoke or ultraviolet rays from the sun).

- From exposure to some viruses (e.g., hepatitis B and human papilloma virus [HPV], or bacteria such as *H. pylori*).

- From chronic inflammation that may be driven by lifestyle (e.g., unhealthy diet and poor nutrition, stress, physical inactivity and lack of exercise, poor sleep habits) and excess body weight (adipose tissue inflammation).

Each person's cancer has a unique combination of genetic changes, and as the cancer continues to grow, additional changes will likely occur. Even within the same tumor, there may be different cells that have different genetic changes. In general, cancer cells have many more genetic changes, such as mutations in DNA, than normal cells. Some of the changes may have nothing to do with the cancer. They may be a result of the cancer, rather than its cause.

Genetic drivers of cancer[3]

Malignant tumors are derived from genetic instability and genetic mutations in regulatory (or "housekeeping") genes which control cell growth and proliferation. There are three types of regulatory genes:

- **Proto-oncogenes** are involved in normal cell growth and division (e.g., HER2). When mutations occur in these genes, they may become cancer-causing genes (oncogenes) that allow uncontrolled cell growth.

- **Tumor suppressor genes** function as regulators of cell growth and division (e.g., p53; BRCA1/2). Cells with certain mutations in tumor suppressor genes may divide in an uncontrolled manner.

- **DNA repair genes** are involved in identifying and repairing damaged DNA. Cells with mutations in these genes survive when they normally would be forced to undergo apoptosis (cell death), and they tend to develop additional mutations in other genes.

Together, mutations to these three types of regulatory genes may cause normal cells to survive beyond their "normal" live span, behave aberrantly, and become cancerous.

Categories of cancer that begin in specific types of cells[4]

Cancers are divided into categories according to the type of cell in which the malignancy originates. There are nine groups and 25 subgroups. On the following pages, we describe the three blood cancers, followed by the six

[1-4]"What Is Cancer?" was originally published by the National Cancer Institute (2021).

solid tumors (in alphabetical order). As you read this section, think about the impact the location and burden of these cancers could have on a person's ability to engage in yoga, and what precautions must be taken to ensure a safe, accessible practice.

Leukemia

Leukemia begins in the blood-forming tissue of the bone marrow. These cancers rarely form solid tumors. Instead, large numbers of abnormal white blood cells (leukemia cells and leukemic blast cells) build up in the blood and bone marrow, and "crowd out" normal blood cells. Normal blood cells include red blood cells, which provide oxygen to tissues; white blood cells, which fight infection; and platelets, which make clots and control bleeding.

When leukemia patients have an abnormally low level of these blood cells, they can develop anemia (low red blood cells) and experience fatigue and shortness of breath. They can also develop neutropenia (low neutrophils, which is a type of white blood cell), which makes the person more prone to develop infections. Patients can also develop thrombocytopenia (low platelet count) and they may bleed more easily.

There are four common types of leukemia:

- Acute myelogenous leukemia (AML)

- Acute lymphoblastic leukemia (ALL)

- Chronic myelogenous leukemia (CML)

- Chronic lymphocytic leukemia (CLL)

They are grouped based on how quickly the disease progresses (acute or chronic) and according to the type of blood cell in which the cancer originates (lymphoid or myeloid).

Lymphoma

Lymphoma begins in lymphocytes (T cells or B cells) which are the disease-fighting white blood cells that are part of the immune system. In lymphoma, abnormal lymphocytes build up in the lymph nodes and lymph vessels, as well as in other organs of the body. There are two main types: Hodgkin lymphoma and non-Hodgkin lymphoma.

Multiple myeloma

Myeloma begins in plasma cells, a type of immune cell that resides in the bone marrow. Large numbers of these abnormal plasma cells, called myeloma cells, build up in the bone marrow. Patients may have a large number of M-protein produced by the myeloma cells, and this can cause kidney dysfunction. Patients may also experience osteolytic bone lesions, and their bones look like Swiss cheese on X-ray. Patients may also have a low red blood cell count (anemia) and high calcium levels in their blood.

Brain and spinal cord tumors

There are different types of brain and spinal cord tumors (they may be malignant or benign). They are named based on the type of neural cell in which they form, and where the tumor first forms in the central nervous system:

- Astrocytic
- Oligodendroglial
- Mixed glioma (glioblastoma)
- Ependymal
- Medulloblastoma
- Pineal
- Parenchymal
- Meningeal
- Germ cell
- Craniopharyngioma (Grade I)

Carcinoma

Carcinomas are the most common type of cancer. They are formed by epithelial cells, the cells that cover the inside and outside surfaces of the body. There are many types of epithelial cells; carcinomas that begin in different epithelial cell types have specific names, as described below:

- Adenocarcinomas form in epithelial cells that produce fluids or mucus. Most breast, colon, and prostate cancers are this type.
- Basal cell carcinomas form in the lower or basal (base) layer of the epidermis, the outer layer of skin.
- Squamous cell carcinomas form in squamous cells, which are epithelial cells that lie just beneath the outer surface of the skin. Squamous cells also line many other organs, including the stomach, intestines, lungs, bladder, and kidneys.
- Transitional cell carcinomas form in a type of epithelial tissue called transitional epithelium, or urothelium. This tissue, which is made up of many layers of epithelial cells that can get bigger and smaller, is found in the linings of the bladder, ureters, part of the kidneys, and a few other organs.

Germ cell tumor

Germ cells begin in the cells that become sperm or eggs. These tumors can occur almost anywhere in the body and can be either malignant or benign.

Melanoma

Melanoma begins in cells that become melanocytes, the specialized cells that make melanin (the pigment that gives skin its color). Most melanomas form on the skin, but melanoma can also form in other pigmented tissues, such as the eye.

Neuroendocrine tumor

Neuroendocrine tumors form from cells that release hormones into the blood, done so in response to signals received from the nervous system. They may be malignant or benign. The tumors may make higher than normal amounts of hormones (such as cortisol and epinephrine) and can cause many different symptoms. They are usually slow-growing and mostly found in the gastrointestinal system, commonly in the rectum and small intestine.

Sarcoma

Sarcomas form in bone and soft tissues, including muscle, fat, blood vessels, lymph vessels, and fibrous tissue (such as tendons and ligaments). The most common kind of bone cancer is osteosarcoma.

The most common types of soft tissue sarcomas are:

- Leiomyosarcoma

- Kaposi sarcoma

- Liposarcoma

- Dermatofibrosarcoma protuberans

Diagnosing cancer

A tumor or mass may be cancerous (malignant) or non-cancerous (benign). Individuals with a tumor or mass may or may not experience symptoms (symptomatic/asymptomatic). Some abnormalities are detected through routine screening procedures such as colonoscopy, pap smear, mammogram, ultrasound, prostate examination, or skin "check" for irregularities and cancerous lesions. Others are discovered during a medical exam investigating specific complaints and symptoms, or perhaps incidentally during tests for other conditions. Primary care physicians are typically the healthcare providers who first discover a suspicious abnormality and order further testing. A medical "work up" includes personal and family medical history and a physical exam, followed by lab tests, imaging tests (scans), or other tests or procedures, including biopsy. A tissue biopsy is often the only way to determine the pathology and confirm a cancer.

Once cancer is diagnosed, the individual is cared for by a team of cancer specialists that may include medical oncologists, radiation oncologists, and surgical oncologists, among others. Each is specialized in one aspect of oncology, but often a multidisciplinary team is utilized to provide optimal care. Patients may also be supported by integrative oncology practitioners, including yoga therapists. Integrative Oncology is defined as:

A patient-centered, evidence-informed field of cancer care that utilizes mind and body practices, natural products, and/or lifestyle modifications from different traditions alongside conventional cancer treatments. Integrative oncology aims to optimize health, quality of life, and clinical outcomes across the cancer care continuum and to empower people to prevent cancer and become active participants before, during, and beyond cancer treatment.

(Witt et al. 2017)

Grading cancer

A pathologist is responsible for looking at tissue samples and determining if they are benign or malignant. They then assign a "grade" to the sample according to how abnormal the cancer cells and tissue look under a microscope when compared to healthy cells. This is done to help predict how fast the cancer will grow and how likely it is to spread. Some cancers have their own system for grading tumors, for example, prostate cancer uses the Gleason scoring system (0–10). However, the majority use a standard Grade 1 to 4 scale, with Grade 1 being the least aggressive and Grade 4 being the most aggressive (Table 4.1).

Staging cancer[5]

The "staging" of cancer refers to the identification of the extent of the disease. Types of staging include:

- **Clinical staging:** The size and extent of cancer is determined by physical examination, imaging tests, and biopsies of affected areas.

- **Pathologic staging:** The size and stage of cancer is determined by a pathologist after a surgery that removes the tumor and explores the size and extent

Table 4.1 Tumor grades*

Grade	Appearance
1	Tumor cells and tissue that look most like healthy cells and tissue. These are well-differentiated tumors and are considered low grade and typically less aggressive and with a better prognosis.
2	Tumor cells and tissue are somewhat abnormal and are moderately differentiated. These are intermediate grade tumors.
3	Tumor cells and tissue look very abnormal and are poorly differentiated, no longer having an architectural structure or pattern. They are considered high grade and aggressive.
4	Tumor cells are highly abnormal and undifferentiated. These are the highest grade and typically grow and spread faster than lower grade tumors. They are generally aggressive.

*Originally published by the National Cancer Institute (2013).

of malignant cells under a microscope. These results are combined with results of clinical staging.

- **Post-neoadjuvant staging:** This determines the extent of cancer that remains upon completion of chemotherapy, hormone therapy, radiation therapy, and other treatments that are given prior to surgery. It also applies in the event no surgery is indicated after chemoradiation and other treatments.

Staging helps to determine the severity of disease and the prognosis. As a tumor changes over time, this new information is added to the original stage. So, the original stage describes the nature of the cancer (even though it may go into remission and there is no longer any evidence of disease [NED]) or the cancer may be upstaged if there is progressive disease. By understanding the extent of a patient/client's disease and its impact on mind, body, spirit, the necessary precautions may be taken to deliver a safe and effective yoga practice.

Systems that describe stage

There are various staging systems. Most include information about where the tumor is located in the body, cell type, tumor size, whether the cancer has spread to nearby lymph nodes or to a different part of the body, and the tumor grade.

General staging system

One popular system followed by medical systems and registries characterizes stages in this way:

- **In situ:** Abnormal cells are present but have not invaded nearby tissue structures.

- **Localized:** Cancer is limited to the place where it started, with no sign that it has spread even though it has invaded normal structures.

- **Regional:** Cancer has spread to nearby lymph nodes, tissues, or organs.

- **Distant:** Cancer has spread to distant parts of the body through the blood or lymphatic systems.

- **Unknown:** There is not enough information to determine the stage.

TNM staging system

A second system is the TNM (Tumor - Node - Metastasis) and is the most widely used pathologic cancer staging system. Most hospitals and medical centers use this system as their main method for cancer reporting, and most pathology reports use this system

---

[5] "Cancer Staging" was orignally published by the National Cancer Institute (2015).

unless the particular cancer being described is staged with its own system (e.g., brain/spinal cord tumors and blood cancers). When cancer is described by the TNM system, there are numbers assigned after each letter that give more details about the cancer as determined by a pathologist. For example, T1N0MX or T3N1M0 (Box 4.1).

BOX 4.1 TNM staging system*

TNM

- T: Refers to the size and extent of the main tumor. The main tumor is usually called the primary tumor.

- N: Refers to the number of nearby lymph nodes that have cancer.

- M: Refers to whether the cancer has metastasized.

Primary tumor (T)

- TX: Main tumor cannot be measured.

- T0: Main tumor cannot be found.

- T1, T2, T3, T4: Refers to the size and/or extent of the main tumor. The higher the number after the T, the larger the tumor or the more it has grown into nearby tissues. "T"s may be further divided to provide more detail, such as T3a and T3b.

Regional lymph nodes (N)

- NX: Cancer in nearby lymph nodes cannot be measured.

- N0: There is no cancer in nearby lymph nodes.

- N1, N2, N3: Refers to the number and location of lymph nodes that contain cancer. The higher the number after the N, the more lymph nodes that contain cancer.

Distant metastasis (M)

- MX: Metastasis cannot be measured.

- M0: Cancer has not spread to other parts of the body.

(continued)

(continued)

- M1: Cancer has spread to other parts of the body.

"Cancer Staging" was originally published by the National Cancer Institute (2015).

AJCC staging system

A third system, the AJCC (American Joint Committee on Cancer) staging system describes it this way:

- **Stage 0:** Abnormal cells are present but have not spread to nearby tissue; also called carcinoma in situ or CIS. CIS is "not all the way to cancer," but may become cancer.

- **Stage 1, 2, 3:** Cancer is present. The higher the number, the larger the cancer tumor and the more it has spread into nearby tissues.

- **Stage 4:** The cancer has spread (metastasized) to distant parts of the body.

Cancer treatment strategies and side effects[6]

There are seven treatments considered to be standards of cancer care: surgery, chemotherapy, radiation, hormone therapy, immunotherapy, targeted therapy, and hematopoietic stem cell transplant. Protocols generally employ one or several, sequentially or concomitantly. These treatments affect not only the disease, but also the body's healthy tissue and organs, causing local and/or systemic side effects that may present as acute, lingering, and late and can affect the whole person – mind, body, spirit. Therefore, many survivors, regardless of cancer status or prognosis, will likely experience ongoing physical, psychological, and social needs that affect their quality of life for many years beyond the initial diagnosis. As you read this section, think about the impact cancer and its treatments could have on a person's ability to engage in yoga, and what precautions must be taken to ensure a safe, accessible practice.

---

[6] "Treatment strategies was originally published by the National Cancer Institute (2015)."

Chapter four

Surgery

The goal of surgery is to remove a cancerous tumor, or as much of it as possible. Procedures may be complex and require radical removal of organs and/or limbs.

Post surgical complications

Side effects depend on the location of surgery and include:

- Hernia
- Lymphedema
- Axillary webbing
- Fibrosis
- Scarring and adhesions
- Range of motion limitations
- Blood clots
- Amputations
- Anesthesia effects
- Pain
- Impact of organ removal on the body systems

Chemotherapy

Chemotherapy drugs are chemicals which are used to kill growing cells, both cancerous and non-cancerous. There are many different chemotherapeutic agents. Categories of chemotherapy drugs include alkylating agents, antimetabolites, antitumor antibiotics, plant alkaloids, and nitrosureas. Chemotherapy may be given as a single drug, or in combination with other chemotherapy drugs, immunotherapy drugs, and/or with other treatments. An example of a chemotherapy regimen is the CAF regimen for breast cancer: Cyclophosphamide (Cytoxan) – Doxorubicin (Adriamycin) – Fluorouracil (5-FU).

Chemotherapy drugs are administered in different ways, including orally, in peripheral veins (intravenous, or IV), or via central vascular access devices (VADs), such as tunneled catheters, PICC (peripherally inserted central catheter) lines, and implanted ports. Central VADs allow repeated and long-term access to the bloodstream for frequent or regular administration of drugs. Chemotherapy is often given with hydration (IV), antiemetics, and/or steroids.

The goals of chemotherapy treatment can be:

- Primary treatment: given to cure the cancer without other treatments.
- Neoadjuvant treatment: given before other treatments, such as surgery or radiation, to shrink a tumor so that the primary treatment is more effective.
- Adjuvant treatment: given after other treatments, such as surgery or radiation therapy, to kill hidden cancer cells.
- Palliative treatment: given to minimize or eliminate a patient's adverse signs and symptoms.

Chemotherapy side effects

While some side effects of chemotherapy are mild, others cause serious complications. They may be acute, long-lasting, or late.

Acute side effects include:

Gastrointestinal:

- Nausea, vomiting
- Burping
- Loss of appetite
- Mouth sores
- Metallic taste in mouth
- Weight loss or gain

(continued)

(continued)

Elimination:

- Diarrhea
- Constipation

Hematologic:

- Low white blood cell (WBC) count (neutropenia) - increased risk of infection and fever (nadir, the lowest point for WBC, is usually 7-14 days after chemotherapy given)
- Low red blood cell (RBC) count (anemia) - increased fatigue and shortness of breath
- Low platelet count (thrombocytopenia) - increased bruising and bleeding

Skin:

- Hair loss
- Finger/toenail discoloration or loss

Sensory:

- Numbness or tingling in the fingers or toes (peripheral neuropathy)
- Pain (including joint)

Long-lasting and/or late developing effects include:

- Cognitive dysfunction ("chemo brain")
- Lung damage
- Heart problems
- Infertility
- Kidney problems
- Nerve damage (peripheral neuropathy)
- Osteoporosis
- Persistent fatigue
- Risk of second cancer from treatment

Radiation

Radiation therapy uses high-powered energy beams, such as photons, to kill cancer cells. Radiation treatment can come from a machine outside the body (external beam radiation), or radiation seeds or rods can be placed inside the body (brachytherapy). Indications for radiation therapy are definitive cure or palliative care. Side effects of radiation are typically site-specific, cumulative, and may be acute or late. (Fatigue is a common side effect that is systemic, not site-specific.)

Radiation side effects

Acute effects include:

General:

- Fatigue

Skin:

- Redness, dermatitis, skin peeling

Brain:

- Alopecia, occasional nausea

Head and neck:

- Dry mouth, mouth sores, dental caries, difficulty swallowing

Chest:

- Cough

Abdomen:

- Nausea and vomiting

Pelvis:

- Diarrhea; urinary or fecal incontinence

Late effects include:

Brain:

- Late cognitive changes

Chest:

- Pneumonitis, late fibrosis

Abdomen:

- Symptoms of gastroesophageal reflux disease (GERD)

(continued)

Pelvis:

- Infertility, menopause, sexual dysfunction, cystitis

Bones:

- Fractures, vertebral collapse

Organs:

- Fibrosis/scarring

Other:

- Spinal cord myelopathy
- Lymphedema

Skin:

- "Radiation recall" reaction

Hormone therapy

Some types of cancers are influenced by hormones that drive or increase the growth of cancer. Removing those hormones from the body by blocking the body's ability to produce them, or by interfering with how the hormones behave may halt cancer cell growth. Most commonly, hormone therapy is used in prostate and breast cancer. To a lesser degree, it is used for adrenal, ovarian, endometrial, thyroid, testicular, and androgen-sensitive salivary cancers.

Hormone therapy side effects

General:

- Fatigue, sleep disturbances, weight gain, injection site pain

Bones:

- Osteoporosis from aging or secondary to surgery or drugs

Gastrointestinal:

- Nausea, anorexia, diarrhea, constipation, liver toxicity, fecal incontinence

Muscle:

- Weakness, arthralgia, myalgia

Genitourinary:

- Urinary incontinence

Cardiac:

- Hypertension, edema, deep vein thrombosis (DVT)

Neurological:

- Mood changes, falls/fractures, seizures

Sexual:

- Decreased libido (sexual desire)

Other:

- Erectile dysfunction, gynecomastia (enlarged breasts), vaginal dryness, hot flashes

Tamoxifen and aromatase inhibitors are examples of hormonal therapies used in the treatment of estrogen positive breast cancer.

Immunotherapy

Immunotherapy uses the body's immune system to fight cancer, helping it "see" and attack the cancer. There are three types:

- Monoclonal antibody therapy
- Immune checkpoint inhibitors
- Adoptive T cell modulators such as CAR-T cell interventions

Immunotherapy side effects

Two types (immune checkpoint inhibitor therapy and CAR-T cell therapies) can trigger a hyperimmune response that targets noninvolved organs of the body, causing serious inflammation to normal tissue such as lungs, liver, colon, skin, and joints.

Understanding Cancer and its Treatment

Targeted therapy

Targeted drug treatments focus on specific abnormalities within cancer cells that allow them to accumulate. They may inhibit signals designed to stimulate proliferation, or they may reactivate cell death pathways.

Targeted therapy side effects

- Skin rash
- Fluid retention
- Diarrhea
- Easy bruising (platelet dysfunction)
- Fatigue

Hematopoietic stem cell transplant

A hematopoietic stem cell transplant (HSCT) (bone marrow transplant) involves replacing diseased, destroyed, or non-functioning hematopoietic cells with healthy hematopoietic progenitor cells (e.g., stem cells). Stem cells are capable of self-renewal, and can mature into a red blood cell (RBC), white blood cell (WBC), or platelet.

HSCT uses bone marrow cells from the person with cancer (autologous), from a donor (allogeneic), or from the twin of the person with cancer (syngeneic). Higher doses of chemotherapy are given, with or without total body irradiation, to treat cancer, eradicate the bone marrow, and cause severe myelosuppression that would be irreversible without the infusion of the stem cells in the HSCT. Due to the high number of potential and actual side effects, patients who are undergoing HSCT are often in the hospital for 4–8 weeks.

Stem cell transplant side effects

- Infections, anemia, and bleeding issues due to severely suppressed hematopoietic system

- Nutritional deficiencies due to severe nausea and vomiting, mouth sores, diarrhea
- Organ toxicity, including lung, cardiac, renal, bladder, liver
- Muscle wasting, deconditioning
- Fascial inflammation, leading to loss of function
- Graft versus host disease (GVHD)
- Side effects from long-term steroids
- Psychological: patient isolation, due to prevention of infection and long hospital stay

Corticosteroids

Steroids are common drugs given episodically to cancer patients to counteract allergic reactions and nausea that can be caused by some chemotherapy drugs.

Steroid side effects

Variables include dosing, range of treatment, type of steroids, and time after stopping.

- Steroid-induced hyperglycemia
- Hypertension
- Cataract formation
- Thinning of skin
- Peptic ulcer disease
- Bone issues (bone loss, osteoporosis, fractures)
- Fragile skin
- Proximal myopathy
- Ruptured tendon
- Weight gain
- Sleep disturbance (insomnia)
- Moodiness

Additional considerations during cancer treatment

Appliances, aids, devices

Some cancer patients/survivors may present with external appliances, aids, or devices that must be accommodated. This includes:

- Port
- PICC (peripherally inserted central catheter) line
- Exterior bags (ostomy/colostomy/ileostomy)
- Tracheotomy
- AICD (automatic implantable cardioverter defibrillator)
- Pacemaker
- Oxygen tank
- Hearing aid
- Walking aids (walker, cane)
- Wheelchair
- Therapy animal
- Filgrastim discharger on arm
- Prosthesis

Respiratory

Many aspects of cancer can affect the respiratory system, including:

- Primary cancer or metastasis to lung
- COPD
- Surgical lung removal
- Radiation to lung or chest area
- Bleomycin therapy
- Pneumonias
- Autoimmune pneumonitis
- Interstitial lung disease
- Chemotherapy

This can lead to shortness of breath, inability to breathe deeply, wheezing, dry cough, fatigue, and steroid use.

Rheumatology

Cancer and its treatment can cause:

- Arthritis and arthralgias
- Musculoskeletal issues
- Rheumatologic issues from immunotherapy
- Joint pain, stiffness, swelling in large and small joints
- Muscle weakness
- Pain
- Decrease in functional status

These problems can lead to loss of motion in joints such as jaw, shoulders, hips, or knees. Adverse effects from radiation therapy will occur in the part of the body that was treated, whereas systemic treatments such as chemotherapy, hormone therapy, and immunotherapy can cause body-wide effects.

Clinical trials

Clinical trials are research studies that evaluate a new medical, surgical, or behavioral intervention. In cancer care, trials are typically used to determine if a treatment is effective or has fewer adverse side effects than standard treatments. The FDA requires Phase I, II, and III clinical trials to be completed, in order to determine efficacy and safety of the new cancer treatment.

Metastatic cancer[7]

When cancer cells travel from the primary tumor to other distant locations in the body (usually via the blood or lymphatic system), the process is called metastasis (from the

Understanding Cancer and its Treatment

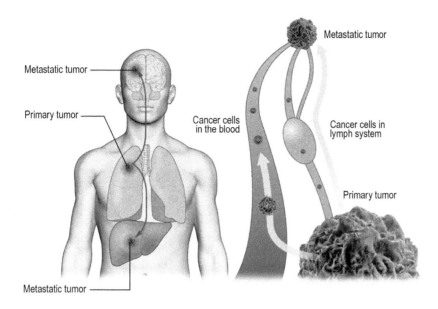

Figure 4.1

Process of metastasis

Reproduced with permission from Janet Penny and Rebecca L. Sturgeon, *Oncology Massage: An integrative approach to cancer care* (Handspring 2021)

Greek word meaning "displacement"). The new tumors are called metastatic tumors and retain the same name as the primary tumor. For example, breast cancer that spreads to the lung is metastatic breast cancer, not lung cancer. Under a microscope, metastatic cancer cells generally look the same as cells of the original cancer and usually have some molecular features in common with the original, such as the presence of specific chromosome changes.

Metastasis is accomplished through a series of steps:

- Growing into, or invading, nearby normal tissue.

- Moving through the walls of nearby lymphatic channels or blood vessels.

- Traveling through the lymphatic system and bloodstream to other parts of the body.

[7]"Metastatic Cancer: When Cancer Spreads" was originally published by the National Cancer Institute (2020a).

- Stopping in small blood vessels at a distant location, invading the blood vessel walls, and moving into the surrounding tissue.

- Growing in this tissue until a tiny tumor forms.

- Causing new blood vessels to grow, which creates a blood supply that allows the metastatic tumor to continue growing (angiogenesis).

Normally, cancer cells that are spreading will die during this process. But, if conditions are favorable for these malignant cells at each step, some will be able to form new tumors in other parts of the body. Metastatic cancer cells can also remain inactive (dormant) at a distant site for many, many years. They may remain forever silent, or they may begin growing again.

While some metastatic cancers can be cured (e.g., testicular, thyroid), in general, the primary goal of treatment is to control and/or stabilize the growth of the cancer or to relieve symptoms caused by it. It is important to note that today in developed countries, many people with metastatic disease are managing their cancer as a chronic condition, thriving, and living for years or decades. This is not the case in under-resourced low-and-middle income countries (LMICs). This is discussed in more detail later in the chapter.

Cancer can spread to almost any part of the body, although different types of cancer are more likely to spread to certain areas than others. The most common sites where cancer spreads are bone, liver, and lung. Table 4.2 shows the most common sites of metastasis, not including the lymph nodes, for some common cancers. As you read this section, think about the impact metastatic cancer could have on a person's ability to engage in yoga, and what precautions must be taken to ensure a safe, accessible practice.

Table 4.2 Common sites where cancer spreads*

Primary cancer type	Main sites of metastasis
Bladder	Bone, liver, lung
Breast	Bone, brain, liver, lung
Colon	Liver, lung, peritoneum
Kidney	Adrenal gland, bone, brain, liver, lung
Lung	Adrenal gland, bone, brain, liver, the other lung
Melanoma	Bone, brain, liver, lung, skin, muscle
Ovary	Liver, lung, peritoneum
Pancreas	Liver, lung, peritoneum
Prostate	Adrenal gland, bone, liver, lung
Rectal	Liver, lung, peritoneum
Uterus	Bone, liver, lung, peritoneum, vagina
Stomach	Liver, lung, peritoneum
Thyroid	Bone, liver, lung

*Originally published by the National Cancer Institute (2020a)

Recurrent cancer[8]

Sometimes cancer returns after frontline treatment has been completed, and after a period during which the cancer could not be detected. A recurrence happens when a small number of cancer cells survive the original treatment and are too small to detect in follow-up tests. Over time they grow and become detectable during regular medical surveillance. When cancer recurs, it is characterized by where it develops and how far it has spread, for example:

- **Local recurrence:** Cancer is in the same place as the original cancer or very close to it.

- **Regional recurrence:** Tumor has grown into lymph nodes or tissue near the original cancer.

- **Distant recurrence or metastasis:** Cancer has spread to organs or tissues far from the original cancer.

Based on this information, a new stage may be assigned to the cancer, and an "r" will be added to the beginning of the new stage, for example, rT4N3M1. The type of treatment for recurrent cancer will depend on the type of cancer, how far it has spread, and the overall health of the patient. In many cases, improved treatments mean cancer has become a chronic disease that people can manage medically while living and thriving for years or decades.

Individuals who have a history of cancer can also develop a new, different kind of cancer (a second primary tumor), sometimes caused by the cancer treatment itself, or due to genetic predisposition. It is important to note that this is different than a *recurrence* of the original cancer and therefore the treatment will be different and will be designed for the new type of cancer that has developed. Individuals may be diagnosed with one or more types of cancer at the same time, or cancers may develop in sequence.

[8]"Recurrent Cancer: When Cancer Comes Back" was originally published by the National Cancer Institute (2020b).

Cancer may recur in a different location but it is still called the *primary* cancer. For example, colon cancer may "come back" in the liver, but the cancer is still called *colon* cancer. The cancer cells are still colon cells, not liver cells.

Cancer health disparity

It is often said that a person's zip code is a bigger predictor of disease than their genetic code (Ducharme & Wolfson 2019). This is especially true in cancer prevention/risk reduction, detection, treatment, clinical trials, and survivorship care. The National Cancer Institute (NCI) defines cancer health disparity as:

Adverse differences in cancer measures such as the number of new cancer cases, the number of cancer deaths, cancer-related health complications, survivorship, quality of life after cancer treatment, screening rates, and stage at diagnosis that exist among certain population groups.

NCI (2020c)

According to the 2020 *Cancer Disparities Progress Report* published by the American Association for Cancer Research (AACR), adverse differences in cancer care exist among groups historically linked to discrimination or exclusion, including racial, ethnic, socioeconomic, gender identity, sexual orientation, age, geographic, and ability (AACR 2021) (Box 4.2). The reasons for health disparity are complex and interrelated, affected by both biological factors (genetic variants that predispose individuals to certain cancers) and social determinants of health (SDoH), which are the conditions in which people are born, grow, live, work, learn, worship, and age.

SDoH domains include:

- Economic stability
- Food insecurity (unhealthy diet/nutrition)
- Access to healthcare (screening, treatment, clinical trials, and survivorship care)
- Environment (child care, transportation, lifestyle behaviors, ability to be physically active, neighborhood influences)
- Education (health literacy, linguistics)
- Social context (discrimination and institutional racism)

By implementing bi-directional initiatives in which all stakeholders work together to co-create solutions, we can begin to:

- Increase education and health literacy among BIPOC[5] and LGBTQIA+[6] populations, as well as in other underrepresented groups.
- Include BIPOC in clinical trials.
- Train and promote more doctors of color.
- Increase access to healthcare (including healthcare that is culturally sensitive).
- Create welcoming and inclusive healthcare environments.
- Use patient pronouns and patient-centered language.
- Address racism and cultural mistrust.
- Educate the medical and healthcare community on bias and institutional racism.

> **BOX 4.2 Examples of racial, geographic, and socioeconomic disparity in cancer care***
>
> **Examples of racial disparities**
>
> - Black women are 39% more likely to die of breast cancer than White women.
> - Black women have double the incidence rate of triple negative breast cancer compared with White American women.
>
> *(continued)*

---

[5]BIPOC = Black, Indigenous, People of Color
[6]LGBTQIA+ = Lesbian, Gay, Bisexual, Transgender, Queer, Intersex, Asexual

BOX 4.2 continued

- Black men have a prostate cancer death rate more than double that of men in other racial groups, and are 111% more likely to die of prostate cancer than White men.

- Native Americans/Alaska Natives are less likely to be up to date with colorectal cancer screening compared to White American adults (64% vs. 48%).

- Hispanic women are 69% more likely to be diagnosed with breast cancer at an advanced stage than White women.

- Asian Pacific Islanders are twice as likely as White Americans to die of stomach cancer.

- Black and Hispanic patients with breast, lung, colorectal, and prostate cancer were almost 30% less likely than White patients to enroll in clinical trials testing treatments for these four types of cancer.

Examples of geographic disparities

- Men living in Appalachia have a lung cancer incidence rate that is 26% higher than that of men living in the remainder of the United States.

- Adolescents living in metropolitan areas have a higher human papillomavirus (HPV) vaccination uptake (65.9%) compared with those in nonmetropolitan areas (50.4%).

- Adults in Massachusetts are significantly more likely to be up to date with colorectal cancer screening than those in Wyoming (76% vs. 58%).

Examples of socioeconomic disparities

- Women in the highest income bracket are significantly more likely to be up to date with cervical cancer screening than women in the lowest income bracket (79% vs. 59%).

- Patients with metastatic bladder cancer who are of low socioeconomic status are 50% less likely to receive chemotherapy compared with those of high socioeconomic status.

(continued)

(continued)

- Adolescents and young adults surviving two or more years after a Hodgkin lymphoma diagnosis who lived in low socioeconomic neighborhoods had a 29% higher likelihood of respiratory system diseases compared with those in high socioeconomic neighborhoods.

In addition, the rates of smoking and alcohol use (which increase cancer risk) are higher among lesbian, gay, and bisexual youths than among heterosexual youths (National Cancer Institute 2020c).

*Data reproduced courtesy American Association of Cancer Research (2021).

As we can see, disparity in cancer care is a critical issue facing our health delivery systems. A commitment to cancer control and survivorship care must include a commitment to health equity in order to achieve optimal health for everyone, giving particular attention to the needs of those most at risk for poor health. Many of our contributing authors have written about disparity and health equity, underscoring the important role yoga and yoga therapy can play in the well-being of underrepresented communities and populations. In Chapter 6, we share their inspiring work.

Action points

Equity vs. equality: There is an important distinction between *equity* and *equality*. We must work toward *equity*.

According to the Milken Institute School of Public Health, George Washington University:

Equality means each individual or group of people is given the same resources or opportunities. Equity recognizes that each person has different circumstances and allocates the exact resources and opportunities needed to reach an equal outcome.

Milken Institute School of Public Health (2020)

Implicit bias: Each of us can test our own racial bias at Project Implicit (https://implicit.harvard.edu/implicit/takeatest.html). The validated Implicit Association Test

(IAT) measures attitudes and beliefs that we may be unwilling or unable to report. Its purpose is to educate the public about bias and to effect positive change (Project Implicit 2011).

Many universities and academic medical centers in the United States offer free online courses and webinars on equity in healthcare, culturally sensitive practices, and the importance of person-centered language. Current programs on diversity, equity, and inclusion in healthcare may be found via Internet search.

The book Why Are Health Disparities Everyone's Problem by Lisa Cooper, MD, MPH is a valuable resource (Cooper 2021).

Conclusion

As we've seen throughout this chapter, there are many challenges inherent in the management of people with cancer and survivors. Our overview of the biology of cancer and its natural history, cancer treatments and side effects, and disparity in cancer care provides context and sets the stage for Chapter 6: The Cancer Care Continuum, in which we look at the side effects of various cancer treatments, their impact on the mind-body, and practical and clinical considerations for yoga and yoga therapy in cancer care. Together, these two chapters inform the delivery of safe and effective yoga and yoga therapy for people with cancer and survivors – many of whom may be medically fragile as a result of cancer, treatments, and comorbid conditions, and therefore at higher risk of injury.

For yoga therapists, the information in this chapter underscores the importance of intake, assessment, patient/client goals and expectations, and individual treatment objectives within the framework of a holistic management plan. And for all yoga teachers and yoga professionals, it illustrates the need to have a working knowledge of the biology of cancer, its natural history, and consequences and toxicities of therapeutic cancer interventions. Given such a foundation, both yoga and yoga therapy can become an essential intervention for bringing people with cancer, survivors, and their caregivers to a place of wellness, regardless of medical condition or prognosis.

Acknowledgments

We credit the National Cancer Institute (NCI) for the cancer-related information presented in the chapter. Information and data are used with permission. Text that is reproduced verbatim, quoted, and/or paraphrased is cited per NCI useage guidelines (cancer.gov). We are grateful for the opportunity to share their information. Secondary sources for the information presented in this chapter include the American Cancer Society (ACS), American Society of Clinical Oncology (ASCO), Centers for Disease Control and Prevention (CDC), and American Association of Cancer Research (AACR).

This chapter was medically reviewed by Gregory Mears, MD, Professor of Medicine, Division of Hematology/Oncology, Columbia University Irving Medical Center and Jeanene "Gigi" Robison, MSN, RN, AOCN, Oncology Education Specialist, St. Elizabeth Healthcare. We are grateful for their important contribution to this book.

References

American Association for Cancer Research, 2021. Cancer Health Disparities. Available at: https://www.aacr.org/patients-caregivers/about-cancer/cancer-health-disparities/.

Ducharme, J., Wolfson, E., 2019. Your zipcode might determine how long you live – and the difference could be decades. *Time.* Available at: https://time.com/5608268/zip-code-health/.

Ferlay, J., Ervik, M., Lam, F., et al., 2020. Global Cancer Observatory: Cancer Today. Lyon: International Agency for Research on Cancer. Available at: https://gco.iarc.fr/today.

Milken Institute School of Public Health, 2020. Equity vs. Equality: What's the Difference? Available at: https://onlinepublichealth.gwu.edu/resources/equity-vs-equality/.

National Cancer Institute, 2013. Tumor Grade. Available at: https://www.cancer.gov/about-cancer/diagnosis-staging/prognosis/tumor-grade-fact-sheet.

National Cancer Institute, 2015. Cancer Staging. Available at: https://www.cancer.gov/about-cancer/diagnosis-staging/staging.

National Cancer Institute, 2020a. Metastatic Cancer: When Cancer Spreads. Available at: https://www.cancer.gov/types/metastatic-cancer.

National Cancer Institute, 2020b. Recurrent Cancer: When Cancer Comes Back. Available at: https://www.cancer.gov/types/recurrent-cancer.

National Cancer Institute, 2020c. Cancer Disparities. Available at: https://www.cancer.gov/about-cancer/understanding/disparities.

National Cancer Institute, 2021. What Is Cancer? Available at: https://www.cancer.gov/about-cancer/understanding/what-is-cancer.

Project Implicit, 2011. Implicit Association Test. Available at: https://implicit.harvard.edu/implicit/takeatest.html.

Siddhartha Mukherjee, S., 2010. *The Emperor of All Maladies: A Biography of Cancer.* Scribner: p. 38.

Sung, H., Ferlay, J., Siegel, R.L., et al., 2021. Global Cancer Statistics 2020: GLOBOCAN estimates of incidence and mortality worldwide for 36 cancers in 185 countries. *CA Cancer J Clin.* 71(3): 209–249.

Witt, C.M., Balneaves, L.G., Cardoso, M.J., et al., 2017. A comprehensive definition for integrative oncology. *JNCI Monographs.* 2017(52).

Further reading
Cancer
Alisangco, J., Sugarman, 2020. Chapter 7: Carcinogenesis. In J.M. Brant (ed.), *Core Curriculum for Oncology Nursing*, 6th ed., pp. 55–63. St Louis, MO: Elsevier.

Eggert, J., 2020, Chapter 10: Genetic Risk Factors. In J.M. Brant (ed.), *Core Curriculum for*

Oncology Nursing, 6th ed., pp. 72–84). St Louis, MO: Elsevier.

Early historical evidence of cancer
Aufderheide, A., 2003. *The Scientific Study of Mummies.* Cambridge University Press; Cambridge.

Boulos, F.S., 1986. Oncology in the Egyptian papyri. In: Retsas, S., (ed) *Palaeo-Oncology: The Antiquity of Cancer.* Farrand Press; London: pp. 35–40.

Hajdu, S.I., 2011. A note from history: landmarks in history of cancer, part 1. *Cancer.* 117(5):1097–1102.

Miller, J.L., 1929. Some diseases of ancient man. *Annals of Medical History 1.* pp. 394–402.

Cancer stigma: global perspective
Adebowale, N., 2021. How Nigeria can reduce cancer-related deaths – health expert. All Africa. Available at: https://allafrica.com/stories/202102040079.html.

Agustina, E., Dodd, R.H., Waller, J., Vrinten, C., 2018. Understanding middle-aged and older adults' first associations with the word "cancer": a mixed methods study in England. *Psychooncology.* 27:309–315.

Lagnado, L., 2008. In some cultures, cancer stirs shame. *Wall Street Journal.* Available at: http://online.wsj.com/article/SB122304682088802359.html.

Neal C., Beckjord E.B., Rechis, R., et al. Cancer stigma and silence around the world: a LIVESTRONG report. LIVESTRONG. Available at: https://www.livestrong.org/sites/default/files/what-we do/reports/lsglobalresearchreport.pdf

Quaife, S.L., Winstanley, K., Robb, K.A., et al., 2015. Socioeconomic inequalities in attitudes towards cancer: an international cancer benchmarking partnership study. *Eur J Cancer Prev.* 24:253–260.

Rosetta, L., 2008. Cancer and the Navajo language. USC Center for Health Journalism. Available at: https://centerforhealthjournalism.org/fellowships/projects/cancer-and-navajo-language.

The Biological Intersection of Yoga and Cancer 5

Leigh Leibel

In solving a problem of this sort, the grand thing is to be able to reason backwards. That is a very useful accomplishment, and a very easy one.

Sherlock Holmes in *A Study in Scarlet*
Sir Arthur Conan Doyle

Yoga has a 5,000-year history providing sustenance and value to its practitioners. But *how* does it work? In recent years, worldwide scientific inquiry into the reasons for its perceived benefits has yielded a great deal of information regarding yoga's impact on our physiology and pathophysiology. Several well-designed clinical trials assessing biomarkers suggest that yoga may improve outcomes such as stress hormone regulation, inflammation, and immune function (Danhauer et al. 2019). The data strongly support the thesis that yoga and related activities such as meditation and mindfulness can be employed in the medical arena to:

- Favorably control aspects of chronic illnesses including cancer (Lin et al. 2018, Milbury et al. 2018, 2019, Rao et al. 2008).

- Help diminish side effects of chronic disorders and their treatments (Danhauer et al. 2019, Mustian et al. 2013, Chandwani et al. 2014, Infante et al. 2014, Raghavendra et al. 2007, Vadiraja et al. 2009, Narayanan et al. 2019).

- Contribute to prevention and risk reduction of chronic illnesses (Cole et al. 2015, Carlson et al. 2014).

- Favorably influence cancer progression, recurrence, and clinical outcomes (Antoni & Dhabar 2019, Surman & Janik 2017).

In this chapter we'll look at the biological intersection of cancer and yoga: the basic science behind DNA and gene expression; the microenvironment and immune system; chronic inflammation; stress and the autonomic nervous system; and the evidence base supporting yoga's favorable effect on these various processes.

DNA and gene expression

Cancer is a very complex set of medical disorders characterized by poorly controlled proliferation of aberrant cells that often have lost their normal functional capacities. This leads to organ damage and invasion of other parts of the body. At the root of cancer genesis is gene malfunction (see Chapter 4).

Most cells in the human body are regulated by genes encoded in their nuclear DNA (red cells and platelets do not have nuclei). All nuclear DNA is identical at birth (except for the DNA of sperm and ova which contain only 50% of the DNA). Whenever a cell divides, nuclear DNA is replicated so that the two daughter cells should have the same genetic apparatus. DNA replication is not a perfect process and mistakes in the coding, called mutations, can occur. Normally, there are control processes to allow for proper repair of the DNA. There are also housekeeping genes that will activate cell death pathways if a newly formed cell does not meet proper standards, very much like the quality control processes on an assembly line. However, mistakes still occur and survive the quality control programs. Over time, a series of mistakes may accrue to a cell that gradually alters its assigned function, and it begins to take on a cancer phenotype (i.e., the observable physical properties of an organism, including appearance, development, and behavior). This is a very gradual process that may take decades to evolve into a fully malignant cell population.

There are many different types of gene errors that can accumulate. Many are trivial and lead to no change in cell function, whereas some alter cell function and can lead to cancer. Normally, only a subset of genes in any given cell group (organ or tissue) is actively expressed to produce the unique functions the cell group is designed to perform. The gene expression can vary over time, often changing in minutes. Think of the genes as musicians in a symphony orchestra. The gene expression of heart cells may be like Beethoven's *Ninth Symphony* whereas the gene expression of pancreas cells may be like Gershwin's *Rhapsody in Blue*.

Typical DNA mutations include some that inappropriately silence a normally active gene for a particular cell type, some that delete a gene, and some that amplify a gene. Usually, one mutation is not enough for cancer to develop. Over time, often years, multiple independent mutations need to accumulate to cause a cell to become cancerous.

Microenvironment and the immune system

Gene mutations may happen by random misadventure (may be innate), but many result from external forces applied to the DNA coming from their microenvironment. Their microenvironment is directly influenced by external forces and events, including lifestyle and behaviors. As one example, the habit of smoking or chewing tobacco leads to the internalization of a number of toxic agents that are capable of damaging DNA by transmission through the microenvironment of the exposed cells and provoking inflammation. Cancers of the lung, bladder, larynx, mouth, esophagus, throat, liver, stomach, pancreas, colon and rectum, cervix, and kidney, and acute myeloid leukemia may develop from exposure to these toxic agents (National Cancer Institute 2017a). Certain infections, notably *H. pylori*, a type of bacteria found in the stomach, can stimulate stomach cancer; human papillomavirus (HPV) can cause cervical, anal, and throat cancer; and hepatitis B can cause liver cancer. All do so by perturbing the immune system in the affected organs, which can then damage DNA from the associated inflammation (van Elsland & Neefjes 2018).

Chronic inflammation

Inflammation may be classified as acute or chronic; it it chronic inflammation that is unhealthy. Inflammatory proteins, called cytokines – although important in acute inflammation to promote healing – are dangerous in the chronic setting as they over-stimulate cell growth and impair DNA repair. For example, morbid obesity (defined by the National Institutes of Health as having a body mass index [BMI] >35 with comorbid conditions) is accompanied by chronic

inflammation because certain cells called macrophages accumulate in visceral fat (fat found inside the abdominal cavity that is wrapped around the internal organs) and are factories for making inflammatory cytokines. Insulin resistance, commonly seen in morbid obesity, causes increased production of insulin, a hormone that has a separate effect stimulating cell growth. The end result is that morbid obesity is linked to an increased incidence of 13 cancers (National Cancer Institute 2017b, Lauby-Secretan et al. 2016).

When talking about cancer-related risk factors, it can be difficult for all parties to communicate about sensitive topics such as weight. Health-related discussions around morbid obesity must occur in a safe and supportive environment and all individuals must be respected regardless of their size, shape, or ability. Importantly, yoga is for everyone and every body, and a regular yoga practice may be prescribed to every person for positive health and well-being, as well as to promote lifestyle and behavior changes. An added bonus is that several well designed randomized controlled trials point to yoga's ability to reduce inflammation (Box 5.1).

BOX 5.1 Yoga's impact on inflammation

Bower et al. found a 12-week restorative Iyengar yoga intervention[1] reduced inflammation-related gene expression in fatigued breast cancer survivors. The investigators conclude these findings "suggest that a targeted yoga program may have beneficial effects on inflammatory activity in this patient population, with potential relevance for behavioral and physical health" (Bower et al. 2014).

Kiecolt-Glaser et al. found *Haṭha* yoga[2] has a favorable influence on inflammation, mood, and fatigue in breast cancer survivors. The investigators conclude "chronic inflammation may fuel declines in physical function leading to frailty and disability. Therefore, if yoga dampens or limits both fatigue and inflammation, then regular practice could have substantial health benefits" (Kiecolt-Glaser et al. 2014).

Rao et al. investigated the effect of an "integrated yoga-based stress reduction program"[3] on sleep quality and neuroendocrine immune response in

(continued)

BOX 5.1 continued

(continued)

metastatic breast cancer patients. Investigators found "a decrease in morning waking cortisol in the yoga group alone following the intervention, and a significant improvement in NK (natural killer) cell percent following intervention in the yoga group compared to the control group. This suggests modulation of neuroendocrine responses and improvement in sleep in patients with advanced breast cancer following the yoga intervention" (Rao et al. 2017).

[1] The Iyengar yoga intervention "emphasized postures, and breathing techniques that focus on passive inversions (i.e., supported upside-down postures in which the head is lower than the heart) and passive backbends (i.e., supported spinal extensions)."

[2] The *Haṭha* yoga intervention consisted of 10 floor poses, 6 standing poses, 3 seated poses, 4 restorative poses, and 4 kinds of breathing practices.

[3] "The yoga practices included in the 'integrated stress-reduction' program consisted of a set of *āsana-s* (postures done with awareness), breathing exercises, *prāṇāyāma* (voluntarily regulated nostril breathing), meditation, and yogic relaxation techniques with imagery. These practices were based on principles of attention diversion, awareness, and relaxation to cope with stressful experiences."

Stress and the autonomic nervous system

Although acute stress is a normal reaction to a threat, chronic stress is unhealthy and makes our bodies more hospitable to cancer growth (Antonini & Dhabhar 2019, Cole et al. 2015, Thaker et al. 2006, Banerjee et al. 2007) (Box 5.2). An imbalance in the autonomic nervous system favoring the sympathetic nervous system over the parasympathetic nervous system causes overproduction of norepinephrine and cortisol. These stress hormones can be damaging to DNA. Such an imbalance is called *allostatic load*, a term coined in 1993 by McEwan and Stellar (McEwen & Stellar 1993). At its most basic, this means "wear and tear" on the body that is accumulated during exposure to repeated

BOX 5.2 Impact of psychosocial stress and stress management on immune responses in cancer patients

In 2019, Antonini and Dhabar conducted research on the impact of psychosocial stress and stress management on immune responses in cancer patients. In their words:

"Chronic stress and adversity are associated with neuroendocrine alterations (sympathetic nervous system [SNS], hypothalamic-pituitary-adrenal axis [HPA]), which can up-regulate inflammation and down-regulate cell-mediated immunity. Immune cells that have undergone such changes may not control cancer cells effectively and may act as stromal cells communicating with the tumor microenvironment and circulating cancer cells to promote tumor growth mechanisms, invasiveness, extravasation into the circulation, and metastasis. Many randomized controlled trials demonstrate physical-, mindfulness- and cognitive-behavioral therapy-based stress management interventions and pharmacologic blockade of stress-related pathways can affect immune parameters in cancer patients and survivors. Importantly, research has now linked stress management-associated changes in immune parameters early in treatment with long-term health outcomes in the context of early-stage breast cancer. Thus, in addition to reducing chronic stress and adversity, stress management intervention can also alter immune cell activity in a manner that may mitigate the biological impact of stress early in treatment, and potentially influence disease progression and clinical outcomes in cancer patients."

(Antonini and Dhabar 2019)

life stressors. According to a systematic review by Guidi et al., allostatic load is associated with poor health outcomes in all populations (Guidi et al. 2020).

Chapter five

Yoga's favorable impact on gene expression, inflammation, and stress

The practice of yoga has been well studied both in India (at yoga research universities such as S-VYASA University in Bengaluru) and in the Western world (at eminent universities and medical centers such as Harvard University and University of Texas MD Anderson Cancer Center). The focus of much of the research is to better understand how yoga may favorably influence chronic illnesses and non-communicable disease (NCD), including cancer. Well-studied topics include yoga's impact on gene expression, yoga's impact on chronic inflammation, and yoga's impact on chronic stress (Bhasin et al. 2013, Cohen et al. 2012, Irwin et al. 2016, Chandwani et al. 2014).

- **Gene expression:** A group at Harvard performed a randomized controlled trial (RCT), the benchmark type of study to demonstrate efficacy, to see if there were favorable alterations in gene expression by employing a meditation practice vs. another leisure activity. The result showed that the meditation practice, but not the other leisure activity, was accompanied by a favorable change in gene expression in white blood cells with down-regulation of genes for inflammation and stress. The change occurred within 20 minutes and the longer the practice, the greater the favorable change (Bhasin et al. 2013).

- **Chronic inflammation and fatigue**: Another group studied the application of a yoga practice to breast cancer survivors and its impact on fatigue and chronic inflammation. They conducted two RCT's, with each demonstrating a regular yoga practice lowered fatigue, increased vitality, and lowered inflammatory cytokines. With more yoga practice (a greater "dose"), the results grew even stronger (Bower et al. 2012, 2014; see Box 5.1).

- **Stress hormones and the HPA axis:** Other groups have carefully studied the impact of a yoga practice on the hypothalamic–pituitary–adrenal (HPA) axis, demonstrating suppression of stress hormones such as cortisol and norepinephrine (Arora & Bhattacharjee 2008). Other studies demonstrate the utility of a yoga practice to suppress the sympathetic nervous system while improving the parasympathetic nervous system response (Cole et al. 2015, Thaker et al. 2006).

An added value to a yoga practice in the cancer arena is its association with a healthy lifestyle and behaviors that minimize the development of of comorbid conditions, obesity, and associated inflammation, now a major cause of cancer both in the developed world and more recently in low-and-middle income countries (LMIC) where Western processed foods are being introduced (Wilson et al. 2020, Kopp 2019).

Conclusion

The study of yoga and its utility in the medical management of chronic illnesses, including cancer, has been very positive. Physiological changes invoked by yoga clearly work against the environmental forces that trigger chronic inflammation and chronic stress, known to damage DNA and promote cancer formation.

Acknowledgment

This chapter has been medically reviewed by Gregory Mears, MD, Professor of Medicine, Division of Hematology/Oncology, Columbia University Irving Medical Center, New York City. We are grateful for his important contribution to our book.

References

Antoni, M.H., Dhabhar, F.S., 2019. The impact of psychosocial stress and stress management on immune responses in patients with cancer. *Cancer*. 125:1417–1431.

Arora, S., Bhattacharjee, J., 2008. Modulation of immune responses in stress by yoga. *International Journal of Yoga*. 1(2):45–55.

Banerjee, B., Vadiraj, H.S., Ram, A., et al., 2007. Effects of an integrated yoga program in modulating psychological stress and radiation-induced genotoxic stress in breast cancer patients undergoing radiotherapy. *Integr Cancer Ther*. 6(3):242–250.

Bhasin, M.K., Dusek, J.A., Chang, B.H., et al., 2013. Relaxation response induces temporal transcriptome changes in energy metabolism, insulin secretion and inflammatory pathways. *PLoS One*. 8(5):e62817. Erratum in: *PLoS One*. 2017 Feb 21;12 (2):e0172873.

Bower, J.E., Garet, D., Sternlieb, B., et al., 2012. Yoga for persistent fatigue in breast cancer survivors: a randomized controlled trial. *Cancer*. 118(15):3766–3775.

Bower, J.E., Greendale, G., Crosswell, A.D., et al., 2014. Yoga reduces inflammatory signaling in fatigued breast cancer survivors: a randomized controlled trial. *Psychoneuroendocrinology*. 43:20–29.

Carlson, L.E., Beattie, T.L., Janine Giese-Davis, J., et al., 2014. Mindfulness-based cancer recovery and supportive-expressive therapy maintain telomere length relative to controls in distressed breast cancer survivors. *Cancer*. 121:476–484.

Chandwani, K.D., Perkins, G., Nagendra, H.R., et al., 2014. Randomized, controlled trial of yoga in women with breast cancer undergoing radiotherapy. *Journal of Clinical Oncology*. 32(10):1058–1065.

Cohen, L., Cole, S.W., Sood, A.K., et al., 2012. Depressive symptoms and cortisol rhythmicity predict survival in patients with renal cell carcinoma: role of inflammatory signaling. *PLoS One*. 7:e42324.

Cole, S.W., Nagaraja, A.S., Lutgendorf, S.K., et al., 2015. Sympathetic nervous system regulation of the tumour microenvironment. *Nat Rev Cancer*. 15:563–572.

Danhauer, S.C., Addington, E.L., Cohen, L., et al., 2019. Yoga for symptom management in oncology: a review of the evidence base and future directions for research. *Cancer*. 125:1979–1989.

Doyle, A.C., 2004 [first published 1887]. *A Study in Scarlet*. Kessinger Publishing; Whitefish, MT: 107.

Guidi, J., Lucente, M., Sonino, N., Fava, G.A., 2020. Allostatic load and its impact on health: a systematic review. *Psychother Psychosom*. 90:11–27.

Infante, J.R., Peran, F., Rayo, J.I., et al., 2014. Levels of immune cells in transcendental meditation practitioners. *Int J Yoga*. 7:147–151.

Irwin, M.R., Olmstead, R., Carroll, J.E., 2016. Sleep disturbance, sleep duration, and inflammation: a systematic review and meta-analysis of cohort studies and experimental sleep deprivation. *Biol Psychiatry*. 80:40–52.

Kiecolt-Glaser, J.K., Bennett, J.M., Andridge, R., et al., 2014. Yoga's impact on inflammation, mood, and fatigue in breast cancer survivors: a randomized controlled trial. *Journal of Clinical Oncology*. 32(10):1040–1049.

Lauby-Secretan, B., Scoccianti, C., Loomis, D., et al., 2016. Body fatness and cancer: viewpoint of the IARC Working Group. *NEJM*. 375(8):794–798.

Lin, P.J., Peppone, L.J., Janelsins, M.C., et al., 2018. Yoga for the management of cancer treatment-related toxicities. *Current Oncology Reports*. 20(1):5.

McEwen, B.S., Stellar, E., 1993. Stress and the individual. Mechanisms leading to disease. *Arch Intern Med*. 153(18):2093–101.

Milbury, K., Mallaiah, S., Mahajan, A., et al., 2018. Yoga program for high-grade glioma patients undergoing radiotherapy and their family caregivers. *Integrative Cancer Therapies*. 17:332–336.

Milbury, K., Liao, Z., Shannon, V., et al., 2019. Dyadic yoga program for patients undergoing thoracic radiotherapy and their family caregivers: results of a pilot randomized controlled trial. *Psychooncology*. 28:615–621.

Mustian, K.M., Sprod, L.K., Janelsins, M., et al., 2013. Multicenter, randomized controlled trial of yoga for sleep quality among cancer survivors. *J Clin Oncol*. 31:3233–3241.

Narayanan, S., Francisco, R., Lopez, G., et al., 2019. Role of yoga across the cancer care continuum: from diagnosis through survivorship. *J Clin Outcomes Manag*. 26:219–228.

National Cancer Institute, 2017a. Tobacco. Available at: https://www.cancer.gov/about-cancer/causes-prevention/risk/tobacco.

National Cancer Institute, 2017b. Obesity and Cancer. Available at: https://www.cancer.gov/about-cancer/causes-prevention/risk/obesity/obesity-fact-sheet.

Raghavendra, R.M., Nagarathna, R., Nagendra, H.R., et al., 2007. Effects of an integrated yoga programme on chemotherapy-induced nausea and emesis in breast cancer patients. *Eur J Cancer Care (Engl)*. 16(6):462–474.

Rao, R.M., Telles, S., Nagendra, H.R., et al., 2008. Effects of yoga on natural killer cell counts in early breast cancer patients undergoing conventional treatment. Comment to: Wachi, M., Koyama, M., Utsuyama, M., 2007. Recreational music-making modulates natural killer cell activity, cytokines, and mood states in corporate employees. *Med Sci Monit*. 13(2): CR57–70 4282. *Med Sci Monit*. 14(2):LE3–LE4.

Rao, R.M., Vadiraja, H.S., Nagaratna, R., et al., 2017. Effect of yoga on sleep quality and neuroendocrine immune response in metastatic breast cancer patients. *Indian Journal of Palliative Care.* 23(3):253–260.

Surman, M., Janik, M.E., 2017. Stress and its molecular consequences in cancer progression. *Postepy Hig Med Dosw (Online).* 71(0):485–499.

Thaker, P.H., Han, L.Y., Kamat, A.A., et al., 2006. Chronic stress promotes tumor growth and angiogenesis in a mouse model of ovarian carcinoma. *Nat Med.* 12:939–944.

Vadiraja, H.S., Rao, M.R., Nagarathna, R., et al., 2009. Effects of yoga program on quality of life and affect in early breast cancer patients undergoing adjuvant radiotherapy: a randomized controlled trial. *Complement Ther Med.* 17(5–6):274–280.

van Elsland, D., Neefjes, J., 2018. Bacterial infections and cancer. *EMBO Reports.* 19(11), e46632.

Yoga in the Cancer Care Continuum

Edited by Leigh Leibel and Anne Pitman

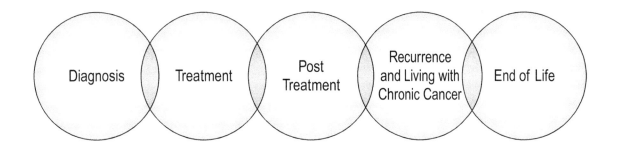

Atha yogānuśāsanam

अथ योगानुशासनम्

Patañjali Yoga Sūtra, 1.1

And now, Yoga.

Introduction
Leigh Leibel

Chapter 6 is the *raison d'être* of this book. It is the *sūtra* – the thread – that weaves the art and science of yoga into a garland of practices across the Cancer Care Continuum. On the pages that follow, 38 yoga therapists and advanced practice yoga teachers from around the world honor stories of illness, giving voice to the joy and suffering of their patients and clients touched by cancer. As readers, we come together to bear witness; we listen with curiosity; we hear their truths; we are solemnly present without judgment or assumption. Through the power of story, we see that our own true north lies with the unique lived experience of each of the patients, survivors, and loved ones for whom these yoga professionals have been privileged to serve. This book would not be possible without them. It is they who teach and inspire us, and it is in their debt that we stand.

The cancer care continuum

In medicine, the term *continuum of care* describes the delivery of healthcare over a period of time. The goal of a continuum model is to provide a patient with *continuity of care* via an organized and integrated system that spans the trajectory of both their wellness and their healthcare. This puts the patient first and provides better coordination and management of their treatment plans, progress, and priorities. A well-known example of the continuum of care model is seen in the field of obstetrics in which mother and child progress from prenatal care to delivery to pediatrics.

An oncology-specific model – the *Cancer Control Continuum* – was developed in 1971 by the National Cancer Institute (NCI), a branch of the National Institutes of Health (NIH) in the United States, to address the complexity of cancer prevention, control, treatment, and survivorship supportive care (National Cancer Institute 2020). It has been widely adopted in other countries. It is a seven-part model that begins with cancer etiology and prevention, and progresses through early detection, diagnosis, treatment, survivorship, and end of life. In this model there are nuances within the treatment and survivorship phases, e.g., *treatment* is characterized as either curative or non-curative (palliative), and *survivorship* describes two different kinds of cancer survivors: individuals with no evidence of disease (NED), and individuals who are living with cancer as a chronic condition or who have had a recurrence of their disease.

Given the importance of continuity in patient-centered care, a continuum framework for the clinical application of yoga in oncology was developed in 2018 to illustrate the optimum delivery of yoga and yoga therapy across all cancer patient populations and treatment intensities.[1] The model was presented at the symposium *"Role of Yoga in Supportive Cancer Care: Mechanism and Practice"* at the 2018 World Cancer Congress: *Strengthen, Inspire, Deliver*, convened by the Union of International Cancer Control (UICC) in Kuala Lumpur, Malaysia, and several weeks later to peers and colleagues at the half-day workshop *"Therapeutic Yoga in Cancer Patients: Research Methodology and Clinical Application"* that was held during the Society for Integrative Oncology (SIO) 15th International Conference, *From Research to Practical Applications*, in Scottsdale, Arizona. It was during this working session that SIO and the International Association of Yoga Therapists (IAYT) came to the table to talk about advancing the field of yoga therapy in healthcare, and to discuss the need to work collaboratively to deliver safe, effective, accessible yoga to people with cancer and survivors.

Under the guidance of leaders in the field (Box 6.1), approximately 30 people attended three consecutive breakfast round tables at the conference to discuss and share ideas. With bilateral support from SIO and IAYT leadership, the SIO Yoga Special Interest Group (SIO Yoga SIG) was launched in 2019 to advance yoga in cancer care. Today, there are 50 active members in the Yoga SIG. More about the group and its partnership projects with IAYT can be found in Chapter 7: Yoga Therapy in Oncologic Care - The Way Forward.

---

[1] The continuum framework was developed by Leigh Leibel as part of a capstone project on yoga in cancer care that was completed during a summer fellowship in cancer prevention and control at the National Cancer Institute (NCI).

BOX 6.1 Thought leaders

- Lorenzo Cohen, PhD, Professor and Director of the Integrative Medicine Program at The University of Texas MD Anderson Cancer Center, Houston (Founding member and President of SIO, 2007-2008).

- Santosh Rao, MD, ABOIM, Medical Director of Integrative Oncology, University Hospitals Connor Whole Health, Medical Oncology, GU Malignancies, Seidman Cancer Center, Cleveland, Ohio (President of SIO, 2023-2025).

- Raghavendra Rao, PhD, Director, Central Council for Research in Yoga and Naturopathy (CCRYN) in New Delhi, India (Co-Chair SIO Yoga SIG, 2019–2021).

- John Kepner, MBA, Executive Director of IAYT, Little Rock, Arkansas (2003-2020).

- Leigh Leibel, MSc, C-IAYT, Columbia University Irving Medical Center, New York City, NY (Co-Chair SIO Yoga SIG, 2019-2022; SIO Board of Trustees, 2019-2023).

The model for the *Yoga in the Cancer Care Continuum* is informed by the NCI model, with modifications. Rather than seven parts, ours is a five-part framework: *Diagnosis, Treatment, Post Treatment, Recurrence, and End of Life.* (Prevention is part of the model; it is beyond the scope of this book.) As we will see throughout this chapter, the continuum highlights the different medical needs of patients during the different phases of care, as well as contraindications to yoga practice. Embedded within the model are six dimensions of healthcare performance: *safety, effectiveness, patient-centeredness, timeliness, efficiency,* and *equity.* These quality aims are adapted from the National Academy of Medicine (formerly Institute of Medicine [IOM]). Their definition of continuity of care in oncology is:

The systematic assurance of uninterrupted, integrated medical and psychosocial care of the pa-

tient, in accord with the patient's wishes, from assessment of symptoms in the pre-diagnostic period, throughout the phase of active treatment, and for the duration of post-treatment monitoring and/or palliative care.

Institute of Medicine (2001)

Editors' notes for this chapter

Chapter structure

This chapter is presented in five sections which correspond with the five phases of the Yoga in the Cancer Care Continuum: 1. Diagnosis, 2. Treatment, 3. Post Treatment, 4. Recurrence, and 5. End of Life. This five-stage continuum is the container in which we have organized and placed the 38 contributing authors' patient/client stories and the editorial backgrounds that precede each one. Each of the five sections begins with a brief introduction to that particular stage of the continuum, followed by the contributor patient/client stories for that stage of care. For medical context, every story is preceded by an editorial overview (called "the background") of the patient/client chief complaint to the yoga therapist or advanced practice yoga teacher.

Woven through the sections are boxes of select yoga practices. These are not presented as prescriptions for the various treatment side-effects and comorbid conditions, but as inspiration in designing an individualized, culturally sensitive yoga program that reflects the patient/client's goals and objectives, and their current medical and health status. We also highlight contraindications and research studies. References and additional reading suggestions are located at the end of each section.

Recruitment and selection of contributing authors

In 2019, we held an open call and invited yoga therapists and advanced practice yoga teachers working in cancer care globally to submit proposals to be considered for inclusion in this book. The objective was to showcase the breadth and depth of yoga practices in cancer care. The open call was promoted internationally through social media and various yoga and yoga therapy associations. Ultimately, we selected 38 yoga therapists and advanced practice yoga teachers from the United States, Canada, Australia, India, and Singapore. These yoga professionals have exceptional expertise working with rich and diverse patient/client and caregiver populations, including age and ability; gender identity and sexual orientation; socioeconomic background; and ethnic and racial backgrounds.

Our 38 contributing authors work with pediatric, adolescent and young adult (AYA), adult, and geriatric populations and their caregivers across all stages of disease and phases of cancer care. They work in a variety of locations, including hospital (in-patient; out-patient; ICU; infusion center; radiation department); clinic; studio; retreat center; in-home; online or via tele-health. Their sessions are delivered one-on-one, in dyads (twosomes), or in small groups. Many are involved in JEDI (justice, equity, diversity, and inclusion), using the tools of yoga to center and amplify the voices of medically underrepresented people worldwide.

Patient/client stories

- The contributing authors are presenting *stories*, not traditional medical case studies. It was their choice whether to use the term "patient" or "client" in their heading and narrative. Typically, yoga therapists who work in hospitals and clinics used the word "patient", while those who work privately or those who are advanced practice yoga teachers used the word "client".

- Throughout the book, we use person-first language when talking about people with cancer; e.g., "people living with cancer", or "people touched by cancer". We use the term "cancer patient" only when we refer to treatment. We also avoid using "battle" language to emphasize someone's experience with cancer as many survivors find it insensitive.

- In accordance with the Health Insurance Portability and Accountability Act (HIPAA) – a United States federal statute that protects patients' personal identifiable information – the names in the stories are false and we deliberately confounded identities for privacy. However, these are real patients and real encounters.

- The interventions and practices described in this chapter are for illustrative purposes only. It is the responsibility of the treating practitioner, yoga therapist, or advanced practice yoga teacher relying on independent expertise and knowledge of the patient/client, to determine the best treatment and method of application for the patient/client.

Diversity and inclusion

- This book follows the *Diversity Style Guide* (DSG) with regard to terms and phrases related to race/ethnicity; religion; sexual orientation; gender identity; age and generation; and physical, mental, and cognitive abilities. According to their website, the DSG is:

    "A resource to help journalists and other media professionals cover a complex, multicultural world with accuracy, authority, and sensitivity. It offers guidance, context, and nuance for media professionals struggling to write about people who are different from themselves and communities different from their own. No one person can determine the correct usage of a word; this guide takes wisdom and advice from leaders in the field who have researched and considered the cultural, political, and linguistic meanings of words. The DSG uses terms with permission" (Diversity Style Guide 2022).

- Per the DSG guidelines, in this book, we describe racial background using the words "Black" and "White," and capitalize both words. However, each contributing author chose the word(s) they use to identify their own race, for example, African American or Black.

- In the headings of each of the patient/client stories, we have included information on age, type and stage

of disease, race/ethnicity, and pronouns.This is medically relevant information for healthcare professionals working with people with cancer and is typically included in a person's medical record. For example, there are inherited genetic variations that play a role in disease development, drug response, and adverse reactions, and genetic variations can differ among different ethnicities. Healthcare providers, including yoga therapists, must consider all relevant information in order to provide high-quality, culturally sensitive, patient-centered care.

- We also acknowledge that health disparities faced by by Black, Indigenous, People of Color (BIPOC) and Lesbian, Gay, Bisexual, Transgender, Queer (LGBTQ+) people are rooted in bias and are often influenced by social determinants of health (see Chapter 4, *Disparity in cancer care*). It is critical that healthcare professionals, including yoga therapists and yoga teachers, create welcoming, inclusive, accessible, culturally sensitive environments for all people. There is also an urgent need for us to conduct more research into racial/ethnic differences in disease manifestation, and to better understand how socioeconomics, ancestry, ethnicity, environmental factors, bias, discrimination, and other factors come into play to influence an individual's health.

Use of sanskrit

- Throughout this book, we acknowledge and honor the traditional roots of Yoga as a system of physical, mental, and spiritual practices originating in ancient India that aim to control and quiet the mind, while recognizing a detached witness-consciousness untouched by suffering (*duḥkha*).

- Sanskrit (*saṃskṛtam*) is the original language of Yoga. In this book, all Sanskrit words are italicized (except for "yoga" which is a recognized loanword permanently adopted from Sanskrit and integrated into the English lexicon) and transliterated from *devanāgari* using the International Alphabet of Sanskrit Transliteration (IAST). In this system, diacritics or accent marks are written above or below a letter to indicate a difference in pronunciation from the unmarked letter. The IAST system allows the loss-less romanization of Indic script so those not familiar with the language can read the text, exactly as if it were in the original script. When writing the words, we follow the rules of Sanskrit grammar that guide us to combine two or more related words into one "compounded" word. Observing this grammatical rule (called *samāsa*), *yoga nidrā* becomes *yoganidrā*; *pañca kośa* becomes *pañcakośa*, and so forth. We also follow the Sanskrit rules of *sandhi* (sound changes within and between words).

- Traditionally, Sanskrit words are not capitalized, but capitalization of the word "yoga" is a debated issue globally. Therefore, in this book, it is the decision of each writer whether (and when) to capitalize the word "yoga". However, yoga will be capitalized when referring to a proper noun or to one of the six Vedic schools (*ṣaḍdarśana*) of Indian philosophy.

Summary

In Chapters 2 through 5, we have discussed the art and science of yoga in cancer care. In this chapter, these concepts are elegantly translated and applied by our 38 contributing authors. Reading their stories, we'll see that yoga – when viewed through the lens of *Yoga in the Cancer Care Continuum* – supports mind, body, and spirit at *every* phase of the cancer journey. The strong and growing evidence supporting yoga's starring role in the field of integrative oncology validates what yoga practitioners have known all along: *Yoga is good medicine.*

Acknowledgment

This chapter has been medically reviewed by Gregory Mears, MD, Professor of Medicine, Division of Hematology/Oncology, Columbia University Irving Medical Center, New York City. We are grateful for his important contribution to our book.

References

Diversity Style Guide, 2022. *Diversity Style Guide*. Available at: https://www.diversitystyleguide.com.

National Cancer Institute, 2020. *Cancer Control Continuum.* Available at: https://cancercontrol.cancer.gov/about-dccps/about-cc/cancer-control-continuum.

Institute of Medicine, 2001. *Crossing the Quality Chasm: A New Health System for the 21st Century.* National Academies Press; Washington, DC.

Taimni, I.K., 2014. *The Science of Yoga: The Yoga-Sutras of Patanjali in Sanskrit.* Theosophical Publishing House; Wheaton, IL.

Section 1 Diagnosis

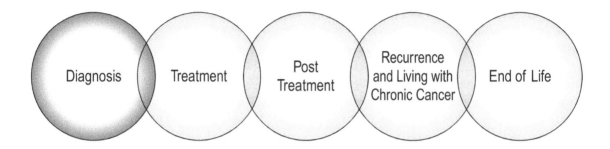

Now it is cancer's turn to be the disease that doesn't knock before it enters the door.

Susan Sontag, *Illness as Metaphor*

Introduction
Leigh Leibel

Diagnosis is the first of the five phases of the Yoga in the Cancer Care Continuum. In this phase of care, an abnormality is discovered through self-examination, routine screening, annual physical examination, during tests for other conditions, or when a person seeks medical attention due to specific symptoms. When this happens, a medical professional will obtain a personal and family medical history and conduct a physical exam, as well as order diagnostic tests, including laboratory and imaging procedures. A biopsy is required to confirm whether an abnormality is benign (noncancerous) or malignant (cancerous); if it is malignant, the person will be referred to oncology – the branch of medicine that specializes in cancer prevention, diagnosis, and treatment. Medical and radiation oncologists and a team of surgeons and specialists will treat the person for cancer, comorbid conditions, and side effects of cancer treatment. In addition, the person may be referred to integrative oncology, the diagnosis-specific field of integrative

medicine that supports people with cancer during treatment and beyond through the use of nonpharmacologic "complementary therapies" such as yoga, qigong, meditation, exercise, nutrition, and acupuncture. According to an educational book released by the American Society of Clinical Oncology (ASCO), "these complementary therapies are evidence-based adjuncts to mainstream care that effectively control physical and emotional symptoms, enhance physical and emotional strength, and provide patients with skills enabling them to help themselves throughout and following mainstream cancer treatment" (Deng & Cassileth 2014).

For most of us, *cancer* may be the most frightening word in medicine. As we saw in Chapter 4, cancer is a fantastically complex disease that has a major impact on our global society. The worldwide cancer burden is expected to increase by about 60% from 2018 to 2040, in part due to increased screening and our growing and aging population (The Cancer Atlas 2022). In 2018, there were 18.1 million new cases globally with 9.5 million cancer-related deaths; by 2040, the number of new cancer cases per year is expected to rise to 29.5 million and the number of cancer-related deaths to 16.4 million (NCI 2022). In 2021, in the United States alone there will be an estimated 1,898,160 new cancer cases; that means that every day in America, approximately 5,200 people will be told they have cancer (Seigel et al. 2021). And it's not just *them*: we are all in this conversation together. Based on 2015–2017 data, approximately 39.5% of men and women worldwide will be diagnosed with cancer at some point during their lifetime: this equates to one in three women and one in two men (NCI 2022).

A cancer diagnosis can be a profound and life-changing experience. It may evoke fear and distress, often leaving a person and their family in shock and facing feelings of disbelief, denial, fear, and anger – all of which are normal reactions to the situation at hand. But it's important to note that the cancer journey is a very personal experience, and every person will react differently to a diagnosis. Certainly, most will react with shock and disbelief, but not everyone will. A cancer diagnosis is perceived and experienced in many ways that are often shaped by broader social or life contexts, however, whatever a person's belief, their desires should be respected by clinicians and healthcare professionals.

Within the diagnosis phase of the continuum there are two stages: the "waiting" period and the "planning" period. In the waiting period (arguably one of the most stressful times of the cancer journey), the person waits for the biopsy and other test results to learn more about the abnormality – is it cancerous or not? If malignancy is confirmed, then the person and their medical team move on to the planning period. This involves staging and grading the cancer; obtaining second or third opinions; identifying treatment options (and their costs and side effects); and developing a disease management plan (See Chapter 4: Understanding Cancer and its Treatment). This can be an emotional time during which people share the news (or decide not to share the news) with family, friends, community, and work associates, as well as begin to deal with practicalities such as arranging for child or elder care and assistance with transportation and daily living. In the United States, securing approvals from health insurance coverage (if people have health insurance) can be an added burden.

The time between diagnosis of cancer to initial treatment is often called "time to treatment". In the United States, the national average for "time to treat" at large academic medical centers is approximately six weeks (Khorana et al. 2019, Abraham & Bolwell 2019). During this often stressful time, highly trained oncology yoga therapists are a valuable and underrecognized resource for people diagnosed with cancer. When introduced to a person early on, a yoga therapist can accompany them across the care continuum, providing continuity of care as the patient moves from diagnosis into treatment. Yoga therapists can also design a *prehabilitation* program to prepare patients for upcoming surgery and chemoradiation therapies, as well as help them develop coping skills to foster well-being, self-compassion, resilience, emotional regulation, and acceptance. Yoga therapy implemented at the time of diagnosis can offer solace and ease, reducing pain and suffering and enhancing quality of life for patients, families, and caregivers.

> It is interesting to note that in the United States, the National Institutes of Health/National Cancer Institute (NIH/NCI) and the American Cancer Society (ACS) consider people with a new cancer diagnosis to be "cancer survivors." They describe a cancer survivor as: "everyone who's ever had cancer, from the time of diagnosis for the rest of their life." Family members are called "co-survivors."
>
> (cancer.org 2022; cancer.gov 2022)

On the following pages, four yoga therapists share stories of working with patients and clients who have been diagnosed with cancer. We'll see how a yoga practice supported them through the initial shock and emotional impact of a diagnosis and helped them adjust to an uncertain future and regain a sense of agency. Through the art of close and deep listening, yoga therapists open themselves to stories of illness – bearing witness to their patients'/clients' lives, giving voice to their vulnerability, celebrating life with Joycean[1] spirit: *"to live, to air, to fall, to triumph, to re-create life out of life."*

---

[1] From *Portrait of the Artist as a Young Man* by James Joyce.

*Patient/client names have been changed and the stories edited to assure confidentiality. Each contributor has chosen whether to use the term "patient" or "client."

1.1 Softening shock after a cancer diagnosis

Background: Shock

Anne Pitman, MSc, E-RYT 500, C-IAYT

There is a lived experience in the words, "You have cancer." Patients often say it is like "having the rug pulled out from under them," or a surreal feeling of being outside of their body and not in the present moment at all. This shocked body pattern, if left uninterrupted, can continue through and beyond treatment.

Although so very challenging in the moment, the human response to "bad news" is intelligently protective. As unpleasant as it may be to embody, fight/flight/freeze or shutdown/collapse, are immediate responsive autonomic nervous system reactions that are meant to help us survive. Early stress responses may appear on a referral as "acute stress reaction" (ASR), "acute stress disorder" (ASD) or "adjustment disorder" (AD) depending, in part, on severity, timing and symptom clusters (Bryant 2018) in the DSM-5-TR (American Psychiatric Association 2022). In clinic, these responses may present as patterns in the body: a pronounced tension at the center of a client's body (throat, chest, and stomach); eyes that are wide, darting, or vacant; the spine stiff, the body held quite still, the breath shallow, rapid or held. This rigid, vigilant, and/or collapsed posture may in itself reinforce a sense of impending danger over time, communicating to the nervous system through afferent means, that even in the absence of immediate threat, we continue to sense threat (Taylor et al. 2010, Tsur et al. 2018 and see Cancer diagnosis through the lens of Polyvagal Theory on p. 18).

One way yoga therapy can help to redress the shock of diagnosis is by offering yogic and somatic "bottom-up" practices, slowly de-patterning the residue of persistent shock; in effect, returning our clients to a full-body sense of safety and agency. These simple, salient, and specific breath and movement practices may go a long way toward helping people be more settled and better able to participate in treatment decisions. Offered in the days and weeks after a diagnosis, clients develop an awareness of their reactions, co-regulate with their therapist (and other trusted humans and resources), and learn to self-regulate, even in the midst of uncertainty. Throughout further cancer treatments and any possible "persistent trauma" over the continuum, these practices and skills may be offered to reduce the incidence of what researchers refer to now as "cancer-related PTSD" (Cordova et al. 2017, Yang et al. 2017).

Client story: Michael

Anne Pitman

Michael (he/his) is a 46-year-old White man who is diagnosed with soft tissue sarcoma.

Michael has recently been diagnosed with a soft tissue sarcoma in his thigh. He hasn't begun treatment and was referred to yoga therapy by his oncologist (with no immediate movement contraindications) for help with shock (possibly ASD) and anxiety. He is not in pain presently, but appears very stiff, shoulders tight, and his breath barely visible. He says he is not eating or sleeping well and can't stop worrying about upcoming treatments and how his family is going to get through the next few months; they are all so concerned. Staring forward he says, "I can't believe this is happening. It's like my body has betrayed me". As he speaks about his teenaged sons, he whispers, "I don't know how to tell them that I might die of this disease. I can't do it." Much time is given to compassionate listening and acknowledging his feelings and worries.

When asked what he is noticing in his body, Michael says he feels an unbelievable tightness in his throat, a feeling of a heavy weight in the center of his chest which "feels like solid rock." When he speaks about the severity of his diagnosis, his breath becomes imperceptible, and he harkens back to that singular moment of diagnosis when he felt the floor fall out beneath him. Referring to that salient moment, he says, "I just went away". We talk simply about shock, the nervous system, and normal human reactions. He leans forward, interested. His breath begins to slow, and his eyes soften.

Michael chooses to practice lying down supine (see Box 6.2), with knees bent and feet on the floor. He is reminded that he could change any movement or breath by visualizing the suggestion instead, or by resting. Practicing side by side, we begin by noticing the body and observing a few exhalations with curiosity. With a practice of simple awareness, we start to roll our heads against the mat very slowly, noticing the sensation of the movement,

wondering how it could be easier, slower, softer. After a few minutes, he feels some trembling inside, and I ask him if he would be willing to turn toward the sensation, to simply witness it. The shaking subsides on its own, and next we bring our arms up, hands to opposite elbow over the chest. As slowly as possible, we begin to rock the elbows side to side, head following arms (not leading), noticing sensations. He remarks when he feels his shoulders begin to "unlock" and pleasant sensations begin to spread across his back. After a few minutes we let our arms gently fall back to the floor, and we pause, observing a few soft exhalations. Suddenly heavier on the floor, he feels his breath ease and deepen. We begin subtle movements again, this time his bent knees rocking slightly side to side. "It feels so good to move like this. I feel like I'm thawing."

After a while, we add the arms again, this time in opposition to the knees, head rolling in the same direction of the legs (see Figure 6.1). We play with moving the eyes, softly, in the opposite direction of the head. "This movement wants to be even slower," he says, letting out a long sigh. After a rest, Michael is invited to move in some way he hasn't yet, as though he could follow the movement his body desires in this moment. He stretches his arms overhead, arches his back and lengthens down to his toes. Slowly, he shakes his hands and pulls his knees up toward his chest, circling his feet.

Following the floor practice, Michael says he feels "restored and unbelievably calm." The tension in his throat and the weight in his chest have all virtually disappeared. His voice sounds stronger and his breath seems both soft and deep. While we sit together again and chat, recounting the inner experience of practice, we add a very subtle seated cat/cow (mārjaryāsana), a "waiting room" practice, something to help him settle his nerves when next at the hospital. He smiles slightly and says with gentle and surprising animation, "I don't know, but I might be ready to talk to my kids." Before he leaves, we pause again and consider the possibility that the feelings of shock and fear may arise again in these next days. He is comforted to know that he can return to any of these simple practices when he can't sleep, and in preparation for upcoming difficult conversations.

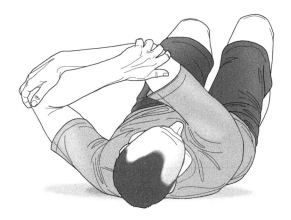

Figure 6.1
Lateral rolling with opposition

We make follow-up appointments to address specific treatment fears by accessing additional yoga practices for nervous system regulation. Referrals are made to a psychotherapist, family counselor, and an acupuncturist for sleep and treatment side effects.

Box 6.2 A three-part interoceptive practice

Anne Pitman

1. Interoceptive movement inquiry

Once trust and safety are established between therapist and client, an interoceptive (relating to stimuli arising within the body) practice can begin, hopefully with the nervous system less defended. With an approach of inquiry, a client makes choices in their movement, guided by internal sensations and preferences. The intent is to explore movements that softly disrupt postural holding patterns, offering an experience of safe mobilization (Sullivan et al. 2018) that is very difficult to come to after a shock.

2. Breath (*prāṇāyāma*)

Although diaphragmatic and/or slow exhalations are said to stimulate the parasympathetic nervous system (Van Diest et al. 2014, Gerritsen & Band 2018, Sullivan et al. 2018), this may not be true for each client, nor such a breath immediately available, depending on their lived experience and allostatic load. The practice begins instead with lateral and/or spinal movements, to stimulate and bring awareness to the trunk and the diaphragm. Through these easeful movements alone, the breath often slows and deepens without prescriptive suggestion.

3. Lateral, spinal, and novel movement

After a shock, most people are initially immobilized, tension quickly gathering around the eyes, head, and spine, preparing the body to fight, flee, freeze, or shutdown/collapse. In this vigilant posture and continued pattern, lateral body movements and movements through the spine do not naturally arise. For this reason, side to side movement (of eyes, spine, and limbs) can signal present-moment-safety to the nervous system, and may, therefore, be preferable to yoga poses that hold the torso and eyes centralized, as this can unintentionally mirror a shocked response. Subtle

(continued)

(continued)

tle side-to-side or wave-like spinal movements, on the floor, against a wall, or while sitting, can become helpful "waiting room" practices when a person is understandably anxious. Trembling and shaking can occur spontaneously as the nervous system releases tension (Ogden & Minton 2000, Levine 2010, Payne & Crane-Godreau 2015, Payne et al. 2015).

Novel movements may also be useful in softening tension (Eddy 2006, Gomes Silva 2014, Mansbach 2016). When a client is feeling steadier, a therapist may offer movements that don't usually "go together" (e.g., eyes and head moving in different directions). Novelty may also be introduced by offering more subtle variations of yoga poses, such as an almost imperceptible seated cat/cow (*mārjaryāsana*) when the client is accustomed to more vigorous movement.

1.2 Prehabilitation for a patient with head and neck cancer

Background: Cancer prehabilitation

Smitha Mallaiah, PhD(c), MSc, C-IAYT

A relatively new model of supportive care in oncology is called *cancer prehabilitation*. This is the concept of supporting people newly diagnosed with cancer by "preparing" them physically and emotionally for their future treatments. The model for cancer prehabilitation (Silver & Baima 2013) is defined as a process on the continuum of care that occurs between the time of cancer diagnosis and the beginning of an acute treatment and includes physical and psychological assessments that:

1. Establish a baseline functional level.

2. Identify impairments.

3. Provide interventions that promote physical and psychological health to reduce the incidence and/or severity of future impairments.

A growing body of scientific evidence supports the concept of preparing people newly diagnosed with cancer for surgery and chemoradiation therapies by optimizing their health prophylactically. Advantages of prehabilitation include improved patient functional outcomes and psychological well-being, as well as reduced postoperative complications. When implemented prior to acute treatments and continued well into survivorship, such a program can offer a solution to the widespread issue of decreased quality of life often experienced after cancer treatment (Lukez & Baima 2020). Prehabilitation is particularly important for people with head and neck cancer since their treatment can be difficult and disfiguring, often causing significant psychological distress and nutritional issues.

Patient story: Mr. Schuler

By Smitha Mallaiah

Mr. Schuler (he/his) is a 65-year-old Black man diagnosed with squamous cell carcinoma of the oral cavity, tongue, and pharynx.

Mr. Schuler has been on medication for 12 years for hyperlipidemia and hypertension. He is accompanied by his wife Mrs. Schuler. They sit down together, and he begins to talk about his symptoms. He is experiencing pain at the site of the tongue lesion, discomfort in chewing, sleep disturbances caused by high anxiety, and a sense of heaviness and discomfort in his chest and abdomen. Mr. Schuler is a former smoker with a 50-pack per month history. He does not have a regular physical exercise or yoga routine, and he eats a typical American diet of meat and potatoes. He endorses feeling guilty, thinking that he brought this disease on himself through smoking and poor lifestyle choices. As he speaks, he begins to tense, his breath changes, and there is a heavy pause in the room. I listen compassionately. We complete the session with goals for yoga therapy. He will have surgery one month from today.

A few days later, he returns to the clinic for what we call a "positive health yoga module," a 90-minute program that he'll attend twice per week before surgery. It includes one-on-one sessions with one of our yoga

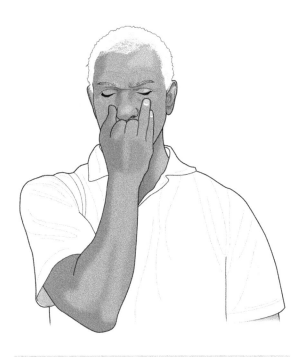

Figure 6.2
Alternate nostril breath (*nāḍīśodhana*)

therapists (Box 6.3) and instruction for daily home practice. Mr. Schuler's program includes these elements:

- To help reduce his anxiety, we use diaphragmatic breathing and alternate nostril breathing (*nāḍīśodhana*, see Figure 6.2) followed by honeybee breath (*bhramarī*), as needed every few hours.

- To prepare for surgery, we build overall physical strength, flexibility, and circulation through various yoga poses like warrior (*vīrabhadrāsana*), triangle (*trikoṇāsana*), and side-angle pose (*utthitapārśvakoṇāsana*).

- We include practices like *mudrā* (hand gestures); *bandha* (internal energetic "locks"); *prāṇāyāma* (breath-work), and other breath energization techniques to help with cardiopulmonary fitness.

- His meditation sessions emphasize mindfulness, concepts of acceptance, appreciation, and gratitude.

- Other bedtime routines include focusing on relaxation practices such as *yoganidrā* (yogic sleep) to help improve sleep quality.

- We refer him to a nutritionist to optimize his nutrition in preparation for surgery.

By the end of 25 days, Mr. Schuler has lost seven pounds, has been sleeping better and improved his energy levels, and can comfortably walk for more than three miles. He feels confident and mentally ready for his upcoming procedure which will be the surgical removal (glossectomy) of less than half of the tongue on his left side, and a neck dissection followed by a flap reconstruction. After surgery, he is discharged in less than four days without complications.

When he returns to the clinic post-surgery he has a smile on his face, thankful he's been able to recover well. His neck, however, is beginning to stiffen from the deep surgical incision. In preparation for the next part of treatment (upcoming radiation therapy), we add to his program:

- Joint loosening (*sūkṣmavyāyāma*) (subtle movements, not literally "loosening"), head and neck exercises, and facial movements to help prevent loss of function, and to facilitate a full range of motion of the neck and facial muscles.

- Swallowing exercises with a neck lock position (*jalandharabandha*), along with sound resonance practices like *A U M* and *Oṃ* to help deepen the relaxation.

Mr. Schuler is apprehensive about radiation, as he is claustrophobic and will have to wear a mask to hold his head still. He practices his yogic relaxation and body scan with guided imagery during radiation treatment. Additionally, he is coached on mindful eating practices to help him connect with food, as he has difficulty tasting and swallowing.

At the end of radiation, even though his skin is very burnt, his neck has full range of motion. He has maintained his weight, remains upbeat, continues with his yoga practices during his recovery, and his symptoms continue to improve. In his own words, "Yoga helped me discover the treasure of happiness within me. I am grateful every day for the gift of life."

BOX 6.3 Yoga therapy model of prehabilitation: a three-step process

Smitha Mallaiah

Sage *Patañjali* lays out the path in the *Patañjali Yoga Sūtra 2.16: heyam duḥkham anāgatam*, translated as "The suffering that is yet to come can be avoided." (Taimni 2014)." The pain already experienced creates an unwanted traumatic memory that exacerbates suffering, but one can prevent it before it develops or worsens. A yoga therapy-based multimodal prehabilitation plan addresses various physical, mental, emotional needs of the patient, filling the gap in care, supporting patients with adjuvant therapy, and preparing them for aggressive treatments.

1. Establish baseline

An established baseline with physical, psychological, and yogic assessments is crucial in developing an individualized prehabilitation plan. (a) At the physical level, we assess the activity tolerance, functional status, muscular strength, and cardiopulmonary fitness. (b) At the psychological level, we screen patients for anxiety, depression, phobias, and negative thought distortions and help them address the issues prophylactically. (c) Finally, we map the baseline on a yogic *pañcakośa* (five layers of human existence), *guṇa* (three psychic compositions that influence mind-body functions), and *doṣa* (three qualities that form essential characteristics of one's constitution) model to create a targeted yoga regimen.

2. Create a personalized yoga therapy plan

Once the baseline is established, the next step is to create a personalized yoga therapy plan to address

(continued)

(continued)

outcomes before the cancer treatment (pre-surgery, radiation, chemotherapy, etc.). At this stage, regular disciplined practice (*abhyāsa*) under an expert yoga therapist can help to adapt the program to the changing needs.

3. Post-cancer assessments and re-evaluation for future yoga therapy

Part of post-treatment assessments is to measure markers of recovery: physical strength, range of motion, and pain (including the recovery time and length of hospital stay). It is best to evaluate the progress and adapt the program for the future. Starting yoga in a prehabilitation model provides continuity throughout cancer care.

1.3 Early detection of breast cancer through interoceptive awareness: a proposition

Background: Interoception

Leigh Leibel

Interoception is the way in which we sense and regulate signals from inside the body such as heartbeat, respiration, and satiety, as well as autonomic nervous system activity related to emotions (Craig 2003). The discrete focus on these internal sensations (both conscious and nonconscious) is achieved when we sense afferent signals sent from visceral organs to the brain and central nervous system, and somatic signals from muscles and skin (Stern et al. 2017). We might call this *body literacy*.

Interoception is involved in many of our body's physiological systems, including cardiorespiratory, gastrointestinal, nociceptive, endocrine, and immune. Interoceptive processes also play important roles in a range of different cognitive and emotional behaviors. This is an exciting new area of research for the National Institutes of Health (NIH). In 2021, NIH launched a multi-year *interoception* research project to better understand its role in human health, and to improve our understanding of the brain-body function (National Institutes of Health 2021).

Awareness of these internal processes can be refined through the practice of yoga and mindfulness, allowing us to be more consciously attuned to body sensations (Mehling et al. 2009). In a traditional *Patañjali* yoga practice, we move our awareness from the gross (the outer practices or *antaraṅga*) to the subtle (the inner practices or *bahiraṅga*). As we move "inward" our minds begin to settle and relax, and we become more aware of our inner rhythms and signals (Farb et al. 2015). To that point, Bessel van der Kolk, MD – a psychiatrist and trauma researcher – has written extensively on the role of yoga in the development of interoception and body-sensing. In his seminal book *The Body Keeps the Score* (van der Kolk 2015), van der Kolk makes a case for yoga as an adjuvant therapy in post-traumatic stress disorder (PTSD) to unite the mind-body complex.

Interoception is often said to lie behind our intuition (e.g., something feels "right" or "wrong"). This poses the question: Can a yoga practice cultivate such an exquisite sensitivity to signals from our inner bodies that we are able to detect disease before the outward manifestation of its signs and symptoms?

Client story: Joana

Sanmay Mukhopadhyay, PhD student, BSc, BTech, MTech, MBA, MSc, PGDYT, C-IAYT

Joana (she/her) is a 41-year-old White woman diagnosed with stage I (ER+PR+HER2+) breast cancer.

Joana started her yoga practice years back when she was studying law at UC Berkeley in California. An avid surfer, she found surfing and yoga were both "sports" that challenged her – forcing her soul, spirit, and mind to "join the game." Her weekend yoga rocked her world. As she told me, "I was inspired by people's strength. By their contortions, by the Sanskrit words spoken. I was transported to a different space and time." As Joana matured in her practice, she gradually moved from power yoga and hip-hop yoga to a more integrative and contemplative kind of mind-body yoga. By chance, she found my traditional Indian yoga classes through her company's wellness program. "Your class looked easy as I was used to doing head stand (*śīrṣāsana*), crow pose (*bakāsana*), no problem. But soon, realization set in that this kind of contemplative yoga was harder – it was very hard for me to focus my mind and turn inward."

During our months of yoga classes together, we practiced quietly. "Stimulate and activate. Energize and relax," I would say as we proceeded through the sequence of *āsana-s* (postures), followed by deep relaxation. "Very gently, very subtly," I suggested. "Situate yourself with space and time. Build your multidimensional awareness." As the instructions energized our yoga space, Joana found a different dimension in her practice. Her stress level came down and slowly, after six months, she started to "get it."

This practice moves from gross to subtle: outside the body, to inside the body (Box 6.4). Space, body, breath, and inner dimensions; the travel continues, as dynamic movement of muscles lead to observation of inner senses. As the practice deepened, we used specific *mudrā-s* (hand gestures, e.g., *cinmudrā/jñānamudrā*; Figure 6.3) to generate pressures at different points in the body; nerve impulses felt and followed. Then, chanting of *mantra-s* (word or phrases), including *bījamantra* (one-syllable sounds, e.g., *AUM, Oṃ, Hum, Vam*) took the mind into a subtle state of awareness in which she explored the idea of *prāṇa* (life-force) moving.

Initially, Joana is confused; utterly focused on her outer spatial dimensions, she has a hard time following her senses. But once the *āsana-s* (postures) become natural, she starts to observe her senses throughout her body. Even after a downward dog (*adhomukhaśvānāsana*) and cobra (*bhujaṅgāsana*) *vinyāsa*, or a specialized dynamic hand to foot pose (*pādāṅguṣṭhāsana*), we would end the practice with a meditative state that combines basal sounds *A, U, M.* Very gently, very subtly. "Almost like a Chopin playing mellifluously throughout the body." She synergized the sensations with the sound vibrations. The sequences include *āsana* focused on breath.

One day in our practice Joana becomes aware of a sensation in her left breast – a dull, nagging pain. Proactive, she immediately calls her gynecologist who sends her straight away for a mammogram. "Yes," the radiologist said, "it is cancer, but we've caught it early. But there is no way the sensation you told me you felt in the breast was connected to this very tiny mass." It was impossible; Joana was imagining it.

The mass is a tiny but aggressive malignancy called HER2+ (human epidermal growth factor receptor 2 positive) breast cancer. It could have taken away her life. But to her surprise, when she meets with her new surgical oncologist, he says that the pain she felt was likely connected to the tumor. "While not directly, the tumor likely hit a nerve that manifested the pain outward."

Joana follows all the modern protocols. A bilateral mastectomy with a d-flap method of reconstruction. "No implants, no foreign objects, all made of my parts… throughout the process, yoga and meditation helped." After 18 months of chemotherapy and Herceptin (trastuzumab) infusions, her scans show no evidence of disease. Her port is removed. She is back to breathing and yoga. She can rest, she can recover.

Today, four years later, we sit together at her oceanfront house. She is now married, the mother of three beautiful boys. Joana reflects, "I have never seen such a breath-focused yoga. I was skeptical but I guess I was older and more receptive. It calmed me down. I remember when we traveled from the outer edges of the cosmos to the cells within…" She laughed. "That stuff is hard, this process was developed using some ancient techniques from India…where the custom is for all the senses, faculties to go deep." "And go deep I did!" Joana says. "I became aware of a sensation in my left breast. It was sort of a dull nagging pain." She could find it whenever she tried to be still, whenever she was still and listening. "But I had listened. I had immediately inquired and had it checked it out. And that saved my life."

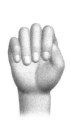

Adhimudrā (Gesture of Primordial Stillness; Core Quality: Stillness)

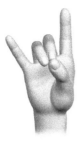

Apānamudrā (Gesture of the Downward Current of Purifying Energy; Core Quality: Purifying Current of Energy)

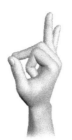

Bhramaramudrā (Gesture of the Bee; Core Quality: Healthy Immunity)

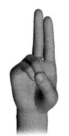

Bhūmudrā (Gesture of the Earth; Core Quality: Stability of the Earth)

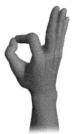

Cinmudrā (Gesture of Consciousness; Core Quality: Surrender to the Divine)/ *Jñānamudrā* (Gesture of Higher Knowledge; Core Quality: Awakening Clear Seeing)

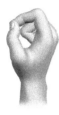

Cinmayamudrā (Gesture of Embodied Knowledge; Core Quality: Security)

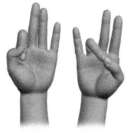

Daṇḍasvāsthyamudrā (Gesture for Healthy Back; Core Quality: Flow of Energy Around Vertebrae)

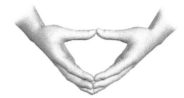

Hākinīmudrā (Gesture of the Goddess *Hakini*; Core Quality: Integration)

Hṛdayamudrā (Gesture of the Spritual Heart; Core Quality: Seeking Divine Refuge)

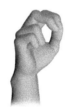

Kuberamudrā (Gesture of the Lord of Wealth; Core Quality: Conservation of Energy)

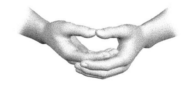

Maṇḍalamudrā (Gesture of the Circle; Core Quality: Spiritual Union)

Añjalimudrā/Namaskāra (Gesture of Reverence; Core Quality: Invoking Divine Union)

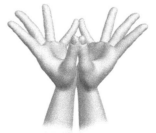

Padmamudrā (Gesture of the Lotus; Core Quality: Unconditional Love)

Figure 6.3
List of *hasta* (hand) *mudrā-s* referenced in the book; source material LePage 2014, Arora 2015

"This very contemplative yoga saved my life. Early detection was key, and then yoga supported me all the way through." Tears of joy trickle down her face, her little boy on her lap. We sit in quiet contemplation. "By training me to be so attuned to my body, I knew something was different, not right. I listened to my inner voice and sought medical guidance which led to rapid treatment. I found my tumor at a very early stage."

Prayatna śaithilya ananta samāpatti bhyam …

"Effortless movement, invite your focus on the body to find sensation, and then expand into infinity."

Patañjali Yoga Sūtra 2.47 (Translated by Sanmay Mukhopadhyay)

BOX 6.4 Five-step interoceptive practice inspired by *taittirīyopaniṣad (yajurveda)*

Sanmay Mukhopadhyay

An interoceptive yoga practice via the five steps (below) facilitates a profound internal connection. The practices allow the mind to prepare and connect internally at a deep level. The instructions are given to generate adequate sensitivity. Specific instructions to observe sensations and *jyoti* (inner light), and the appropriate usage of sound vibrations may help the client attain a heightened "intuition" about the body and enable them to sense pain or discomfort at an early stage.

Further, specialized usage of *mantra-s* (repeated word, sound, phrase) and deep chanting helped the client manage anxiety, depression, acute pain, and disturbed sleep.

1. **Align the geometry:** Invokes a series of supine, standing, prone, and sitting postures (*āsana-s*) in relationship with the outside world; eyes are closed to "feel" for the proprioception (Van der Kolk 2015) that establishes a balance with space and body correlation.

2. **Calming of breath:** Invokes mindful breathing along with *āsana-s*, activating vagal stimulation resulting in calming of the mind. Longer exhalation activates the parasympathetic nervous system; yogic practices trigger neurotransmitters that release serotonin, dopamine, and endorphins (Sarkar 2017, Farb 2015).

3. **Tāṇḍava** (the sacred dance-drama of India performed with vigorous, brisk movements): Invokes dynamic practices that stimulate the fascia (Schleip & Jäger 2012), generating sensations. A mental focus to observe these senses follows. This cycle of stimulation and relaxation enables deeper rest and increased sensitivity (Taimni 2014, Farb 2015, Katz & Egenes 2015, Nagendra et al. 2010).

4. **Deeper dive:** This technique allows us to delve into the subtler layers of sensitization. The client is invited to relax in *śavāsana* (corpse pose). Client chants soothing sounds (*A, U, M*) and follows the gaps in between the sounds. This practice increases the sensitivity that allows the client to listen to the signals from the autonomic nervous/efferent system (Stern et al. 2017, Price & Hooven 2018) via the neural pathways.

5. **Cellular awareness:** This includes meditation in *śavāsana* (corpse pose) following special instructions created to enable observation of senses like heartbeat (García-Cordero et al. 2017), pulse, and flow of sensations. Instructions then guide the client into a focused deep dive using *prāṇa* (life-force, imagine and feel the cells). This is followed by a "mental expansion" (Taimni 2014, García-Cordero et al. 2017) and relaxing into an "expansive state."

1.4 Humming to unravel anger after a cancer diagnosis

Background: Anger

Leigh Leibel

Anger is a common reaction to a cancer diagnosis that is often experienced by patients and their caregivers. It is a situation-appropriate response to a life-altering medical diagnosis, particularly when a person is facing difficult decisions regarding treatment and goals of care, or if pain and other side effects are not adequately managed (Kübler-Ross et al. 1972, Holland et al. 1987, Julkunen et al. 2009, Philip et al. 2007). But when anger is unregulated and it begins to interfere with day-to-day functioning, a person may experience higher levels of pain (Gerhart et al. 2015) and have difficulty engaging social support systems (Greenwood et al. 2003). Unhealthy responses to anger include an inability to express difficult emotions and/or engagement in harmful behaviors, both of which can affect mood and may lead to depression (Cancer.Net 2022). On the other hand, there are times when people may find that expressing anger in a healthy way may help them find strength to deal with difficult treatments. Yoga and yoga therapy offers strategies to help people identify and address things that cause them to feel angry, and help them find healthy ways to express how they're feeling and to help them cope and manage stress.

Client story: Julie

Maryam Ovissi, E-RYT 500, C-IAYT

Julie (she/her) is a 55-year-old Latina woman diagnosed with stage III cervical cancer.

Julie is married with no children, and was recently diagnosed with cervical cancer, stage III. Her treatment plan includes total hysterectomy, adjuvant chemotherapy, and radiation. She is a "hot yoga" fan who loves practicing the set sequence of *āsana* (postures) performed in a heated room, but her oncologist advised against this kind of yoga practice during forthcoming chemotherapy and radiation; she is also feeling very fatigued and doesn't have much stamina. Her oncology nurse has suggested a gentler possibility – yoga therapy.

I begin working with her to help her prepare for surgery and chemotherapy treatment. Julie has signed up for ten one-hour yoga therapy sessions and walks into our first session enthusiastic and curious. I offer the option of a chair or a mat on the floor and she chooses the latter and unrolls her mat. As we talk, I ask her about her relationship, if any, with breath, movement practices, and meditation. "All I have done is hot yoga," she says. "I know the set sequence but nothing specific about the breath or meditation. I really need to learn how to cope with the anger I am experiencing on this journey with cancer." I ask her if she would like me to know more about her anger. "Yes, I'm angry I got cancer," she says. "Especially after experiencing severe traumas and sexual abuse in my life back in South America. I don't deserve cancer. I have been angry since the day they told me I have cancer – and I'm still angry today."

I see on her intake form that she is currently seeing a psychotherapist for a clinical diagnosis of PTSD. I make a mental note to ask her permission to reach out to her therapist to find out how I can best support their work together. I also begin to think about the many yoga-centered practices I might offer as an adjunct to her therapy – interventions that could help her feel safe and better able to regulate her feelings.

> When working with a client who has experienced trauma, it is important that a yoga therapist work in conjunction with a licensed mental health professional to maximize healing. "Breakthroughs" can happen in yoga that are beyond a yoga therapist's scope of practice. A licensed mental health professional can help the client process the insights.
>
> L.L.

As she tells me about her anger, I see she is becoming visibly red in the face; her eyes fixed in an intense stare, she appears to be entering a hyper-aroused state. I breathe, waiting, acknowledging her feelings. We sit in an atmosphere of nonjudgment without needing anything to change.

I ask if the anger occurred immediately after the diagnosis. "Yes," she offers. "I was at home by myself and received the call. Immediately, I felt anger rise up in me.

I went into 'let's do what we need to do' mode. Of course, I don't want to be angry, but this is what I am feeling. Can I change this, even if I want to? Can I find ways to move this anger?" She also shares with me that she never acknowledged this anger from the beginning of the journey because she felt she had to be "strong" and "stay positive."

Given her response, my number one intention for the yoga therapy sessions is to offer Julie tools to safely manage her anger and return to her peaceful center. We decide to focus on humming practices. Humming will expose her to the power of self-created sounds. It also naturally lengthens the exhale and invites diaphragmic activation and helps quiet the chatter of the mind. Julie is not familiar with *mantra* (repeated words, sounds, phrases) work, so humming is an alternative that will allow her to safely explore sound without it being attached to any specific culture.

> Chanting may be unfamiliar to people being exposed to yoga therapy for the first time. Humming may be more accessible. Bee breath (*bhramarī*) has a similar effect and is a yogic practice traditionally used to quiet the mind.
>
> M.O.

For the first few sessions we focus on humming and breath-work (*prāṇāyāma*). But understanding that she is accustomed to the set movements in hot yoga to help her manage the intensity of her feelings, in subsequent classes I offer her a series of practices that combine movement and humming. She chooses tree pose (*vṛkṣāsana*), cat/cow (*mārjaryāsana*), and some seated variations. Throughout our sessions, I invite an exploration of sensations and heart rate. We enjoy practicing together – sometimes humming with movement, and sometimes humming between movements – and ultimately, pausing, resting in the present moment.

The various humming techniques remain foundational practices for Julie during each of our ten sessions together. She records the practices on her phone and continues to practice them at home. I suggest she practices every other day, but after the first week she says that she is doing them daily. There are some weeks where she feels more fatigued and opts to do just one of the three practices – it is her choice which one. The power of choice is very important for Julie and keeping the power of choice front and center is a basic principle of trauma-informed practice.

As she begins to use the yogic tools more and more, she feels more in control of herself. While anger is a natural part of life, throughout our weeks together, Julie says she spends significantly less time suppressing her anger. Humming has become her anchor, a consistent companion to ground her whenever she begins to feel unsafe, and whenever she feels her anger rising. She combines this with other compassionate practices, along with the tools she learns in her ongoing sessions with her psychotherapist, allowing her to feel calmly empowered as she moves through her medical treatment and beyond. "The feelings of anger have softened significantly," Julie shares. "Who knew I could find this sense of peace without hot yoga."

Today, Julie is on a journey of recovery having completed her treatment. She enjoys group classes and has cultivated a home practice. Humming has become a great companion to connect back to herself and help her feel empowered to handle all that comes her way. Understanding that the delivery of the cancer diagnosis was quite traumatic for her has helped Julie create a compassionate plan when she begins to feel unsafe. She now recognizes that tools like humming can be a good way for her to navigate any obstacle that comes her way.

> It is important that we not tell our clients how they *should* feel, or even if they *should* shift their feelings/perspective. The client must have the desire to make a change, even if it feels impossible to them in the moment.
>
> M.O.

National Cancer Institute (NCI), 2022. Cancer Statistics. Available at: https://www.cancer.gov/about-cancer/understanding/statistics/.

Siegel, R.L., Miller, K.D., Fuchs, H., Jemal, A., 2021. Cancer statistics. *CA Cancer J Clin.* 71:7–33.

Sontag, S., 1990. *Illness as Metaphor and AIDS and its Metaphors.* Picador; New York, NY: p. 5.

The Cancer Atlas, 2022. Cancer Statistics. Available at: https://canceratlas.cancer.org/the-burden/the-burden-of-cancer/.

1.1 Softening shock after a cancer diagnosis

Bryant, R.A., 2018. The current evidence for acute stress disorder. *Current Psychiatry Reports* 20(12):111. https://doi.org/10.1007/s11920-018-0976-x

Cordova, M.J., Riba, M.B., Spiegel, D., 2017. Post-traumatic stress disorder and cancer. *The Lancet Psychiatry.* 4(4):330–338.

Eddy, M., 2006. The practical application of Body-Mind Centering® (BMC) in dance pedagogy. *Journal of Dance Education.* 6(3):86–91.

Gerritsen, R.J.S., Band, G.P.H., 2018. Breath of life: the respiratory vagal stimulation model of contemplative activity. *Frontiers in Human Neuroscience.* 12:397.

Gomes Silva, S.M., 2014. *Engaging Touch & Movement in Somatic Experiencing® Trauma Resolution Approach.* Available at: engaging-touch-and-movement-in-se-trama-resolution-approach-dissertation-bySoniaGomes-2014.pdf.

Levine, P.A., 2010. *In an Unspoken Voice: How the Body Releases Trauma and Restores Goodness.* North Atlantic Books; Berkeley, CA.

Mansbach, A., 2016. Becoming ourselves: Feldenkrais and Foucault on soma and culture. *Feldenkrais Research Journal.* 5.

Ogden, P., Minton, K., 2000. Sensorimotor psychotherapy: one method for processing traumatic memory. *Traumatology.* 6(3):149–173.

Payne, P., Crane-Godreau, M.A., 2015. The preparatory set: a novel approach to understanding stress, trauma, and the bodymind therapies. *Frontiers in Human Neuroscience.* 9:178.

Payne, P., Levine, P.A., Crane-Godreau, M.A., 2015. Somatic experiencing: using interoception and

---

Research: neurohemodynamic correlates of "*Oṃ*" chanting

People may feel a sense of vibration when they hum or when they chant *Oṃ*. These two practices can stimulate the vagus nerve and affect the brain. In an Indian study published in the *International Journal of Yoga* that looked at the neurohemodyamic correlates of *Oṃ* chanting using functional magnetic resonance imaging (fMRI), "significant deactivation was observed bilaterally during *Oṃ* chanting in comparison to the resting brain state in the brain's bilateral orbitofrontal, anterior cingulate, parahippocampal gyri, thalami, and hippocampi. The right amygdala also demonstrated significant deactivation; however, no significant activation was observed during *Oṃ* chanting. In contrast, neither activation nor deactivation occurred in these brain regions during the comparative task (which was the "ssss" pronunciation)". The investigators conclude chanting causes limbic deactivitation. They note that because vagus nerve stimulation is used in depression and epilepsy, *Oṃ* chanting could have a role in clinical practice (Kalyani et al. 2011).

L.L.

Section 1 references

Introduction

Abraham, J., Bolwell, B.J., 2019. Time to Treatment. ASCO Post. Available at: https://ascopost.com/issues/december-25-2019/time-to-treatment-is-a-priority/.

Deng, G., Cassileth, B., 2014. Integrative oncology: an overview. *American Society of Clinical Oncology Educational Book* 34: 233–242.

Khorana, A.A., Tullio, K., Elson, P., et al., 2019. Time to initial cancer treatment in the United States and association with survival over time: an observational study. *PLoS One.* 14:e0215108.

Joyce, J., 1916. *A Portrait of the Artist as a Young Man.* New York, NY: B.W. Huebsch.

proprioception as core elements of trauma therapy. *Frontiers in Psychology*. 6:93.

Sullivan, M.B., Erb, M., Schmalzl, L., et al., 2018. Yoga therapy and polyvagal theory: the convergence of traditional wisdom and contemporary neuroscience for self-regulation and resilience. *Frontiers in Human Neuroscience*. 12:67.

Taylor, A.G., Goehler, L.E., Galper, D.I., et al., 2010. Top-down and bottom-up mechanisms in mind-body medicine: development of an integrative framework for psychophysiological research. *Explore: The Journal of Science and Healing*. 6(1):29–41.

Tsur, N., Defrin, R., Lahav, Y., Solomon, Z., 2018. The traumatized body: long-term PTSD and its implications for the orientation towards bodily signals. *Psychiatry Res*. 261:281–289.

Van Diest, I., Leuven, K.U., Vansteenwegen, D., 2014. Inhalation/exhalation ratio modulates the effect of slow breathing on heart rate variability and relaxation. *Applied Psychophysiology and Biofeedback*. 39(3–4):171–180.

Yang, J., Guo, J., Jiang, X., 2017. Executive function in cancer patients with posttraumatic stress disorder. *International Journal of Psychiatry in Medicine*. 52(2):137–146.

1.2 Prehabilitation for a patient with head and neck cancer

Lukez, A., Baima, J., 2020. The role and scope of prehabilitation in cancer care. *Seminars in Oncology Nursing*. 36(1):150976.

Silver, J.K., Baima, J., 2013. Cancer prehabilitation: an opportunity to decrease treatment-related morbidity, increase cancer treatment options, and improve physical and psychological health outcomes. *American Journal of Physical Medicine and Rehabilitation*. 92(8):715–727.

1.3 Early detection of cancer through interoceptive awareness – a proposition

Craig, A.D., 2003. Interoception: the sense of the physiological condition of the body. *Current Opinion in Neurobiology*. 13(4):500–505.

Farb, N., Daubenmier, J., Price, C.J., et al., 2015. Interoception, contemplative practice, and health. *Frontiers in Psychology*. 6:763.

García-Cordero, I., Esteves, S., Mikulan, E.P., et al., 2017. Attention, in and out: scalp-level and intracranial EEG correlates of interoception and exteroception. *Frontiers in Neuroscience*. 11:411.

Katz, V., Egenes, T., 2015. *The Upanishads: A New Translation*. Tarcher Corner Stone Edition/Penguin.

Le Page, J., Le Page, L., 2014. *Mudras for Healing and Transformation*. Integrative Yoga Therapy.

Mehling, W.E., Gopisetty, V., Daubenmier, J., et al., 2009. Body awareness: construct and self-report measures. PLoS ONE. 4(5):e5614.

Mudra *The Sacred Secret*, 2015. Indu Arora, Yogsadhna LLC.

Nagendra, H.R., Nagarathna, R., Telles, S., 2010. *Yoga and Cancer*. Swami Vivekananda Yoga Prakashana; Bangalore, pp. 18–34.

National Institutes of Health, 2021. NIH Research Projects on Interoception to Improve Understanding of Brain-Body Function. Available at: https://www.nih.gov/news-events/news-releases/nih-research-projects-interoception-improve-understanding-brain-body-function.

Price, C.J., Hooven, C., 2018. Interoceptive awareness skills for emotion regulation: theory and approach of mindful awareness in body-oriented therapy (MABT). *Frontiers in Psychology*. 9:798.

Sarkar, D., 2017. *Yoga therapy, Ayurveda, and Western Medicine*. Nataraja Books Publishing: pp. 90, 96–210, 878.

Schleip, R., Jäger, H., Klingler, W., 2012. What is 'fascia'? A review of different nomenclatures. *J Bodyw Mov Ther*. 16(4):496–502.

Stern, E.R., Grimaldi, S.J., Muratore, A., et al., 2017. Neural correlates of interoception: effects of interoceptive focus and relationship to dimensional measures of body awareness. *Human Brain Mapping*. 38(12):6068–6082.

Taimni, I.K., 2014. *The Science of Yoga: The Yoga Sutras of Patanjali in Sanskrit*. Theosophical Publishing House; Wheaton, IL: pp. v-viii, 87, 88, 205, 258–267; 205–291; 307–347; 410–411.

Van der Kolk, B.A., 2015. *The Body Keeps the Score: Brain, Mind and Body in the Healing of Trauma*. Penguin Books: pp. 89–106; 249; 265–278; 416.

1.4 Humming to unravel anger after cancer diagnosis

Cancer.Net, 2022. Coping with Anger. Available at: https://www.cancer.net/coping-with-cancer/managing-emotions/coping-with-anger.

Gerhart, J.I., Sanchez Varela, V., Burns, J.W., et al., 2015. Anger, provider responses, and pain: prospective analysis of stem cell transplant patients. *Health Psychol.* 34(3):197–206.

Greenwood, K.A., Thurston, R., Rumble, M., et al., 2003. Anger and persistent pain: current status and future directions. *Pain.* 103(1–2):1–5.

Holland, J.C., Geary, N., Marchini, A., Tross, S., 1987. An international survey of physician attitudes and practice in regard to revealing the diagnosis of cancer. *Cancer Invest.* 5:151e154.

Julkunen, J., Gustavsson-Lilius, M., Hietanen, P., 2009. Anger expression, partner support, and quality of life in cancer patients. *J Psychosom Res.* 66:235e244.

Kalyani, B.G., Venkatasubramanian, G., Arasappa, R., et al., 2011. Neurohemodynamic correlates of 'OM' chanting: a pilot functional magnetic resonance imaging study. *Int J Yoga.* 4:3–6.

Kübler-Ross, E., Wessler, S., Avioli, L.V., 1972. On death and dying. *JAMA.* 10;221(2):174–179.

Philip, J., Gold, M., Schwarz, M., Komesaroff, P., 2007. Anger in palliative care: a clinical approach. *Intern Med J.* 37:49e55.

Section 2 Treatment

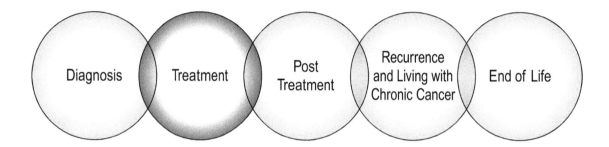

Will they cure me, or won't they?

Aleksandr Solzhenitsyn, *Cancer Ward*

Introduction
Leigh Leibel

Treatment is the second of the five phases of the Yoga in the Cancer Care Continuum. In Phase One, the cancer is diagnosed, staged, and the treatment plan designed. In Phase Two, the patient begins *treatment* for their disease, thereby joining a unique and often fragile medical population.

As we saw in Chapter 4, the standard therapies for treating cancer (surgery, chemotherapy, radiation, immunotherapy, targeted therapy, hormone therapy, and hematopoeietic stem cell transplant) affect both cancer cells and healthy cells. The side effects may be systemic and/or local and often harsh. Consequently, many patients and their families turn to yoga and other nonpharmacologic integrative therapies to support mind, body, and spirit during this acute phase of cancer care. In addition to the holistic benefits of a yogic lifestyle, it is well established in the scientific literature that yoga interventions (including postural and restorative poses, breathing, mindfulness, and meditation)

can mitigate adverse side effects of medical treatments and improve patient quality of life (Danhauer et al. 2019, Milbury et al. 2018, 2019, Lin et al, 2018, Mustian et al. 2013).

Global burden of cancer

So, how many people are in active cancer treatment? In 2020, there were 19.3 million people worldwide being treated for cancer, and in 2040, that number is predicted to increase to more than 30 million (IARC 2020). In the United States alone, in 2020 there were an estimated 1,806,590 new cases of cancer diagnosed (NCI 2021). There are many reasons for the increase in cancer incidence: improved early detection and longer actuarial lifespans, but also as a result of the global obesity epidemic and risk-provoking lifestyle behaviors such as physical inactivity, diets high in fat and sugar, smoking, and alcohol use (NCI 2021).

Minimize harms and maximize benefits of yoga for patients in active cancer treatment

Yoga is an ancient practice that research shows can improve the physical and psychological well-being of people with cancer. The paradox is yoga can also cause harm if treatment-induced changes in immune, neurological, and musculoskeletal functions, as well as psychological conditions aren't observed and addressed during every yoga session. For this reason, in addition to all the safety and injury prevention strategies routinely applied to healthy populations, yoga therapists and advanced practice yoga teachers must also apply additional considerations and precautions specific to the cancer population. Yoga professionals should be fluent in the wide variety of cancer treatment options that can put individuals at risk for short- and long-term side effects and understand cancer-specific safety and injury precautions. While everyone's risk is different, many factors synergize to influence the incidence and severity of adverse effects, including type of cancer and its treatment, genetics, age, gender, lifestyle, and comorbid health conditions.

Awareness that a person with cancer may have a variety of side effects during treatment, reinforced by advanced training in oncology yoga, allows both the yoga therapist and the advanced practice yoga teacher to design programs to address a patient's symptomatology, as well as work with them to modify the risk of morbidity, mortality, recurrence, and to improve clinical outcomes and quality of life. In so doing, the art and science of yoga beautifully come into play during an individual's cancer journey.

Holistic healing

As cancer treatment progresses over months, perhaps years, patients and their caregivers are the authorities on their bodies and illness experiences. Through a yoga therapist's compassionate and reflective listening, their stories are seen and heard; their lived experience honored. When all parties come together to understand the nature of suffering and implication of the patient's symptomatology, a more meaningful patient/client–clinician relationship and clinical approach can emerge. The union of heart and hands reminds us that when caring for an individual with a cancer diagnosis, a yoga ther-

apist sees the patient/client and their family as individuals, not as their disease. Holistic healing is the unity of both the patient/client's and clinician's wellness: hand in heart, heart in hand. This is the magic of yoga therapy in patient-centered cancer care.

On the following pages, thirteen yoga therapists share stories of working with their patients and clients who are undergoing treatment for cancer. We'll see how incorporating yoga helped them manage the difficult side effects of cancer and its treatment and provide calm and ease in their lives.

Topline considerations for yoga therapists working in active cancer treatment

- Secure patient informed consent; work within your licensed or certified scope of practice; refer patient to other healthcare practitioners as warranted; and adhere to regional and institutional regulations regarding confidentiality of patient medical information.

- Understand the specifics of the patient's cancer diagnosis and the treatment they receive. A new patient treatment form can be helpful in this regard.

- Understand the side effects associated with the patient's cancer surgery and treatment, taking into consideration numerous cancer-specific safety considerations such as changes in the immune, neurological, and musculoskeletal functions.

- Understand the body systems (cardiovascular, musculoskeletal, nervous, endocrine, and immune) adversely affected by cancer and cancer treatment that may have positive or negative implications for the patient's yoga practice.

(continued)

Conclusion

- Understand this information within the context of the patient's overall health (pre-morbid conditions), fitness level, mental health, and spiritual well-being before the cancer diagnosis.

- Tailor treatments to address these effects, as well as work on modifying each patient's risk to not only reduce the risk of morbidity, mortality, or recurrence, but also enhance quality of life.

- Update and reevaluate at every session. A patient's cancer treatments and conditions are constantly changing.

- Document every yoga therapy session. This is important for planning the next session and showing patients and their healthcare team how they are progressing. It is also important for risk management in event of an emergency.

- Seek interdisciplinary expertise, including consult-liaison psychiatry and physical therapy/physiatry clinical judgments, among others.

- Develop emergency procedures to ensure a quick response to, and accurate documentation of incidents.

Contributing authors to Section 2*

*Patient/client names have been changed and the stories edited to assure confidentiality. Each contributor has chosen whether to use the term "patient" or "client."

2.1 Yoga in pediatric oncology: helping a child connect to his personal power

Background: Pediatric oncology

Tonia Kulp, MS, E-RYT 500, C-IAYT and Leigh Leibel

Every 1.3 minutes a child somewhere in the world will be diagnosed with cancer. More than 400,000 children worldwide receive a cancer diagnosis each year; it is a leading cause of morbidity and mortality in the 0–14 age group (ACCO 2021, Steliarova-Foucher et al. 2017). Most of these children will face unique challenges not only during cancer treatment, but often for the rest of their lives. Indeed, given the significant effects of aggressive treatments delivered at a time when young bodies are growing and brains developing, it is said that pediatric cancer "is for life." According to the American Childhood Cancer Organization (ACCO), two-thirds of children worldwide who survive cancer will face at least one chronic health condition, and one quarter will face a late effect classified as severe or life-threatening. This includes heart damage, second cancers, lung damage, infertility, cognitive impairment, growth deficits, hearing loss, and more (ACCO 2021).

> The most common pediatric cancers in the United States include leukemia, brain and other nervous system, and lymphoma, with increasing incidence trends for all three from 2001 to 2017 (NCI 2021).

It's therefore no surprise a pediatric cancer diagnosis triggers shock and fear throughout the entire family unit. Parents desperately try to hold it together as they face life's greatest fear – losing a child. Everything is new, information comes fast, the pace is relentless. Emotions of shock, grief, fear, anxiety, guilt, and panic lead to increased stress within the family unit that can continue through treatment and over the course of the year after diagnosis (Mu et al. 2015). In a study of 125 families with a pediatric cancer diagnosis, all par-

ents except one reported post-traumatic stress symptoms (Kazak & Baxt 2007). And yes, siblings are very much affected, too. Given this, it is important for a yoga therapist to design practices not only for the child with cancer, but also their parents and siblings, as well as provide long-term support implemented through a model of traumatic stress.

Patient story: Christopher

Tonia Kulp

Christopher (he/his) is a seven-year-old White boy diagnosed with Ewing sarcoma, a common childhood cancer that forms in bone and soft tissue.

Christopher is a beautiful, blond boy recently diagnosed with cancer. The news was a complete shock to his family – his mother Deb, father Mark, and sister Beth. The sore on Christopher's left thigh, which he lightheartedly named "Razzle," was not the bug bite the family originally thought. The mass was Ewing sarcoma, and the unexpected diagnosis would immediately thrust this young athlete into the dark world of needle sticks and IVs (intravenous needles or tubes) full of lifesaving but toxic drugs, and treatment side effects such as nausea, mouth sores, headaches, physical pain, and extreme anxiety.

Christopher enters the day hospital in tears. His arms cover his chest, fiercely protective of the new hole in his body where his port (a device placed under the skin that is used to draw blood and give treatments) resides. There is a constant stream of healthcare providers who today will see 15 children just like Christopher. They will need to access his port, draw blood for labs, and hook him up to the IV pole to face his new reality. Christopher is inconsolable and Deb, who appears in shock herself, is trying desperately to hold it together. Christopher holds his penguin close, his tear-stained face buried deep in the stuffed animal's fur. His breath is shallow, and Deb's matches his rhythm.

I enter Room 6 quietly and softly close the door behind me. I dress differently from the rest of the clinical staff, wearing a tie-dyed T-shirt in lieu of scrubs. I introduce myself and put my hand on Deb's shoulder. She jumps. "Hi, Mom." I kneel down to hopefully catch Christopher's eye, but he is not ready. "Hi, Christopher, my name is Tonia. I am sorry that you are so upset. I'm not going to ask you any questions, but if it is OK with you and Mom, I am here to read a story. Sometimes these stories help us to relax when we are feeling nervous or scared. You can listen if you'd like, hug your penguin, and just rest." I slowly begin.

The story of the beautiful white star starts with its rays shining gently over Christopher's face, drying his tears and relaxing his eyes. The starlight eventually makes its way all the way down to Christopher's toes and by that time his crying has stopped. The sweet, scared boy is calm. He looks up, red eyes and puffy face and asks for another story.

We talk for a few minutes. His penguin's name is Ricky. He asks to hold the Hoberman sphere (a breathing ball popular with children to help them calm and connect to their breath). We take a few breaths together and imagine our bellies filling like balloons. "I like blue balloons," he says slowly. "Me, too," I respond. His breath has deepened. His mother's shoulders soften. The transfer of energy between mom and son is powerful to witness. The sweet introduction to meditation and *prāṇāyāma* (breath-work) will kick-off Christopher's journey into yoga therapy.

Christopher's first week in clinic was long, but by day five he is making progress. When Megan, his nurse approaches to flush he knows the taste is coming. "Wait," he yells. "I am going to buzz. Once my buzz gets good then you can flush." Christopher closes his eyes, inhales to five and exhales with a low hum … *bhramarī* (humming bee breath) has never sounded so beautiful.

Four weeks later and it is time for Christopher's lumbar puncture. I am invited in and kneel at the side of the bed, and we breathe, rehearsing for what is to come. Chris recalls his *mantra* (repeated word, sound, or phrase) of the day, "I am brave," and we repeat with

each inhale and exhale. Christopher is ready for sedation, he is empowered. He says to Mom, "I've got this."

Months later I ask Christopher what has been the hardest part of treatment to which he responds, "my mouth sores." We giggle at the absurdity of his former request for salty crackers and lemonade. "Can you think of anything that would feel worse on mouth sores?" I blow up a blue hospital glove, and we begin inhaling as our fingers trace each part of the glove, inhaling up the thumb, exhaling down, laughing at the memory of lemonade and salty crackers.

Another day, and Christopher is feeling well. His shoulders round in an effort to protect his port. Deb talks openly about the dark days but how they all can see a light ahead. She tells me that Christopher has been doing his "*Oṃ*-work." Yesterday she found him, hands shaped like a bowl, just sitting. "When his blood counts go up (and his immune system is strong enough for him to go out in a public space), he wants to try puppy yoga. He's found a class near home."

"Chris, let's try moving today, what do you say?" He nods okay as we roll out the mats. Lizzie, another patient, asks to grab the hospital blankets out of the warmer and we start to stack them like tubes. Restorative fish (*matsyāsana*) with warm blankets. Kids buzzing like bees, arms outstretched in star-pose (*utthitatāḍāsana*) (Figure 6.4), no regard to their ports or their lines. Just kids, humming and breathing, together.

And a final, favorite memory just before maintenance therapy begins, and right before ringing the chime (a patient ritual in many infusion centers that signals chemotherapy treatment has been completed). We borrow craft paper from Child Life (healthcare professionals who are trained in the development and psychological needs of children and help them cope with medical issues) and take enough for Chris and his sister Beth. We sit on the hospital floor, drawing our silhouettes. We reflect on memories from this long journey, each gets a symbol, a color, a feeling. "Razzle," Christopher's pet

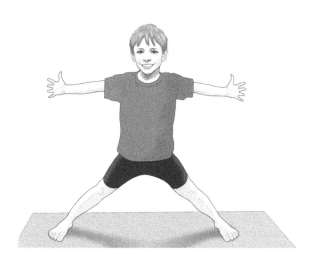

Figure 6.4
Star pose (*utthitatāḍāsana*)

name for that bump that started this whole ordeal gets a color, a feeling, a place, and an X right on top. "He doesn't look as scary now as he did in the beginning." Mom, dad, and sister, each with a different emotion on their face. How far they've come. Diagnosis to maintenance, reflecting on and embracing all of the physical and emotional "razzles" they met with on the way. This was just a small part of brave Christopher's journey.

2.2 Yoga for scan anxiety after a brain cancer diagnosis

Background: Scan anxiety

Leigh Leibel

Physicians routinely prescribe radiologic imaging procedures such as computerized tomography (CT); positron emission tomography (PET); magnetic resonance imaging (MRI); X-ray; mammogram; and ultrasound-guided biopsy to diagnose and/or stage a primary cancer, metastasis, recurrence, and/or for cancer surveillance. For many people, these scans provoke debilitating fear and anxiety (Abreu et al. 2017). This is often called *scanxiety*, a term coined by lung cancer survivor Bruce Feiler who characterized the anxiety as "arising from

emotional roulette...land on red, we're in for another trip to Cancerland; land on black, we have a few more months of freedom" (Feiler 2011). Though a popular topic on social media and forums, the prevalence of scanxiety is not well-described in the literature; however, a 2006 study of long-term breast, prostate, and colorectal survivors found 36–44% of them are affected by this kind of anxiety (Deimling et al. 2006). In various qualitative descriptions, patients reported that their anxiety symptoms worsen in the days before a scan appointment, reach a peak while waiting for the results, and then lessen immediately afterward (Thompson et al. 2010). However, another study found the distress from a scan may last well beyond the scan itself (Bates et al. 2017) – in other words, being told that a scan shows no evidence of disease progression might not be as reassuring as previously assumed. Scan-associated distress thus has the potential to have a significant and lasting impact on a patient/survivor's overall quality of life, affecting both the individual and their loved ones. A yoga therapist has many choices in the yogic toolbox to help mitigate a patient's fear and anxiety during cancer care.

> It is well known among radiation oncologists, radiation therapists, dosimetrists, and physicists that "high levels of patient anxiety affect ^{18}F-FDG biodistribution (e.g., uptake of ^{18}F-FDG in muscles or brown adipose tissue) during PET/CT scans, and this can interfere with the accuracy of cancer results, causing false-positives and complicating the medical diagnosis" (Abreu 2017). The adjunct use of yoga as a non-pharmacologic anxiolytic is warranted.

Patient story: Theresa

Sadie Grossman, MS, E-RYT 500, C-IAYT

Theresa (they/their) is a 35-year-old Latina woman diagnosed with glioblastoma, an aggressive form of brain cancer.

Theresa's story begins with a spontaneous seizure while they and their wife are sleeping. Prior to this, they exhibit no common warning signs of a brain tumor such as headaches, nausea, dizziness; they were asymptomatic. Three days after a biopsy and the accompanying shock of a cancer diagnosis – a time marked by the rapid pace and nature of the medical machine – Theresa was on the surgical table for the removal of their life-threatening brain tumor. Rapidly undertaking oral chemotherapy, followed by a type of radiation called intensity-modulated radiation therapy (IMRT), the immediate *lifesaving* yet *life-altering* treatment for this terrifying diagnosis continues. This storm rattles their life into surprise, with their thoughts catapulting into an unforeseen/unknown future. Theresa finds our hospital's integrative therapy group through their nurse navigator and seeks my work specifically via a personal recommendation. At this time, yoga therapy is the only integrative modality used and this work will serve as their introduction to integrative oncology.

I ask Theresa, "What brings you joy?" They reply, "The face of my son." From here, we instantly know what images will keep them grounded as treatment steadily moves along. I ask if they would like to try meditation, and invite them to feel heavy eyelids and a weighted body, to trust that the earth can and will hold them, giving weight to their own weight. I invite them to bring attention to the parts of their body which touch the air and the space above and for them to trust that they are full of light. We proceed through Theresa's systemic body relaxation, traveling from the forehead, landing at heart. Pausing here, I suggest that they visualize the face of their son, feel the sensation of love only his smile provides, and to notice how that feeling seeps through their body. We finish this meditation, remaining in reclined goddess pose (*suptabaddhakoṇāsana*) and drawing our consciousness to the sounds of the vibrant hospital around us. We embrace these noises, invite them in, and begin to add breath awareness as a layer to this experience. In the face of "noise," can our response be wider, longer, more controlled breath?

During intake, Theresa has told me about their strong spiritual base, so we integrate their personal rosary to bridge the gap between their already existing spiritual practice and their diagnosis. Applying Theresa's love of prayer repetition and acknowledging that the MRI machine is their location of trauma triggers during treatment and scans, we set a specific image in their mind which will provide a focus. MRI machines are excruciatingly loud and often terrifying, therefore we consider the machine as workers on a construction site. "I am a house. These workers are here to help. The sounds are a symphony of healing hands repairing my home." We repeat silently, linking each sentence with a cycle of breath. We invite images of construction workers to fill their mind. By using the circumstances of the present moment, we are able to create a sense of calm during a storm of a situation which was once fear-based paralysis. Changing the story behind the noise allows us to find freedom within the confines of our circumstances. Theresa not only expects loud noises now but welcomes them as helpers. Theresa's homework is to notice when their mind paints pictures of dis-ease and come back to their body as their home, medicine and machines as helpers, and this diagnosis as an opportunity to show their son all the colors of what it is to be human.

Theresa attends weekly yoga therapy sessions and daily radiation treatments, and as we progress steadily with our work, they notice clear differences in their heart rate, breath capacity, and ability to walk into the clinic without pausing. They now have a specialized positive thought to interrupt their anxiety of scans. When approached by a medical professional, they are able to silently remind themself they are helpers, healers, coupling that thought with breath. Survivorship has only strengthened Theresa's resolve for the importance of yoga in their life, for this diagnosis requires quarterly scans. As of today, their mindful MRI remains an impactful and important part of their life.

2.3 Titrating effort and ease for cancer fatigue

Considerations when working with a person diagnosed with glioblastoma brain cancer

Patients may experience fatigue, sleep disturbance, depression, radiation dermatitis, low blood counts, headaches, nausea, vomiting, hearing loss, seizures, personality changes, anger, and trouble with memory or speech as a result of disease or treatment. Some of these side effects may appear immediately while others present late.

- Practice should occur in a safe space free of fall-risk.

- Practices should be demonstrated with simple, slow, and repeated instructions.

- Care must be taken with head and neck positions (ask the person what is comfortable for them).

- No inversions.

- Use props as necessary to enhance the experience.

- Dim the lights; use music cautiously.

- Avoid seizure and stimulus-specific triggers, like flashing lights or noises.

At each session, always ask the patient what feels good for them, today.

L.L.

In 2019, researchers at the University of Texas MD Anderson Cancer Center conducted a pilot randomized controlled trial (RCT) to look at the feasibility and efficacy of a dyadic yoga intervention for supportive care of glioma patients undergoing radiation treatment and their caregivers. Investigators

(continued)

(continued)
concluded it is feasible, well-received, and beneficial (Milbury et al. 2019).

L.L.

Background: Cancer-related fatigue

Lórien Neargarder, BSME, E-RYT 500, C-IAYT and Leigh Leibel

Cancer-related fatigue (CRF) is a prevalent and disabling side effect of cancer and its treatment. CRF is more than just being "tired." The National Comprehensive Cancer Network (NCCN) characterizes this type of fatigue as "a distressing, persistent, subjective sense of physical, emotional, and/or cognitive tiredness or exhaustion related to cancer or cancer treatment that is not proportional to recent activity and interferes with usual functioning" (NCCN 2018). It commonly occurs in symptom clusters that include pain, distress, anemia, and sleep disturbance.

CRF is very common among people with cancer. A 2008 United States national survey of people undergoing chemotherapy or radiation found as many as 80% reported CRF symptoms that affected their quality of life (Henry et al. 2008). And while many people are inclined to reduce their activity when they feel tired, a large body of research suggests exercise can help decrease CRF (Patel et al. 2019). Exercise includes active forms of postural yoga, and for those who are deconditioned and weak, there is restorative Iyengar yoga. A 2014 randomized controlled trial showed that restorative yoga postures can mitigate cancer-related fatigue in patients with breast cancer (Bower et al. 2012).

Most importantly for the field of yoga therapy, the NCCN 2022 Clinical Guidelines for Management of Cancer-Related Fatigue recommend yoga as a category one (highest evidence) nonpharmacologic intervention for people with cancer during active treatment and post treatment survivorship (NCCN 2022). Yoga is a boon for the fatigued, and can mitigate a patient's accompanying symptoms of pain, distress, and insomnia.

Client story: Joyce

Lórien Neargarder

Joyce (she/her) is a 73-year-old White woman diagnosed with metastatic cancer of undetermined origin; her oncologist is treating it as primary ovarian cancer.

My first thought when I see my new client is that she is the most fatigued and physically limited student I have met outside of a hospital, and I think to myself what an effort it must have taken her just to meet me. Joyce is in her seventies, has strong family and community support and is dealing with an ambiguous cancer diagnosis. She went to the doctor when she developed fatigue, shortness of breath, abdominal bloating, and loss of appetite – all symptoms of ovarian cancer. She explains to me that her doctors are using an ovarian cancer protocol to treat her, even though they cannot say whether or not her metastatic cancer originated there. During her first chemotherapy cycle she lost too much weight, and her doctors have paused her treatment until she becomes stronger.

> Ovarian cancer symptoms include fatigue, shortness of breath, abdominal bloating, loss of appetite, feeling "full" after a few bites of food, gastrointestinal and elimination issues, gynecological issues, and pain in the abdomen, pelvis, back, or during sexual intercourse. If any of these symptoms persist for two or more weeks, consult with a physician.
>
> L.L.

Joyce shows me her port (a device placed under the skin that is used to draw blood and give treatments) located near her left collarbone and describes her 8-inch vertical scar that begins above the belly button and extends to the pubic bone. This is a result of surgical staging and debulking (removing as much of the cancer as possible), which is the standard of care for ovarian cancer. Patients who have had this kind of surgery are

at high risk of hernia, so I make a note to modify practices that might affect the abdomen and incision, and to accommodate the area around the port.

I ask Joyce about breathing and she tells me she has a pleural effusion which makes it difficult to breathe and adds to her fatigue. A pleural effusion is an accumulation of fluid in the space surrounding the lung that is confirmed by imaging and managed with thoracentesis (surgical procedure) or drains. This condition can impact a yoga practice because the lungs can't expand normally due to fluid compression. I can see how this breathlessness and fatigue affect Joyce. She says she can take only a few steps without her walker and shares that she recently fell and was too weak to get off the floor. She adds that she cannot hold herself upright for very long and is soon slumping in her chair.

Although her cancer is metastatic, her medical records confirm there are no lesions to the spine and bones (or osteoporosis) that would contraindicate certain movements. So, through trial and error, we discover a position that feels restorative for her, a seated variation of child's pose (*bālāsana*). I position a bolster on a chair opposite hers so that when she rests her head and chest on it there is no pressure against the port. She tells me how good this feels to stretch. We try a few more movements and postures, but she returns to this pose when the others prove difficult. She has tender spots on her back from remaining sedentary over the past three months and she tells me this pose helps.

At our second meeting, Joyce arrives with a bit more energy. She completed more cycles of her chemotherapy, which reduced some of the disease-related fatigue. (Chemotherapy can reduce fatigue caused by the cancer, but paradoxically, the chemotherapy drugs can also cause fatigue.) Lately she has a better appetite and has put on a little bit of weight but is still tired and worries about fluid retention in her lungs, abdomen, and ankles. I set up the chairs for her version of child's pose (*bālāsana*) and she tells me she's been stretching in bed in the morning and demonstrates her flexibility by setting her feet onto the chair opposite her and folding into a variation of butterfly pose (*baddhakoṇāsana*). She holds this posture for a few breaths and then moves into the child's pose (*bālāsana*) variation, this time without the bolster on the seat of the chair in front of her. When she is ready, I invite her to come out of it and we discuss how to practice at home with her own furniture.

At our third session, Joyce gets to the floor and back up without any assistance; she can now walk one mile unaided, though slowly. She tells me she was feeling more vigorous but then missed her last chemotherapy infusion when the date fell during the holidays and is again feeling drained. She is frustrated that she needs these medications to support her quality of life and I ask what bothers her most. She responds, "I think I'm most afraid of not getting back to the life I'm used to living. I know losing my life is possible, too. But I'm just not thinking of that right now." I guide her into child's pose (*bālāsana*), this time from the floor. After a few minutes here I ask her to recline back against a bolster propped at an incline. This is the first partial-supine position she's been able to practice with me and it takes a few minutes for us to support her body with blankets so that her back is comfortable, arms are supported, and head is adequately elevated. I observe her breath in the posture for a few moments and I tell her about the Japanese art of *kintsugi*, where broken pottery is mended and the seams of the broken pieces are honored by mixing glue with gold, resulting in a new piece even more beautiful than the original. I ask her to travel through her body to find her scars (inside and out), discomforts, and disconnections, and imagine these areas filled with gold, like the seams in a piece of beautiful Japanese pottery.

After this guidance I take a few moments to observe her breathing. It is now visibly deeper and slower. After a few more minutes here I ask her how it feels to breathe. "Really good," she replies with a big smile on her face and a twinkle in her eye. As she helps me put the props away, she remarks that she feels energized after our session, "Not like I drank a caffeinated drink," she

explains. "Calmer than that. I guess it's a bit more like myself before all of this started."

2.4 Embracing the challenges: axillary web syndrome – an underrecognized consequence of breast cancer surgery

Background: Axillary web syndrome

Christa Eppinghaus, MS, PT, CLT, C-IAYT

Axillary web syndrome (AWS), also known as cording, may develop in women, man, and non-binary people as a side effect of sentinel lymph node biopsy, axillary node dissection, and breast cancer surgery. The defining characteristic of the condition is a visible web located in the axilla of the affected surgical side (Figure 6.5). The web/cords usually become more visibly taut and painful with shoulder abduction, but there may be times when the cording is not visible, yet the symptoms are still present. In addition to presentation in the axilla, cords may also be seen:

- Along the entire medial aspect of the affected arm into the wrist and hand, causing pain and restriction at any point along the continuum (some people may have close to full range of motion [ROM] but still suffer from tightness in the involved extremity).

- In the breast, posterior chest wall, or abdominal wall.

- On the antecubital fossa of the medial aspect of the elbow.

The incidence of AWS reported in the literature is somewhere between 6% and 72% (Torres et al. 2009) and is frequently overlooked in the early postoperative phase unless healthcare practitioners are aware of the condition. Typically, AWS occurs within the first 8 weeks after axillary surgery and symptoms resolve within the first 12 weeks postoperatively (Yeung et al. 2014); however, some studies have reported its appearance well beyond that time (O'Toole et al. 2013).

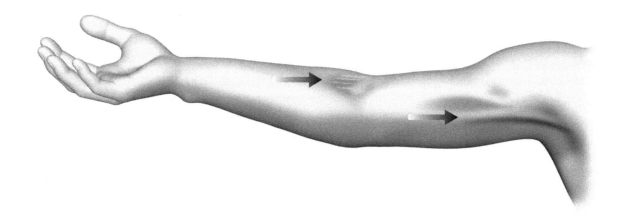

Figure 6.5
Axillary web syndrome

A 2015 study found that *prophylactic* contralateral mastectomy in women (a surgical option for those genetically at high-risk for breast cancer, e.g., BRCA I and II) can also lead to AWS (Koehler et al. 2015).

L.L.

Immediate effects of AWS are:

- Decreased ROM and/or pain in any of the following: shoulder abduction and flexion, elbow extension, and wrist extension.

- Decreased functional movement of the shoulder girdle and upper extremity.

- Limitation with activities of daily living.

- Pain, anxiety, and depression.

- Low quality of life.

- (Long-term effects are unknown.)

There is no definitive treatment, but yoga therapy can assist in reducing anxiety and depression, as well as assist physiatrists, physical and occupational therapists, and sports medicine trainers with an individual's physical limitations.

Client story: Luna
Christa Eppinghaus

Luna (she/her) is a 42-year-old Latina woman diagnosed with early-stage HER2+ breast cancer.

Luna's breast cancer was found during a work-up for pneumonia. Her cancer has a favorable prognosis due to its early stage and the availability of therapies for HER2 amplification.

Even though her cancer is at an early stage, she has an extensive medical history that I had to consider when designing her therapy plan: a month after diagnosis, Luna started five months of Taxotere (docetaxel) and carboplatin chemotherapies delivered in a three-week cycle, along with Herceptin (trastuzumab) and Perjeta (pertuzumab) (targeted therapies for HER2 amplification). One month after she completed chemotherapy, she had a left breast mastectomy with removal of three lymph nodes. She was subsequently diagnosed with AWS and a frozen shoulder, and physical therapy was initiated two months after surgery secondary to decreased left shoulder function, decreased ROM, and pain. She received physical therapy one to two times a week for four months, and upon completion, her physical therapist referred her to yoga therapy to continue her holistic healing process.

This medical history was important for me to know due to the side effects of each of the drugs (e.g., risk for chemotherapy-induced peripheral neuropathy, cognitive dysfunction, and cardiac issues); the impact of her breast surgery on her upper body (possible physical limitations, lymphedema risk, AWS, and frozen shoulder); the medical diagnoses (any comorbid conditions); and the work she was doing with other therapists (and therefore the need to coordinate care so as not to duplicate movements and overtax her body). I modified our practices accordingly and reviewed progress at each session.

Her immediate goals for yoga therapy were to improve ROM of the left shoulder, build strength, exercise, and find peace and relaxation to prepare for the reconstructive surgery. We worked together for four sessions over a one-month period prior to reconstruction. She returned eight months later, post-surgery, presenting with neck and arm stiffness/tightness, decreased shoulder ROM bilaterally, abnormal movement patterns of the shoulder girdle complex, fatigue, and stress. We worked together once a month for an additional four months to address persistent left shoulder restrictions and pain from the left mastectomy, as well as decreased ROM and pain of the right shoulder secondary to port (a device placed under the skin that is used to draw blood and give treatments) placement. Therapy included postures targeting the upper body, restorative yoga poses, and various breathing techniques, as well as a type of isometric (somatic) movement called pandiculation (the nervous system's natural way of waking up our sensorimotor system and preparing us for movement), followed by gentle somatic movement flows coordinated with the breath. These techniques were utilized to increase body

awareness and normalize movement patterns, leading to improved function and decreased pain for this client.

In addition to yoga therapy which focused on her specific issues, Luna attended group yoga classes at a local cancer center and participated in Livestrong at the YMCA, a 12-week physical activity program designed to get survivors back on their feet. The shoulder exercises – specifically pandiculation – helped tremendously to improve her ROM, as Luna said, approaching 100% back to normal.

> One of the risk factors for lymphedema is axillary webbing syndrome (AWS). Recognizing the clinical characteristics of AWS and immediately referring to a lymphedema specialist can lead to early detection, prevention, and/or rehabilitation for those affected by the condition.
>
> L.L.

2.5 Cancer while Black: role of yoga in trauma stewardship and advocacy during breast cancer
Background: The role of community in cancer care disparity

Marsha D. Banks-Harold, BSEE, TCTSY-F, E-RYT 500, YACEP, RPYT, RCYT, C-IAYT and Leigh Leibel

Cancer while Black is a metaphor for what it means to be a Black person with cancer in America, carrying the historical trauma of systemic and structural racism across generations (Cure Today 2021). The stark reality is that in the United States, almost 60% of Black people feel they are treated less fairly while receiving medical health treatment compared to only 26% of White people (Cure Today 2021). According to the National Cancer Institute, Black people are more likely to die of most cancers than any other racial group (NCI 2020, ACS 2022). The statistics are egregious and staggering. The *2020 Cancer Disparities Progress Report* published by the

American Association for Cancer Research (AACR) says in the United States, Black men, for example, are 111% more likely to die of prostate cancer than White men, and Black women are 39% more likely to die of breast cancer than White women (AACR 2020). The report describes many more examples of inequity and disparity.

> Sitting with the reality that one has cancer is not an easy journey. Neither is racism.

We now know from research on collective trauma that racism-induced inter-generational pain and the trauma of oppression is stored within the human body as allostatic load. This term describes the physiologic burden of chronic stress that can negatively impact health at the cellular or biological levels (Akinyemiju et al. 2020). Higher levels of allostatic load have been associated with increased risk of cancer-specific mortality among both Black and White populations (Akinyemiju et al. 2020).

For many Black women, the trauma of a breast cancer diagnosis adds to their preexisting trauma caused by racism. This can leave many women feeling isolated, devalued, unheard, unseen, and unsupported. Many express an intuitive need for community and advocacy in order to begin the healing process and return to wellness. This innate wisdom is reinforced by the work of Bessel van der Kolk, MD, a psychiatrist, post-traumatic stress researcher, and author of *The Body Keeps the Score: Brain, Mind, and Body in the Healing of Trauma*. Van der Kolk says, "Having a good support network constitutes the single most powerful protection against becoming traumatized ... To recover, the mind, body, and brain need to be convinced that it is safe to let go" (Van der Kolk 2015).

To best create a supportive and compassionate community for those affected by collective trauma, there must be both trauma stewardship and servant leadership. In her 2010 book, *Trauma Stewardship: An Everyday Guide to Caring for Self While Caring for Others*, trauma expert Laura Van Dernoot Lipsky defines trauma stewardship as "the overall practice of caring for oneself in order to remain effective at – and avoid negative effects of – caring for others" (Van Dernoot Lipsky & Burk 2010).

The foundation of trauma stewardship is self-care, which is a critical aspect of successful advocacy work. It taps into the very essence of an individual's calling to serve and be a servant leader. When the servant leader practices self-care, they may be better able to focus on the most sacred opportunity to work collaboratively with all people to foster a safe and compassionate environment that can lead to empowerment, transformation, and healing for both themselves and their clients.

Accepting the calling to be a servant leader is the first step in preparing oneself to advocate for people with cancer and survivors who have experienced racial trauma, bias, and microaggression, as well as for other people who may not be seen or heard. This work is not for the faint of heart. It requires the highest level of commitment and willingness to serve from the most humbling perspective. Christine Courtois, PhD, editor of *Treating Complex Traumatic Stress Disorders in Adults* says:

The opportunity to assist another human being in engaging in the most fundamental acts of learning and psychological growth, after that person has been denied that opportunity by fate and trauma, also is a sacred trust that requires the extraordinary mental, emotional, spiritual, and ethical dedication from both therapist and client.

Courtois & Ford (2020)

Facilitating trauma stewardship and advocacy through yoga (Box 6.5) is a gift that yields many rewards. It allows healers and caregivers to not only take care of themselves, but also selflessly serve others. Supporting the emotional, psychological, spiritual, and physical well-being of members of the compassionate community through the practice of yoga empowers all people – healers, caregivers, and their clients – to better face the often-overwhelming traumas they confront every day and to move toward holistic healing and recovery through love, compassion, and fellowship.

BOX 6.5 Advocacy and trauma stewardship: Yoga as a catalyst to empower Black people with cancer

Marsha D. Banks-Harold

Yoga therapists can facilitate compassionate yoga therapy sessions by building relationships among people who are interconnected by the experience of cancer. This "sharing" fosters a sense of community and passion for advocacy that may result in a less traumatic experience for everyone.

The FCCE acronym guides us: *Facilitate and Collaborate to create a Community of Empowerment:*

Facilitation

The ability of the yoga therapist to facilitate this sharing experience is based on their ability to intuitively connect with clients and to simultaneously connect clients with each other. According to Mark Stephens, an award-winning writer of scholarly yoga books, "Other teachers share their knowledge and insight with students while encouraging students to explore in ways that fully empower the student to learn from the experience and to adapt the practices in ways that make sense to them" (Stephens 2017).

The facilitated experience is comforting and stimulates a feeling of internal aspiration for the client to continue the new post-cancer diagnosis journey of life. To that point, Stephens continues, "The teacher-as-facilitator role and the qualities of kindness and compassion help form the foundation of healthy relationships in which adaptive practices are fully explored in support of a client's goals and aspirations" (Stephens 2017).

Collaboration

The collaborative effort between the yoga therapist and the client is critical in the healing process. This collaborative process allows both parties to practice acceptance and gratitude for the gift of gaining new perspectives on situations or experiences that may appear daunting. The collaborative/shared experience is further enhanced when the clients, with the common diagnosis of cancer, explore *āsana* (posture), *prāṇāyāma* (breath-work), and meditation integrated with the lifestyle management guidelines found in yoga philosophy.

Community

Creating community is manifested through the principles of building therapeutic relationships. Stephens says, "The center of our practice is in the heart, in how we hold space with a client to foster healing resonance. This begins with the quality of our communication and overall interaction with clients" (Stephens 2017).

Holding space for our clients in a group yoga therapy session is seen during the intake process where the yoga therapist offers each of the clients the opportunity to share where they find themselves physically, intellectually, emotionally, and spiritually. This process of sharing stimulates the innate ability of clients to empathize, connect, and be compassionate with the yoga therapist and community members.

Empowerment

Empowerment is embodied in making a safe, inclusive, accessible, adaptive, and diverse community where those who have the common diagnosis of cancer (and the impact of trauma) can collectively benefit from sharing similar experiences, while reaping the benefits of mitigating physical, intellectual, emotional, and spiritual imbalances. Community provides the opportunity to connect and fellowship with people who share similar experiences. This community connection is a powerful element of the recovery process.

Client story: Asor, Victoria, Jessie, and Zenzele

Marsha D. Banks-Harold

Asor (she/her), Victoria (she/her), Jessie (they/their), and Zenzele (she/her) are Black women diagnosed with various types and stages of breast cancer who come together weekly in a community yoga therapy session.

Asor, a woman of faith, has been living with breast cancer for 12 years prior to seeking out the physical aspects of yoga. She has been living Yoga all her life but has just recently decided to try a yoga therapy session upon her retirement. She recognizes that she has thrived over the years because her family, friends, and church members increased their level of support for her when she was diagnosed with cancer. At this point in her journey, she is craving community to cope with living with the cancer diagnosis, to connect, and share with others impacted by cancer, and to honor the sacredness of life regardless of any diagnosis.

Upon joining our group yoga therapy sessions, Asor quickly recognizes similar advocacy and community building skills that she honors, present in the yoga therapist. She feels right at home, empowered, and immediately connected to the other clients. Asor is excited to expand her community to include her new friends. She becomes a role model, supporting women newly diagnosed with cancer and who are just starting their wellness journeys. After each yoga therapy session, each of the community members supports each other by sharing their life experiences and how much everyone really values the time that they have spent together.

Asor's positive essence is contagious and inspires others in the yoga therapy sessions to build relationships in the same capacity. Victoria, a newer client just diagnosed with stage IV cancer, upon connecting with Asor, takes it upon herself to pay forward the sense of community by building relationships with other clients recently diagnosed with cancer. Victoria personally holds space for Jessie, as Jessie journeys from their initial cancer diagnosis to the final chemotherapy and radiation sessions. The community gathers socially to support the success of both Victoria and Jessie and all the other clients who have similar medical conditions.

Finally, Zenzele, a woman staying in the hospital where weekly yoga therapy sessions are offered, shows up one evening unannounced to the group session. She arrives physically drained and supported by a security guard aiding her in her quest to find the group yoga therapy session. Upon her entrance into the space, the yoga therapist immediately pauses the session and compassionately greets the new client. Zenzele shares that she desperately needs community support. The others respond immediately by obtaining a chair and blankets. They honor the pause by holding space for their new friend. By the end of the session, she expresses how grateful she is for the received support. Outside of the group session, the yoga therapist continues to serve as a sounding board for Zenzele and advocates for her by connecting her with other community members who are instrumental in locating housing and alternative practices to support her healing journey.

Community presents in all forms and shapes. Ultimately, the acceptance of the calling to serve rings louder than any other calling, permitting yoga therapists to empower those who crave the benefits of advocacy and community.

2.6 Yoga and lymphedema secondary to cancer treatment: the priority is *ahiṃsā* or "do no harm"

Background: Lymphedema secondary to cancer treatment – role of yoga

Annette Loudon, MMedSc, AAYT, YA, Fitness Australia, ALA, C-IAYT

Yoga can be safe for those with secondary lymphedema after cancer treatment if certain principles are adhered to and rigorously observed, in conjunction with treatment by specialized lymphedema therapists. With these precautions, yoga has been shown to have benefit in lymphedema management. To create an effective and safe yoga practice for our clients, we must ensure they follow the current gold standard* recommendations for the treatment of secondary lymphedema to which we apply our knowledge of therapeutic yoga. To do this it is vital we understand the:

- Function of the lymphatic system.

- Lymphedema secondary to cancer: effects and treatment protocol.

- Current evidence base of exercise for those with secondary lymphedema.

- Current evidence base of yoga for those with secondary lymphedema.

* The current gold standard is complete decongestive therapy (CDT), which includes manual lymph drainage (MLD), compression therapy, decongestive and breathing exercises, and skin and nail care.

Yoga therapists can help provide health benefits, self-care, and empowerment for people with secondary lymphedema by combining these principles/current evidence with our focus on slow and full breathing, balancing the sympathetic nervous system (SNS) and parasympathetic nervous system (PNS), improving heart rate variability, and creating effective fascial integration.

Function of the lymphatic system

The lymphatic system, or lymphoid system, is an organ system that is part of the immune system and circulatory system. It comprises a large network of lymphatic vessels, lymph nodes, lymphatic or lymphoid organs, and lymphoid tissues. The vessels carry a clear fluid called "lymph" back towards the heart, for re-circulation to all parts of the body. Our lymphatic system, which lies within our fascia, is pumped by breathing, muscle movement, and smooth muscle contraction within the lymphatic vessels. These actions cause "debris," such as fats, viruses, proteins, and bacteria, to be picked up

from the lymph fluid in lymphatic capillaries. Lymph is then transported in a one-way valve system to larger lymphatic vessels before proceeding to local, and then regional, lymph nodes.

The functions of the lymphatic system complement the bloodstream functions:

First, it returns lymph from the tissues back into the bloodstream and regulates the fluid volume of the body. From the lymph nodes, the fluid now flows to two major lymphatic vessels that take the cleared lymph back to the venous system at the subclavian veins, located at the medial collar bones.

Second, it filters pathogens from the blood. Lymph nodes play a major role in our overall healthy immune response and function. They activate immune cells such as NK (natural killer) cells and lymphocytes to rid the lymph of harmful bacteria and viruses.

Lymphedema secondary to cancer: effects and treatment protocol

Due to disruption to the lymphatic transport system, some people will experience swelling known as secondary lymphedema. This can emerge during, soon after, or many years after cancer treatment. Secondary lymphedema can occur in the arm, chest, head and neck, leg, trunk, and genitals.

Risk factors include:

Treatment-related:

- Surgical lymph node dissection, multiple lymph nodes removed, delayed surgical wound healing

- Radiation therapy: location and formation of scars or fibrosis

Cancer diagnosis-related:

- Tumor invasion and/or advanced disease

- Infection: affected extremity, concurrent illness

- Traumatic injury to affected extremity

Non-cancer related:

- Prolonged immobilization

- Long-distance travel

- Air travel with suboptimal cabin pressure

- Poor nutrition

- Thrombophlebitis

- Skin inflammation or disorders

- Obesity/elevated body mass index (BMI)

- Genetics may be influential

Effects

Over time, secondary lymphedema creates changes in the tissue, including a deposition of adipose tissue. If left untreated, fibrosis occurs and the oxygen-deprived tissue can become a breeding area for bacteria, leading to infections such as cellulitis (International Society of Lymphology 2016). As well as the swelling, some may experience other symptoms such as aches, tingling, and temperature changes in the limb or affected area. Altered movement patterns can occur.

For many, the diagnosis of secondary lymphedema impacts them psychologically. It may create shock and disbelief, for which they feel unprepared. Some people say that living with the lifelong treatment of lymphedema and threat of infection is worse than their cancer treatment. Feelings of shame and loss of body image, compounded by the cost of necessary lifelong treatment (e.g., wearing compression garments), can lead to altered identity and lowered well-being. Some people with secondary lymphedema in the head and neck area will walk only at night due to embarrassment. People with secondary lymphedema in the genitals may also feel embarrassed or may be too ashamed to seek medical help. In addition, some people may need to change their jobs due to their altered appearance or abilities, which can further erode their sense of self (Fu et al. 2013).

Treatment protocol

Treatment by qualified lymphedema therapists focuses on specialized manual lymphatic drainage (MLD) based on clearing the lymph from proximal to distal, creating alternative lymphatic pathways, and reducing the fibrotic tissue. These specialists also teach their clients specific lymph clearing exercises, diaphragmatic breathing, and other self-management techniques. Lymphedema therapists provide precision-fitted compression garments to optimize pressure changes for the lymph to flow in daily life (which are ideally replaced every six months). An example of the recommended clearing stages for arm lymphedema is shown in Figure 6.6, and recommended self-management techniques are noted in the following gray box.

Recommended self-management techniques

Include:

- Monitoring of affected limb for changes or infection

- Regular lymphatic self-massage

- Healthy lifestyle and weight control

- Skin care; prevention of abrasion and cuts as an entry point for infection

Avoid:

- Extreme temperatures

- Holding affected limb in one position for too long

- Overuse of affected limb

- Constriction by clothing or jewelry (e.g., tight rings, tight bra straps)

- Cuts, bites, or injury to affected limb

As recommended by the Australasian Lymphology Association (2020)

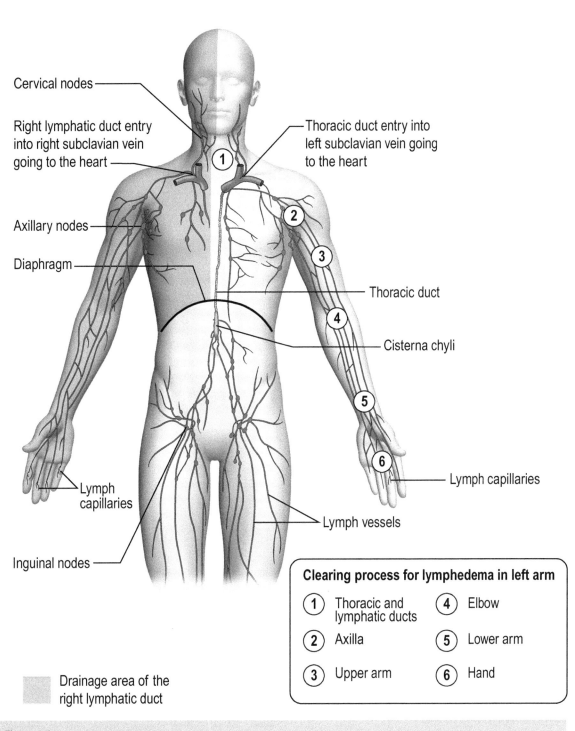

Cervical nodes

Right lymphatic duct entry into right subclavian vein going to the heart

Thoracic duct entry into left subclavian vein going to the heart

Axillary nodes

Diaphragm

Thoracic duct

Cisterna chyli

Lymph capillaries

Lymph capillaries

Lymph vessels

Inguinal nodes

Clearing process for lymphedema in left arm

1 Thoracic and lymphatic ducts   4 Elbow

2 Axilla   5 Lower arm

3 Upper arm   6 Hand

Drainage area of the right lymphatic duct

Figure 6.6
Lymph node ducts and clearing method

Recent advances

The good news is that evidence-based research is leading to greater understanding of how the lymphatic system works, and providing hope for more effective treatment and self-management regimens. For example, imaging techniques are uncovering more precise lymphatic pathways and drainage patterns (Suami & Scaglioni 2018, Barbieux et al. 2019). Surgical interventions are being investigated, as well. Early intervention is providing better outcomes by measuring limbs before and at regular intervals after surgery (Australasian Lymphology Association 2019), leading to decreased swelling and perhaps lymphedema prevention.

Current evidence base of exercise for those with secondary lymphedema

Exercise, once contraindicated, is now recommended, with the caveat that it is personalized and monitored with slow warm-up and cool-down. Dr Kathryn Schmitz, a leading researcher in exercise oncology, conducted a 2009 study (Physical Activity and Lymphedema [The PAL Trial]) in breast cancer survivors that showed that those with lymphedema could benefit from gradual, closely supervised weight training – a finding that challenged the conventional wisdom that people with lymphedema should avoid weight-bearing exercise. While most exercise studies have been carried out for those with breast cancer-related lymphedema (BCRL) and include aerobic and resistance-type exercise along with yoga, tai-chi, and water-based exercise (Olsson Möller et al. 2019, Bauman et al. 2018), there is currently a lack of sufficient evidence for the effect of exercise on secondary lymphedema from other cancers (Singh et al. 2016).

Current evidence base of yoga for those with secondary lymphedema

Most of the studies on yoga and secondary lymphedema have been conducted specifically in breast cancer populations. These studies have found positive results for this group of people. These yoga practices have been based on lymphatic clearing techniques, reducing fibrotic tissue, and improving quality of life. In conjunction with this is the gradual and progressive restoration of mobility, stability, kinematic movement patterns, and strength. Two 8-week randomized pilot trials (Loudon et al. 2014, 2016) have reported no adverse effects and some benefits for those with BCRL. Benefits reported from these two pilot trials are symptom and fibrotic tissue reduction (Loudon et al. 2014) and stabilization of pelvis and shoulder (Loudon et al. 2016). A third pilot study by Pasyar et al. reported improved quality of life (Pasyar et al. 2019).

A 2021 systematic review conducted by Saraswathi et al. on yoga therapy in the management of breast cancer-related lymphedema (BCRL) looked at seven studies. They found there was evidence of "moderate robustness" to affirm the safety and efficacy of a yoga intervention in BCRL. Quality of life, range of motion, and musculoskeletal symptoms showed improvement in all the studies. The authors recommend further long-term trials involving a large sample-size in order to develop and standardize yoga intervention guidelines for BCRL patients.

A protocol based on Satyananda yoga has been developed by Loudon et al. for those with BCRL, which the authors report has also had benefits for those with secondary lymphedema from other cancers, as well as for the immune system (Loudon et al. 2017). One non-randomized prevention study of breast cancer survivors has been published based on Ashtanga-based yoga resulting in no adverse effects (Mazor et al. 2019). Evidence for other cancers is lacking. However, a study of a large cohort of people in Kerala, India, with secondary lower-limb lymphedema caused by filariasis that used a yoga-based lymphatic clearing protocol as part of a larger treatment regimen, has reported reduction in swelling and improved pelvic stabilization (Aggithaya et al. 2015).

A vetted source of information on lymphedema is the National Lymphedema Network, based in the United States (www.lymphnet.org), or in Canada, The Canadian Lymphedema Framework (www.canadalymph.ca). The International Lymphedema Framework is at www.ilf.org, and many countries also have their own lymphedema associations with excellent resources where you may find physical therapists trained in lymphedema issues, as well as various position papers and educational videos.

Vital considerations for the yoga professional

Yoga is a self-management technique; it is not a cure for lymphedema. Yoga professionals must have knowledge of the lymphatic system, lymphedema, its effects and treatment, and refer patients/clients to an appropriate medical professional when necessary. It is essential to:

- Ensure clients follow current "gold standard" recommendations for those with secondary lymphedema, which is complete decongestive therapy (CDT) which includes manual lymph drainage (MLD), compression therapy, decongestive and breathing exercises, and skin and nail care.

- Ensure lymphedema treatment is being conducted by qualified personnel.

- Individualize and supervise progressive yoga practices. Start gradually, increase cautiously, and stop for pain, increased swelling, or discomfort.

- Consider the location of the lymphedema.

- Ensure slow warm-up and slow cool-down, and slow movement patterns.

- Clear proximal to distal lymph drainage areas, and then distally.

- Monitor and provide for all health considera-

(continued)

(continued)

tions (e.g., diabetes, heart disease, neuropathy, arthritis, osteoporosis, etc.), as well as lymphedema.

- Follow usual precautions for metastatic cancer.

- Check for anything in the yoga studio that could cause skin abrasion.

- Maintain a stable room temperature.

- Request clients not wear anything too tight (e.g., rings, bra straps).

- Slowly build up to postures that are "held" or are weight-bearing. Sudden increase in an individual's usual exercise duration or intensity may trigger or worsen lymphedema.

- Avoid excessive repetitions involving the affected limb/area.

- Ensure students wear a compression garment during or immediately after the yoga session, if advised by their lymphedema specialist.

Contraindications

- Hot yoga.

- Too much, too soon.

- Avoid prolonged restriction in affected area. For example, during relaxation, ensure graded elevation of limb: for example, with neck lymphedema, while lying down, do not compress the neck, but have it in neutral with chest and head gently inclined.

Yoga for secondary lymphedema in practice

Our aims in yoga are to:

- Optimize lymphatic clearing through movement.

- Not overload the lymphatic system.

(continued)

(continued)

- Potentially reduce the swelling.

- Create mobile and soft fascial tissue for ease of flow of the lymph, and prevent or soften fibrotic tissue.

- Create improved and progressive mobility and stability of affected limbs.

- Create improved whole body kinematic movement patterns and strength.

- Improve quality of life.

How can we structure a yoga session for someone with secondary lymphedema?

- Slow warm-up and slow cool-down are essential.

- The slow, full yoga breath will create pressure changes and empty the lymph from the lower to the upper body, and return the lymph to the venous system.

- Pauses after the inhalation and exhalation can enhance these pressure changes.

- Slow diaphragmatic breathing at the beginning of, during, and at the end of a session will continually clear the lymphatic system.

- Use postures and practices to empty the lymphatic system from proximal to distal, then distally, so the lymph from the extremities will have a clear path to flow.

- Lymph moves slowly: focus on slow movements and repeat the same movement perhaps 4–7 times to ensure emptying of the specific area.

- Include periods of rest after each series of movements, as lymph will continue to flow from each area.

- Periods of rest will ensure effective lymph flow

(continued)

(continued)

and emptying of one area before proceeding to the next area.

- Isometric muscle contraction on inhalation will create pressure changes for the lymph to flow on exhalation – high pressure to low pressure.

- Elevation of the affected limb before, during, and at the end of a session will aid lymphatic flow.

- Relaxation, with affected limb elevated, at the end of a session.

- Compression garments/gauntlet fitted by a lymphedema specialist, should be used as instructed during and after a yoga session.

Client story: Mira

Annette Loudon

Mira (she/her) is a 45-year-old White woman diagnosed with bowel cancer. She has a permanent colostomy. She is showing early signs of treatment-induced lower extremity lymphedema.

Mira is a former refugee, having lived through and finally escaping a civil war. English is a second language for her. She lives now where I practice, on a remote island off Australia's mainland. She is referred to me by a friend. She asks to see me privately, six weeks after surgery for bowel cancer. She asks if the swelling, heaviness, and discomfort in her leg could be lymphedema, a condition she has learned about from trawling the internet. Despite having 48 lymph nodes removed from her groin during surgery, no one has spoken to her about the signs of lymphedema. She wears, she tells me, a colostomy bag, which she has enclosed in a self-made, beautifully embroidered cotton bag; a touching example of her self-care after this traumatic period. Soft-spoken, she tells me how she doesn't want to socialize, and continues to experience low energy and heavy fatigue. I am moved by the heartfelt description of her extreme homesickness during her treatment: a consequence faced by most rural people needing cancer treatment far from home. This feeling is heightened by her previous experience in a civil war, as well as having to communicate in a second language in a stressful medical situation. She is hopeful yoga may help her. I congratulate her on her self-discernment and reassure her that her current feelings are not at all unusual.

My first duty of care is to refer Mira to the local lymphedema therapist, whom we phone on the spot to make her initial appointment. Early intervention, I tell her, can prevent the condition from worsening. In fact, had I known her prior to surgery, I would have started a lower limb lymphatic clearing sequence and immediately referred her to a lymphedema therapist. I explain that we can do some gentle practices to support her lymphatic and immune systems (hopefully helping her to feel a little better in the process) until she gets her eight-week medical clearance to resume exercise and is able to engage in a more comprehensive, more active yoga practice. Her surgeon has instructed her to walk daily, do daily gentle yoga and non-weightbearing activities, such as cooking, but nothing as vigorous as laundry.

First, I show Mira how to elevate her legs on a wall or chair with her buttocks on a cushion (a modified *viparītakaraṇi*), a posture she can do before her daily walk. This will help reduce the lower limb swelling before the stimulation of walking. In this position, we practice *praṇavadarśana*: which is three-part yoga breath (*dīrghaprāṇāyāma*), followed by full yoga breath using the appropriate *mudrā* (see Figure 6.3) for each part for the movement of the ribs and lungs: for example, *cinmudrā* (gesture of consciousness) for lower lungs; *cinmayamudrā* (gesture of awareness) for middle lungs; *adhimudrā* (gesture of primordial stillness) for upper lungs; and *brahmamudrā* (gesture of the divine) for full yoga breath. I explain how this will help to clear the lymphatic system back into the venous sys-

tem before her walk, restore elasticity to the connective tissue, balance the nervous system, and improve all the systems of her body. I ask her to repeat the elevated position after her walk to assist in emptying the lymph fluid from the legs that walking will have created. Here she can add some slow, full, plantar- and dorsi-flexion of her ankles in time with her breath to further facilitate the movement of lymph fluid. I record a short body scan for her to listen to in this posture to activate her parasympathetic nervous system (PNS), allow the flow of lymph to continue to slow down, and to promote her interoception.

She is interested in *mantra* (word, phrase or sound) repetition, so we repeat our *praṇavadarśana* practice, voicing *A-U-M* together. The use of *mantra*, with the full yoga breath, is intended to enhance lymphatic clearing from the lower body to the upper body and empty the lymphatic system back into the venous system. It will help calm her nervous system, and prepare her deeper abdominal muscles for further training once she has been given full medical clearance for active practice. I record an individualized *yoganidrā* (yogic sleep) for her and show her how to elevate her legs slightly while she listens. I know a regular practice of *yoganidrā* may help calm her reactions and emotions related to the difficulties and traumas she has experienced in her life and during her cancer treatment. This practice is her favorite, she tells me one day, due to its easeful relaxation.

I check in with Mira by phone the next day, and a week later. I am always vigilant in monitoring the effect of yoga on a swollen limb, due to the possibility of infection. She has also given me permission to contact her lymphdema specialist, so she can be kept up to date on our yoga practice. Mira has done everything I suggested and has had no negative effects. Most importantly, she perceives a decrease in her swelling. Her enthusiasm for the practices is evident in her voice. She feels she is helping herself and regaining some degree of empowerment over her healing. I am thrilled that she has incorporated parts of the practice into her daily life. For example, leg elevation before and after cooking the evening meal, *yoganidrā* at various times during the day, and *praṇavadarśana* before sleeping. She is creating her own therapy.

As the months go by and Mira's rehabilitation continues, we work together to create a progressive lymph clearing and lower body stabilizing sequence. After eight months she bravely starts attending a small weekly class, where we continue to refine her personalized sequence. The *saṅgha* (community) of the class creates a gentle return to socialization. Five years later, Mira has the leg swelling under good professional and personal self-management care and continues with her yoga. She still loves her *yoganidrā*.

Client story: Georgina

Annette Loudon

Georgina (she/her) is a 50-year-old White woman diagnosed with recurrent breast cancer and clinically confirmed pre-existing upper limb lymphedema due to her previous breast cancer surgery.

Georgina, a dedicated yoga practitioner, has asked to see me privately, rather than speak during a cancer-care class that she has been attending for years. Her fear shows on her face as she tells me that she has recently been given a diagnosis of recurrent breast cancer, in the same breast as last time. She is afraid that her existing arm lymphedema (from a lumpectomy and axilla clearance eight years ago) will become worse. Currently, she wears a compression sleeve, goes to a lymphedema therapist every eight weeks, and manages her condition with self-massage and skin care. Her arm swelling is impacted by heat, but elevation helps. She follows a lymphatic clearing protocol in our yoga class and naturally puts her fingers into *varuṇamudrā* (see Figure 6.3), even when watching television. Georgina reminds me that eight years ago, the diagnosis of secondary lymphedema was the worst part of her first cancer experience. Despite this, her lymphedema care is optimal, and her doctor has cleared her for yoga therapy.

Together, we prepare a 30-minute sequence that she can do daily (Box 6.6). Our aim is to maintain optimal lymphatic clearing and prepare her lymphatic system and fascial tissue for her upcoming surgery and radiation in three weeks. As is often the case with people preparing for treatment, she did this sequence two or three times a day until her surgery. The sequence begins and finishes with the full yoga breath combined with contraction of pelvic floor and transversus abdominis on the exhalation, and release/relaxation of these areas on the inhalation: all to facilitate the movement of lymphatic fluid into the venous system. A *mantra* is also added which will have the same effect. We add an *A-U-M mantra* to encourage this engagement and to help ground and calm her. We then do slow and focused physical practices based on clearing the lymph, proximal to distal, then distal to proximal again. This will prepare the connective tissue in her chest, upper back, and arm for the surgery and radiation that will follow. We also strengthen her lower body and abdominal area to create a strong base of support and optimize lymphatic clearing. I record the breathing practice and a *yoganidrā* (yogic sleep) for her use now and from the moment she wakes up after surgery, in the hospital. Our students tell us they love to hear a familiar voice at this time. Georgina enjoys visualization and exploring the *cakra* systems (in yogic philosophy, these are the energy centers), and so these features overlie the program: working with *maṇipūra* (solar plexus) for grounding and courage, *anāhata* (heart) for acceptance and self-compassion, and *viśuddhi* (throat) for acknowledgement of her own level of discernment.

When I meet Georgina, weeks afterward, she tells me that the sequence we worked on together gave her the best possible chance of preparing both her body and mind for surgery and radiation. Her treatment went well, and the lymphedema of her affected arm did not worsen. To this day, she continues to advocate for yoga as a self-management tool and/or preventive technique for those with, or at risk of, secondary lymphedema from cancer treatment.

BOX 6.6 30-minute yoga practice for secondary upper limb lymphedema

Annette Loudon

Each series of movements is repeated 4–7 times, slowly and with awareness, and followed by a period of rest – to avoid overloading the lymphatic system (which will continue to pump for at least two minutes after each series of movements) and to allow for interoception. To promote lymphatic drainage of the arm in all movements, make a fist while inhaling, and release the hand on the exhalation. (See Figure 6.6 for the order of lymphatic emptying.)

Lying supine

- Full yoga breath with voiced *mantra* (such as A-U-M). Purpose: to empty the lymph system to the venous system, enable elasticity of the tissue, and cultivate calm. Rest.

- Neck rotation with outward rotation of opposite arm. Repeat on both sides. Purpose: to further empty the lymph system at the neck, warm up the upper body, create gentle movement of fascia through the chest, arm, and neck, and connect with *anāhata (heart) cakra*. Rest.

- Shoulder rotations. Purpose: to empty the axilla and soften fascia in chest and upper back. Rest.

- Contraction of pelvic floor, transversus abdominis, and rectus abdominis on exhalation. Combine with arm movements: abduction toward the floor, with bent elbows on inhalation, adduction with straight arms above chest. Purpose: to empty whole lymphatic system, empty cubitals at elbow, cultivate pelvic strength and connect to *maṇipūra* and courage. Rest.

Kneeling

- Thoracic rotation, extending both arms to the side (with outer rotation), one arm at high diagonal, one arm low diagonal, neck rotating toward the low side. Repeat on other side. Purpose: to create integrated fascial functioning, open the chest, empty lymphatic fluid from the whole arm, and connect with *prāṇic* frontal channel. Rest.

Standing

- Side bend variation with left hand sliding down left leg, right hand sliding from right hip towards right armpit with elbow bent. Repeat other side. Purpose: to empty nodes along the ribs, soften tissue, and empty lymphatic fluid from arm. Rest.

- Slow cat (*mārjaryāsana*) variation with shoulder blade retraction (and outward rotation of arms) on inhalation and shoulder protraction (and internal rotation of the arms) on exhalation. Purpose: to empty lymphatic system to venous system, create stability in lower body, connect to outer world on inhalation and inner world on exhalation. Rest.

- Tree posture (*vṛkṣāsana*) with arm elevation and gentle movement of hands and fingers, while balancing on each leg. Purpose: to empty lymph down the arms, promote steadiness and balance, and to begin cool-down. Rest.

Sitting or lying

- Alternate nostril breath (*nāḍīśodhana*) in comfortable seated posture. Purpose: to continue cool down while activating parasympathetic nervous system (PNS), to slow down lymph flow and connect to self. Rest.

- Relaxation with affected arm elevated in a comfortable supported position. Purpose: to complete PNS activation while lymph continues to empty down the affected arm and create a deep sense of calm.

- Full yoga breath and voiced *Oṃ mantra*. Purpose: to empty lymph system back to venous system and create a sense of connection to something greater than oneself.

2.7 Delivering yoga therapy in the chemotherapy infusion center: expanding the reach of mind-body therapies to patients in clinical settings

Background: Chemotherapy infusion center

Tina Walter, BA, C-IAYT and Leigh Leibel

Imagine a busy infusion center where cancer patients receive systemic anti-cancer drugs delivered directly to the bloodstream via catheter inserted in a port (a device placed under the skin that is used to draw blood and give treatments), central line, or a vein in the arm, hand, or thigh. Each patient has their own IV (intravenous) pole with numerous hanging bags that could include some or all of the following: chemotherapy, immunotherapy, antiemetic/anti-vomiting and pain medications, saline for hydration, and perhaps Benadryl (diphenhydramine) and dexamethasone for allergic reactions. Amidst the cacophony of environmental sounds – transfusion pump alarms, a patient in distress from an allergic reaction to Taxotere (docetaxel), cell phones, test results, and visits from medical staff and family – it can be anything but calm. Now picture that same unit with a yoga therapist leading a patient through guided imagery or a gentle "head and neck movement" series to lessen tension. Maybe another patient is led in a relaxation technique called *yoganidrā* (yogic sleep), accompanied by soft music; all creating a tranquil, peaceful space.

Patients usually spend 30 minutes to 10 hours in the infusion center (the time spent in the chair is dependent on the number of drugs given and their dosage protocols, as well as the time it takes for routine pre-chemotherapy blood draws and results, and for the drug to be prepped by the pharmacy). This is an ideal time to deliver a yoga therapy session; in fact, it is often a patient's first introduction to yoga. Offering yoga therapy during infusion provides the oncology patient population convenient access to the breadth of practices which may otherwise be unattainable due to barriers (e.g., fatigue, scheduling, or transportation), thereby preventing patients from attending sessions or classes (Sohl et al. 2016). Importantly, yoga interventions can lessen a patient's symptom burden (e.g., reduce pain and anxiety, or teach a home remedy for sleep or pre-surgical coping mechanisms).

A yoga therapist working in an outpatient infusion center works within an integrative team of specialists, personalizing one-on-one yoga sessions in a manner which addresses a patient's specific goals in relation to the side effects and symptoms of their disease. After initial assessment, modifications and adjustments in the yoga instruction are made based on information about the patient's illness and the description of their personal experience with cancer. Ideally, pre–post assessments and qualitative data are captured to show efficacy of intervention and validate the work of yoga therapists.

Providing yoga interventions in a busy outpatient unit presents many challenges, from completing the intervention before the anti-allergic pre-med Benadryl is administered and causes drowsiness, to the distractions of people crying in the next pod, to some patients' "get in and get out" mentality. Interruptions often include medication administration, IV maintenance, treatments, and visits from medical staff and family. For example, if the registered nurse (RN) enters the patient's room/bay during a yoga intervention and needs time with the patient, the yoga therapist excuses themselves and returns to the patient after the required nursing tasks are completed. Flexibility of the yoga therapist is key, while adhering to the clinical needs of the patient and staff.

Some vitamins and herbal supplements can affect and interact with chemotherapy. For example, some varieties of the ginseng plant are estrogenic and contraindicated for people being treated for hormone-positive cancers. A yoga therapist must never step out of their scope of practice to recommend, suggest, or share vitamins or herbal supplements with people undergoing cancer treatment.

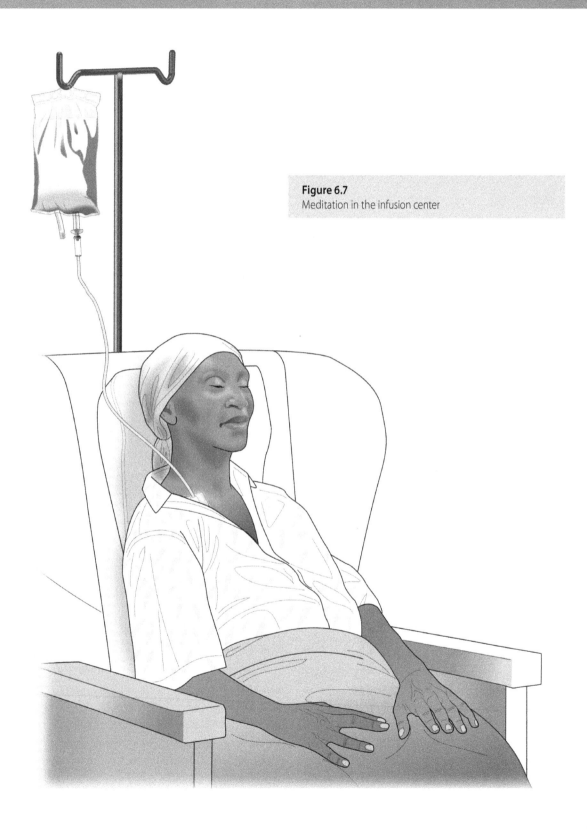

Figure 6.7
Meditation in the infusion center

If a patient complains of pain in the area of the catheter, port, or veins, call the nurse ASAP. Some chemotherapy drugs can cause damage if they leak.

Patient story: Karen

Tina Walter

Karen (she/her) is a 48-year-old Black woman diagnosed with colorectal cancer who has a temporary ileostomy.

I meet Karen during her first chemotherapy treatment. Two months prior, she had undergone colorectal surgery to remove part of her colon and 24 lymph nodes, followed by immediate reconstruction. This has left her with a temporary ileostomy (to give the bowel time to heal) that is to be reversed after she completes chemotherapy. A schoolteacher and mother of two disabled children, she begins by talking about her fears, and she identifies anxiety as her biggest issue. On this first day of chemotherapy, Karen has tears in her eyes as she tells me she is worried how she is going to take care of her 20-year-old daughter, who has severe autism and seizure disorder. "All I can think about is just how sick am I going to be, and whether I can take care of my children." Karen also says that she is very sensitive by nature and can feel the needle being inserted into her port, which is causing lots of anxiety. She reports a pain level of seven, and an anxiety level of ten. This is measured by the pre–post assessment tool (Likert scale: 0 = no pain/anxiety; 10 = highest level of pain/anxiety) the nurses and I created so that I could document patient changes.

I begin by helping her verbalize exactly what she fears regarding the chemotherapy, and then help her reframe that thinking. I guide her in a practice I call the *organic weave*, inviting her to notice her strength and energy (Box 6.7). We use guided imagery to imagine the port as a "vessel of goodness" and direct softness and ideas of healing into the areas where she is experiencing pain. Afterward, Karen reports that her pain has dropped to two, and anxiety to four. She says she feels less stressed, and an increased feeling of peace and quiet. Her introduction to yoga, made in the infusion center, led to her attending yoga therapy-for-cancer classes weekly, which she has now been doing for over a year. Karen continues to use the relaxation and guided imagery regularly to help control her anxiety while at work and at home.

BOX 6.7 Organic Weave: a relaxation practice for patients undergoing anti-cancer infusion

Tina Walter

- To begin, invite the patient to find a relaxed position in the chemotherapy chair (see Figure 6.7) and let go of "trying too hard." Because noise is typically a factor in the chemo unit and directly affects relaxation, very special attention is given to hearing, processing, and releasing sounds.

- Next, verbally guide the patient in a whole-body relaxation, beginning with awareness from the crown of the head to eventually reaching legs and feet. The patient is cued to notice sensations and feelings present in the physical, emotional, energetic, and thinking self.

- The patient is encouraged to give themselves permission to relax throughout the practice without needing to fix or change anything and are guided to instead meet these places in their body with friendliness, or at least acceptance without judgment.

- Using the mind, the senses, and the imagination consciously and intentionally, instruct patients to notice "organic wholeness" by weaving together all parts of the breath and the physical body. Culminating this sense of wholeness, the patient can notice vitality and how all energy moves toward healing and well-being.

- Finally, the patient may be invited to imagine breath as healing energy, and cultivate the idea of letting it touch every cell, every organ of the body.

2.8 Coming of age with cancer: adolescents and young adults (AYAs)

Background: Adolescents and young adults with cancer

Amelia Coffaro, BA, RYT 500, C-IAYT

What does it mean to be an adolescent or young adult (AYA) with cancer? AYAs face a life interrupted and an entirely new way of experiencing and navigating the world. For the 89,500 young people in the United States between the ages of 15 and 39 diagnosed with cancer each year (American Cancer Society), the added and complex layers of stress shape the experience of "coming of age" with cancer. While overall survival rates continue to improve in this population, AYAs continue to face unique quality-of-life issues, and issues around health disparity (Box 6.8). There is a call for holistic, mindfulness-based and multidisciplinary care for this population (Lidington et al. 2021, Van der Gucht 2017). In the following pages we describe how a yoga therapist can best meet the needs of an AYA population across the cancer continuum by embracing a therapeutic approach to yoga and supporting unique mental health needs.

BOX 6.8 Unique quality of life issues faced by AYA populations, during and after cancer treatment

Amelia Coffaro

As distinct from younger and older people facing cancer, and depending on their diagnosis, AYAs experience:

- Conflicting needs for support and autonomy (Aubin at al, 2019).

- Financial difficulties and interruptions in education, career trajectory, and employment (Cavallo 2019, Park & Rosenstein 2015).

- Dissatisfaction with body image, difficulty in establishing intimate relationships, sexual

---

dysfunction, and increased fertility concerns (Cavallo 2019, Lidington et al. 2021, Park & Rosenstein 2015).

- Higher incidence of fatigue, and greater risk of post-traumatic stress, anxiety, and depression due to disruptions in developmental trajectory, greater symptom burden, higher levels of pain during treatment, and increased likelihood of developing aggressive disease (Cavallo 2019, Park & Rosenstein 2015).

- Unmet psychological needs and health system/information needs leading to higher incidence of "cancer-related distress" (Sender et al. 2020).

- Outcome disparity, with survival rates higher for some cancers and significantly worse for others, such as leukemias and triple negative breast cancer (Keegan et al. 2016, Park & Rosenstein 2015).

- Greater need for information regarding prognosis and side effects of treatment, and more support around decision-making and facing mortality (Figeroa Gray et al. 2018).

- Increased feelings of isolation and susceptibility to suicidal ideation, and completed suicide (Park & Rosenstein 2015).

How yoga therapy can support AYAs

Amelia Coffaro and Anne Pitman

Embrace a therapeutic approach to yoga

Educate AYAs on therapeutic yoga

- AYAs commonly report having no previous experience with yoga, or only limited experience with more strenuous "power" variations, usually done in a heated room. As they discover new physical limitations during cancer treatment, yoga therapists can educate young adults on the benefits of honoring their bodies and embracing a more therapeutic approach to yoga that includes gentle movements and practices beyond the physical.

Highlight acceptance

- When AYAs struggle with losing their identity, or conversely see "cancer patient" as their only identity, yoga therapy offers them the opportunity to practice acceptance, nonjudgment, and the ability to see beyond the cancer experience, to their essence.

Engage in steady practice

- Yoga therapy is an accessible tool for sustainable well-being for AYAs from diagnosis and throughout survivorship. For AYAs living with advanced cancer and limited expected survival, yoga therapy can provide a sense of comfort and support for the unique needs of young adults in end-of-life care.

Focus on self-compassion

- A practice of self-compassion can support AYAs who may be critical of themselves when experiencing the upheaval of cancer, during the developmental years of their life. Teachers trained in Mindful Self-Compassion can support AYAs in learning to be mindful of intense and difficult emotions, such as fear, anger, and sadness, and learn tools like cultivating a kind inner voice, associated with positive psychological strengths (Neff 2019).

Encourage peer connection

- Through yoga therapy compassion practices, AYAs can learn how to relate more deeply to other AYAs, or to friends that may have come and gone from their lives during cancer. AYAs often report that relationships with other survivors are vital. Only 50% of AYAs rated support from family and friends as a top five need, while 100% rated connecting with other survivors as a top five need (Zebrak et al. 2006).

Hear their voice

- Empower AYAs to use their voice throughout their cancer experience to make decisions and to advocate for themselves.

Support mental health needs

Screen for distress

- AYAs are inconsistently screened for cancer-related distress, including comorbid depression and anxiety. As a result, their mental health needs are often overlooked by healthcare providers (Sanson-Daly & Wakefield 2013). Feelings of depression, anxiety, and post-traumatic stress can influence factors such as adherence to treatment, completion of therapy, quality of care, and overall outcomes.

Think creatively

- Forming one's identity, making new relationships, and other "regular" developmental tasks can be challenging when removed from the "normal" stream of life. Yet AYAs sometimes hesitate to participate in individual psychotherapeutic treatment. Creative and flexible psychosocial support programs are needed to engage this population, especially those with limited expected survival (Knox et al. 2016).

Ease off on expectations

- Many AYAs feel isolated trying to "keep up" after a setback with cancer. They sometimes become competitive with themselves when trying to rebuild their lives. Support AYAs by helping them to take their time, and mindfully manage the pressure of returning to normal life.

Gather them in

- Further research, access to clinical trials, and clinical expertise in treating AYA populations is needed (Coccia 2019). Creative and extensive somatic-based mental health resources are needed in order to encourage the regular use of yoga therapy practices across the cancer care continuum.

Patient story: Claire

Amelia Coffaro

Claire (she/her) is a 28-year-old White woman diagnosed with triple negative breast cancer.

Claire and I meet in the infusion center during the second month of her chemotherapy treatment for breast cancer. After checking in at the nurses' station to get an overview of the daily patient schedule, the nurse hints to me that Claire, seated in bay three by the window, likes yoga and may be interested in meeting me. As I approach her chair, I see her wrapped in a beautiful, bright shawl, staring out the window as she awaits her pre-meds.

"Hello, Claire. My name is Amelia, and I am the Yoga Therapist here at the hospital. Your nurse said you might be interested in meeting me." With a warm smile on her face, she invites me to sit down. Just as we begin to settle in and talk, the nurse walks over with Claire's pre-meds. "Name and date of birth?" she asks. Claire responds and I notice her fingers tighten their grasp on the arms of the chair in anticipation of having her port accessed next. "Cold spray?" asks the nurse. "Always," says Claire. She closes her eyes, turns her head away and holds her breath as the nurse first makes the poke and then secures the needle in place with an adhesive bandage. "You're all set!" the nurse says joyfully, almost innocently unaware of what the next several hours and days will bring for Claire, to no fault of her own. Claire lets out a big exhale and her face relaxes. We return to our conversation, making small talk: what it's like to be one of the only young people sitting in the infusion center week after week; the routine of packing the cooler of snacks she brings for herself every time she comes to treatment; the discomfort of the cold cap therapy (an FDA-approved frozen gel cap that covers the head and causes vasoconstriction of the scalp to minimize hair loss during chemotherapy). Claire is trying to prevent hair loss to maintain as much normalcy in her life as possible.

After we have the chance to get to know one another a bit, we shift our attention to yoga, and begin the pre-intervention symptom scale she and the nurses created. Today, Claire is rating moderate-to-severe levels of fatigue, and high levels of anxiety and distress, as well as other symptoms of which she notes are sleep-related. Since it's our first time working together, and since Claire reported her only experience is with hot yoga, I consider simple practices that also allow her to experience the benefits in a short period of time, with the goal of encouraging further exploration and implementation at home for regular practice.

"I always have a poor sleep the night before and after chemo," she says. "Even after several months, I feel anxious before my treatments – I worry about my future, the big picture, both with cancer and my life outside of cancer. And then the days after treatment, I start to feel a little depressed – I'm tired, I have no energy or motivation to do anything sometimes. All of this has happened so fast – one day I went to the doctor for an exam and the next thing you know, I have breast cancer. And I just got married two months ago so this is how I'm starting my marriage." I thank her for sharing with me, and before I get the chance to ask Claire what she feels in her body at that moment, I can see her eyes become heavy and start to slowly blink, a sure sign that Benadryl is now taking effect. Based on what she reports during the pre-intervention scale, I briefly explain the practice of *yoganidrā* (yogic sleep) and asks if she is interested in the guided experience. Claire nods yes, and we begin.

I invite her to find as much comfort in her chemo chair as possible. She pulls a quilt over herself that her friends made for her, and within a few moments Claire is settled and voluntarily closes her eyes, resting her palms on her abdomen. As she continues to settle in the chair, her shoulders round slightly inward, in an almost protective mechanism, and her breath is short and quick, primarily restricted to the chest. I take note of the physical and mental *tamasic* (lethargic) and *rajasic* (restless) qualities Claire is presenting that are commonly associated with chemotherapy side effects like depression, extreme fatigue, and anxiety. I begin by inviting Claire to bring her awareness to her breath, to simply notice her breath as it is without trying to change it. AYAs commonly present with maladaptive breathing patterns and a sense of bracing in the body, due to the stress and shock of a diagnosis, followed by the start, duration, and anxiety of treatment.

I decide to first work with Claire on developing breath awareness and share with her that deepening her awareness of how she's breathing will not only support her in developing a healthy breathing rhythm to help her body relax, but also educate her that in moments that feel scary or isolating, the breath is a tool she can use to empower herself, by slowing down to stay in and move through the challenges that frequent the path of AYA cancer experiences. "Slow deep breaths are the new power yoga," she says. We look at one another and quietly chuckle with a shared sense of understanding for a life that was once and is no longer.

After a few rounds of breath, I guide her to bring her awareness to her feet and begin leading her through *yoganidrā*. For AYAs with often fast-paced lives in modern day society, and who are faced with learning to slow down during cancer treatment and recovery, the practice of *yoganidrā* in the infusion center offers a new opportunity to deepen states of rest needed for the journey ahead. By the time I reach her arms and see Claire is not responding to the cues, I realize that she may be sleeping, but continue to guide the practice anyway, as the experience of Benadryl alone can feel like a state between sleeping, and wakefulness. I finish the practice and realize that indeed, she is very fatigued and has fallen asleep. Instead of waking her, I leave a note on her chairside table saying it was nice to meet her and thanked her for her willingness to participate.

Three weeks have passed, and I again see Claire in the infusion center; she's now almost halfway through her chemotherapy. Today, she is joined by her brother who is playing a game of checkers with her when I arrive. I greet Claire and she apologizes for falling asleep during our time together a few weeks ago, but I reassure her that this is OK, and a sign from her body that she was tired. She smiles with a sense of reassurance, and tells me, "But wow, the relaxation helped so much, and I slept great that night!" She also notes that the practice was hard to remember and do on her own in the days that followed and shares with me that she tried acupuncture for the first time to help with neuropathy in her feet and hands.

During our check in, Claire again reports moderate to severe levels of fatigue, anxiety, and distress. This time she shares she's feeling somewhat stressed about work. "I'm taking on less in work and life, but today I feel particularly anxious about my upcoming surgery and the decision on what type of surgery I'll opt for. If I just remove one breast, I have a certain percentage of recurrence, and if I remove both, my risk reduces, but I won't be able to breast feed future children. And then there's the question of reconstruction – should I do it? Should I not? And if I do, where do they take the skin from? What is it going to feel like waking up from surgery? To look at my chest for the first time after they take my breasts away? Will my husband ever look at me the same way? I guess I don't really care either way, I just want to have cancer out of my body and be healthy again."

I hear her anxiety through her rambling thoughts, and see Claire's body start to tighten, her eyes moving quickly from one side to the other as she anxiously thinks through her thoughts out loud. "Sorry," she says, "it's hard to believe that just six months ago I was traveling around the world for my job and now I am faced with these decisions. How is that possible? Not to mention I am still not sleeping well, and this Benadryl makes me feel like I am numb in my own body. When I look in the mirror, I feel like I don't even know who I am sometimes. And then some days I feel bad because I have so much to be grateful for. My friends, family...my life.

Sorry again. How did I go off on that tangent?" I reassure her that there is no reason to apologize and validate for her that this experience is overwhelming, almost like whiplash, and scary in a way that brings so many conflicting emotions to the surface. We share a few quiet breaths together. "I'm looking forward to some practice today," she says. "I need it."

Claire's brother decides to participate in the practices today, too. He clears the game away from the chairside table and settles himself in the chair next to her. Before we start, I grab a warm blanket to cover her and a pillow to support her neck. Claire reaches for the controls on the side of the chair and reclines all the way back, her legs slightly elevated, and chest and shoulders gently open. Even though Claire reports a high level of fatigue from disrupted sleep due to treatment side effects like hot flashes and nausea, my intention for our time together is to lead her through practices that address the underlying, visible anxiety that is present. We begin again with a guided *yoganidrā* first, a passive/active practice to give the body a chance to experience deep rest and the mind to quiet without Claire having to make too much effort. Slowly I observe her body soften, the tension in her face melt away, and the breath become slow and smooth. As we near the end of the *yoganidrā*, the nurse finally arrives with pre-meds – it's a hurry up and wait kind of morning in the infusion center today – but kindly waits until Claire is more fully alert to ask her name and date of birth before connecting her to the infusion, an agreement Claire made with the nurse before we started practice. I gently ring the tingsha bells and guide Claire and her brother out of the relaxation. The nurse reapproaches, and in a soft voice asks her for her information to begin the pre-med. Claire turns her head towards the nurse, opens her eyes, and gives her name and date of birth. As the nurse connects the line, Claire turns her head back to a resting position, closes her eyes and says, "I feel like a child in a rowboat on still water, dipping my hand in, feeling so at peace with myself and the world. To know I can feel this way even in this stressful environment gives me hope. I never knew I could do this for myself."

2.9 Yoga to enhance caregiver connectedness during lung cancer treatment

Background: Role of caregivers in cancer care

Smitha Mallaiah, PhD(c), MSc, C-IAYT

A cancer diagnosis affects the entire family unit. As a person begins cancer treatment, their loved ones often take on a primary caregiving role and are integral to their well-being and recovery. Many consider it a privilege to care for their loved one, yet research shows that the tremendous daily stress of caring for an ill family member can take a serious toll on emotional and physical health (Bevans & Sternberg 2012). Fatigue, worry, sadness, anxiety, and sleeping problems are just some of the common challenges facing carers. The burden is significant. Research shows long-term stress suppresses the immune system and increases the chance of developing chronic health problems such as heart disease or high blood pressure, and may also accelerate existing health conditions (Antoni & Dhabhar 2019). Therefore, there is a profound need to include caregivers in mind-body interventions to promote long-term cancer adjustment. Most yoga programs in cancer populations have targeted only people with cancer and not their caregivers.

Many people newly diagnosed with cancer and family caregivers are motivated to make lifestyle changes to improve cancer-related outcomes. Yoga, with its variety of practices that address mind, body, and soul can beautifully support the physical, emotional, and spiritual needs of a person with cancer and prepare them for aggressive treatments ahead. The yoga tradition draws from India's beautiful and rich cultural heritage of *sanātanadharma* (duties or virtues). In Indian philosophy, Śiva – the first Yogi – is known to have taught Yoga to his wife *Pārvatī*. *Śiva*, as a symbol of union, merged himself with *Pārvatī* to become *ardhanārīśvara* – half male and half female. The concepts of *ardhanārīśvara* are a representation of opposite equivalents, honoring differences, acceptance, and above all, unconditional love. Emotional interdependence, where the feelings of one person are related to the feelings of another person, is often seen as a key characteristic of close relationships. Yoga therapy tools such as postures (*āsana*), breath-work (*prāṇāyāma*), and meditation (*dhyāna*) can be modified to include both patient and caregiver and enhance their interconnectedness through various aspects of practice.

Patient story: Mr. R

Smitha Mallaiah

Mr. R (he/his) is a 65-year-old White man diagnosed with lung cancer. His wife Mrs. R is in attendance as his primary caregiver.

Mr. R has been married for 30 years and his wife is his cancer caregiver. The cancer diagnosis is definitely a shock. His wife (like many other caregivers) is actively engaged in the treatment decisions and also a firm believer that healthy lifestyle, including healthy eating, exercise, and stress management can put her husband on track for a better outcome. In our first session they are arguing about this:

Mrs. R: *You should change your eating habits; you should drink the green smoothie I make.*

Mr. R: *I don't like the vegetables, it tastes like grass.*

Mrs. R: *You should be on an anti-cancer diet to help yourself and our family.*

Mr. R: *You are the one who was eating the more unhealthier diet.*

Mrs. R: *But guess what honey? You are the one with cancer.*

Mr. R: *Yeah, that's right. Thank you for reminding me.*

And he slowly tears up, frustrated. Mrs. R tears up, too, but right now they are not ready to face or console each other. There is a long silence in the room, followed by Mrs. R talking about her worst fears for herself and her husband. Mr. R has smoked for over 20 years without his wife knowing about it, but he did quit smoking four months ago after his diagnosis. He also enjoys his meat and sugar-heavy meals. Mrs. R feels he betrayed her trust and blames his lifestyle and choices for cancer. This has become the core of their disagreement and it trickles down into all areas of their relationship, from eating to cancer treatment. Our couple's yoga program is intended to target the needs of them *both* with a focus on their interconnectedness (see Box 6.9).

When I invited them to practice, they did not want to face each other. For the next several weeks we began each session with a short discussion (*vijñānamayakośa* [sheath of wisdom]; see Chapter 2, *Yoga philosophy*) on various tools of yoga therapy with an emphasis on meditations that included nonjudgmental awareness of self, tolerance, acceptance, appreciation, and unconditional love for self and one another. When we practiced tolerance and acceptance of self, Mr. R said, "I am struggling to accept myself fully, knowing how I have neglected and abused my body, I don't know how I expected you to fully accept me. I am sorry, forgive me." Mrs. R said she felt a sense of relief.

After going through a few couple's yoga sessions, the two felt less on edge, more accepting of each other, and are learning to support each other. They attended two to three weekly sessions (60 minutes each) over the course of the five to six weeks of Mr. R's radiotherapy. The program consisted of four main components from S-VYASA tradition:

1. "Joint loosening" (gentle stretching – *sūkṣmavyāyāma*) with breath synchronization.

2. Postures (*āsana*) and a deep relaxation technique.

3. Breath energization (*prāṇāyāma*) with sound resonance.

4. Meditation (*dhyāna*).

On the day they practiced meditation on unconditional love, Mrs. R reflected, "I am reminded of our marriage promise we made for each other. I am so much in love with you again. Yoga has been our only island of hope and calm through our cancer treatment." Tears rolled down their cheeks, with a kiss followed by a long hug.

BOX 6.9 Considerations for designing a couple's yoga practice
Smitha Mallaiah

- **Client's position:** Instead of facing the therapist/teacher, invite both the patient and caregiver to face each other. They begin by looking into each other's eyes and take a few moments to connect at the start of the session. There is no need to say or do anything, just be present for each other.

- **Interdependence in postures:** Help the patient and caregiver not only to learn the postures themselves, but also help each other through postures. This can mean giving support physically in triangle pose (*trikoṇāsana*) or tree pose (*vṛkṣāsana*); and make sure both parties give and receive support. In this way they both have something to offer each other while practicing. *(continued)*

(continued)

- **Breath matching:** Breathing can be one of the simplest, yet profound practices to help couples connect. Looking into each other's eyes, they slowly start matching their breaths: taking an inhalation to match their partner's breath, and the same as they exhale. If couples prefer, they can sit back-to-back (Figure 6.8), and start slowly breathing, focusing on their own breath. After a few rounds, they can try to match their partner's breath. This can be carried out through all the *prāṇāyāma* practices, and the therapist can facilitate this process.

- **Meditation:** Slowing down the mind (toward silence and mindfulness) can prove to be great tools for helping couples to center themselves, and better connect with their partners. In yoga therapy, *Bhakti Yoga* (Yoga of Devotion) is one of the main tools for emotion culture (how emotions are influenced by yogic philosophy). In the *Nārada Bhakti Sūtra-s*,

(continued)

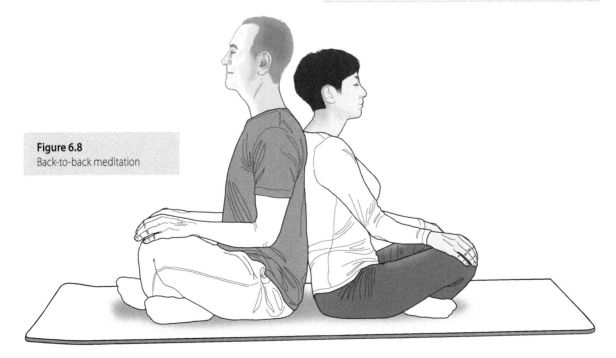

Figure 6.8
Back-to-back meditation

BOX 6.9 continued

Sage Nārada talks about *paramaprema* or the highest form of unconditional love, and has laid down the path from tolerance, acceptance, and appreciation to a sense of wonder in love. This concept, and loving kindness towards each other, can be very empowering and apt for working with couples.

2.10 *Prāṇic* Energization Technique (PET): can it improve symptoms associated with "chemo brain"?

Background: Chemotherapy-related cognitive dysfunction – "chemo brain"

Suveena Guglani, PhD student, MSc, C-IAYT and Leigh Leibel

Cancer and its treatments can adversely affect a wide range of mental processes, from attention and focus to working memory (Brezden et al. 2000). This cancer-related cognitive dysfunction (CRCD) can be debilitating, enduring, and may negatively affect the psychosocial functioning and quality of life of patients (Ahles et al. 2002). It is reported by 17–75% of patients (Jean-Pierre 2010), and its severity has been correlated with the treatment dose (van Dam et al. 1998). CRCD has been attributed to many factors, both physical and psychological. Physical factors include genetic predisposition, failure of blood–brain barrier integrity, cancer treatment-related brain toxicity, DNA damage, reduction in estrogen and testosterone levels, effects of cytokines in the brain, microvasculature obstruction, and infarction of brain tissue (O'Shaughnessy 2003, Cleeland 2003). Psychological factors include cancer-related fatigue, anxiety, and depression (Staat & Segatore 2005). There is no solution for this common and difficult side effect of cancer treatment, and researchers continue to look for answers. One area that researchers are looking at is the impact of breath on cognitive function. We share several yogic-based breathing studies below:

- A study by Zauner et al. (2002) shows that the brain needs oxygenation to function at its peak, and a series of deep breathing sequences can provide the oxygen needed to promote brain healing.

- Research conducted at Northwestern University in Chicago found that the rhythm of cyclic breathing coordinates electrical activity across a network of brain regions associated with smell, memory, and emotions, and can enhance their functioning (Zelano 2016).

- A study at Sri Aurobindo College in Indore, India details the effect of *prāṇāyāma* (breath-work) on the cognitive functions of a group of medical students in which they showed distinct improvement of cognitive dysfunction caused by stress and anxiety (Jain 2016).

- *Prāṇāyāma* can also help to increase the parasympathetic response and improve the processing of sensory information at the level of the thalamus, accompanied by the experience of alertness and reinvigoration (Jerath et al. 2006).

- In India, researchers are investigating an advanced meditation technique called *Prāṇic* Energization Technique (PET) in a variety of settings and populations. The technique involves breath regulation, chanting, and visualization. In one randomized controlled trial that looked at the effect of PET on the healing of fresh bone fractures, researchers found PET as an add-on practice showed significant improvements in ratings of pain, tenderness, fracture line density, and bridging of cortices, compared to patients given standard treatment alone (Oswal et al. 2011).

Both the PET technique and various *prāṇāyāma* practices warrant further investigation in cancer populations for patient symptom management.

Patient story: Diane

Suveena Guglani

Diane (she/her) is a 38-year-old White woman diagnosed with early-stage DCIS breast cancer.

Diane has been recently diagnosed with stage Ib ductal carcinoma in situ (DCIS) breast cancer, pT1cN1a, 1 of 2 nodes positive. Her doctor has prescribed chemotherapy. When we meet, she is undergoing her second round of chemotherapy cycle and is already reporting symptoms of forgetfulness and having a high level of stress and anxiety. She complains of forgetting appointments, walking into a room and wondering why she is there, and not being able to remember which floor her doctor's office is on. All symptoms point to "chemo brain." She seems resigned to the fact that her cancer treatment is affecting her life and ability to function. She says that she maintains a healthy lifestyle, exercises, and pays attention to what she eats. She mentions that her symptoms make her feel inadequate and helpless, and she is considering taking a leave of absence from work. I ask her about her support system, and she indicates that she has a husband and sister who accompany her to medical appointments.

I explain to her that I am conducting a yoga research study at the hospital that involves deep breathing-focused sequences that have been shown to provide some relief for the symptoms mentioned above. She looks skeptical. I show her the data indicating an improvement in anxiety and stress in many of the patients, and explain this is a practice she could do while waiting or receiving her infusion in the chemotherapy suite. She could also practice this before going to bed. She asks for more details, and after some discussion, indicates she is ready to try. I mention to her that as with anything, disciplined practice is essential to see measurable improvement. She seems hopeful that this is something she might be able to manage.

We start her deep breathing practices. She experiences a sense of deep relaxation after the first one and thinks that she should be able to continue with this at home. She asks if I could continue to provide her the practice when she comes for her future infusion sessions. We see each other weekly for six weeks. After several weeks of working with the protocol (called PET or *Prāṇic* Energization Technique; Box 6.10) she feels relaxed, calmer, and reports improvement in sleep quality, anxiety, and depression. Her quantitative scores measured by various validated questionnaires confirm that improvement.[1] Her executive function also shows an improvement, and we discuss the possible underlying mechanism that might have led to this improvement. We discuss the possibility of the symptoms getting worse as the treatment progresses, and how she can continue to use the breathing to help with controlling the anxiety and depression. She completes her cycles of chemotherapy and reports she has started to rely on this method to combat fatigue and forgetfulness and that it has helped with anger management as well. We promise to stay in touch, and she completes her chemotherapy, followed by radiation therapy. The cycle continues as Diane steps off the carousel, and another Diane steps up to begin the journey from cancer diagnosis to wellness.

> ### BOX 6.10 Steps for *Prāṇic* Energization Technique (PET)
>
> **Suveena Guglani**
>
> PET is an advanced yogic technique that summons *prāṇaśakti* (life energy) to energize the entire body. This was developed at S-VYASA Yoga University in Bengaluru, India, pioneered under the expert guidance of Dr. H. R. Nagendra and Dr. Nagarathna. Their research shows every system and organ of the body can be revitalized by this process, and it can strengthen the immune system (Nagendra et al. 2005).
>
> *(continued)*

---

[1]Edmonton Symptom Assessment System (ESAS-r), Pittsburgh Sleep Quality Index (PSQI), Hospital Anxiety and Depression Scale (HADS-A), Center for Epidemiologic Studies–Depression scale (CES-D), General Anxiety Disorder (GAD-7)

BOX 6.10 continued

1. Breath awareness and balancing of breath

- In a supine position, observe the breath at the tip of the nostrils. Let the breathing be totally natural without any manipulation.

- Feel the cool air entering the nostrils and the warm air coming out.

- Trace the cool air from the tip of the nose through the nasal tract, throat, trachea, bronchi, and lungs and the warm air back from the lungs, bronchi, trachea, throat, nasal tract, and tip of the nose.

2. Recognition of the energy breath (*vyāna; one of the five prāna-s*))

- Gently adopt *cinmudrā* (see Figure 6.3 for *mudrā-s*) by touching the tips of the index fingers to the tips of the thumbs. Observe the pulse, heartbeat, and their synchronization. Press and release the index finger and the thumb without losing contact and feel the nerve impulses going along the hand to the brain. Continue for a few rounds and then gently stop the practice.

- Adopt *cinmayamudrā* by placing the tips of the index finger and the thumb together and folding the remaining fingers to touch the palms. Press and release all fingers without losing contact with the thumb and the palms and feel the nerve impulses rising to the brain. Let the face be smiling and the whole body relaxed.

- Gently move to the next *mudrā* (hand gesture) by folding the thumb and closing the remaining fingers over the thumb forming *adhimudrā*. Press and release and feel the avalanche of nerve impulses to the brain.

- Next, adopt *namaskāramudrā* by joining the palms, and feel the pulse and the heartbeat. Press and release the palms, and feel the nerve impulses from the hand moving towards the brain. Chant *ṃ-kāra* and feel the vibrations and resonance.

- Now slowly separate the palms and move them

(continued)

(continued)

- away from each other and then join them again. Continue this movement for a few rounds and feel the space between the palms getting sensitized. Experience *vyāna* (energy breath) in that space. Now rotate the palms clockwise and anticlockwise churning the *vyāna*. Repeat this for a few rounds.

3. Movement and rotation of the energy breath (*vyāna*)

- Now place the palms on the knees and start moving the *vyāna* from the right heel, calf muscle, from under the thigh, right buttock, right lower back and all along the way up to the shoulder. Then move the *vyāna* from the fingers to the palms, wrist, forearm, upper arms, and shoulder, and join this *vyāna* at the shoulder level below the neck along with the *vyāna* which was brought from the heels. Then move it upwards from the back of the head, and coming down to the right forehead, right eye, and right nostril, down to the right side of the neck, chest and abdomen, further down to the right pelvis, thigh, knee, and shin, right up to the toes. Also move the *vyāna* downwards from the shoulders up to the fingers. Repeat the same on the left side and then both sides.

4. Balancing and energization

- We shall now move the *vyāna* from the higher density regions to the lower density regions. For this, please compare the right side of the body with the left side, and the front side with the back side. Recognize the imbalance, then move the *vyāna* from the higher density regions to the lower density regions. After this practice, you may feel balanced and energized.

5. Silence

- Feel the *vyāna* around the body expanding and diffusing into the infinite blue sky. Experience the expansive silence and the associated bliss. Try to remain in this blissful and expansive state for as long as you can.

6. Resolve

- Now take a resolve. A resolve is a positive state-

(continued)

ment with minimum words. Resolve needs to be in the present continuous tense in your own mother language, e.g., "I am blissful," "My immune system is very powerful." Repeat the resolve nine times with utmost faith.

2.11 Creating *saṅgha* through videoconferencing

Background: Telehealth

Stella Snyder, PhD student, MS, C-IAYT

The COVID-19 pandemic was an inflection point that caused yoga therapists and teachers around the world to pivot, and offer their classes through the "Zoom Room" and other online equivalents. For many people with cancer this was advantageous, as they found they could practice without leaving the comfort of home, which was especially relevant for patients with immune issues. However, social isolation and other psychosocial issues already experienced by the cancer population became magnified in the face of self-quarantine, and the social distancing required to mitigate viral infection. But the question remained, how can we create *saṅgha* on Zoom?

Our cancer clinic found that a series of yoga therapy sessions for both the patient and their primary caregiver (a "dyad" or twosome) can provide an intimate space for healing during cancer treatment and create a sense of connection and support. It is an opportunity for the dyad to express emotions and thoughts to each other. They attend sessions together and this helps provide additional support with issues such as modifications and alignment. An additional benefit is that they both learn yogic techniques to help manage stress and anxiety.

Patient story: Adam and John

Stella Snyder

Adam (he/him) is a 34-year-old White man diagnosed with late-stage head and neck cancer. His partner John is in attendance as his caregiver.

Adam and John have come to our cancer center from out of state. They are staying in a local Airbnb while Adam receives five weeks of proton beam therapy (a form of radiation) with concurrent chemotherapy for his stage IV head and neck cancer. John has some experience with meditation and is the driving force behind Adam's participation in yoga therapy, which due to COVID-19, is now delivered exclusively online. The couple uses the Zoom platform on their personal laptop for our 15 private yoga therapy sessions (see Figure 6.9). They are one-hour long sessions spread out over the duration of the radiation treatment (around three yoga therapy sessions per week). The sessions are introduced and instructed through videoconference, and they mostly participate from their bedroom in the Airbnb. The wireless connection is strongest there, and it provides a quiet, private space for the practice. We always begin our sessions with joint loosening movements (*sūkṣmavyāyāma*) (gentle stretching) in chairs, then move to standing postures, and then use the bed for guided relaxation – *prāṇāyāma* (breath-work), imagery, and meditation. Adam and John are encouraged to practice at home, in between sessions, and recordings are provided.

As Adam goes through radiation treatment, he becomes weaker, and modifications to this practice are made. The videoconference yoga therapy sessions still create a space where they feel comfortable engaging and sharing. Adam has anxiety around his radiation mask, a common issue amongst patients with head and neck cancer. The face mask used for radiation to the head and neck area must fit very closely, to stabilize the area during treatment. For most patients, this face mask can cause feelings of claustrophobia, as well as fear of choking on saliva or mucus. Benzodiazepines are commonly used for these anxieties. (In our cancer clinic we have observed that some of the patients with cancer who participate in our yoga therapy sessions are eventually able to replace their anxiety medication with calming *prāṇāyāma* techniques or imagery practices.) Adam also has had a close friend that died due to choking on thickened mucus while receiving similar radiation treatment, which intensifies his anxiety. This comes up in our second session. On the Zoom screen,

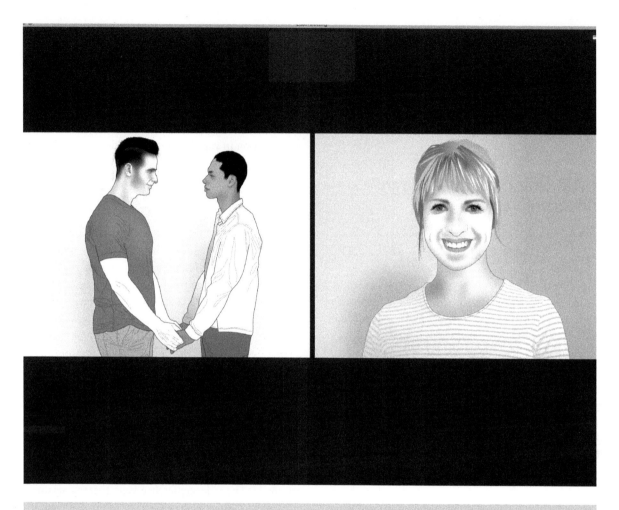

Figure 6.9
Telehealth yoga therapy

Adam and John tear up as they describe the trauma of losing their friend, as Adam expresses his heightened fear of choking during his treatment. I express sympathy to the couple for the loss of a friend and offer the idea of honoring that friend in some way while Adam is going through treatment.

This will provide the opportunity to practice cognitive reframing, or yogic philosophy's *pratipakṣabhāvāna* (the practice of cultivating thoughts to transform perceptions and experience). If Adam reframes the memory of his friend as something that will provide strength and support during treatment, it may reduce his fear and anxiety. Adam does eventually happily tell me that he's eliminated Ativan (lorazepam) from his pre-treatment routine, and instead uses imagery of his friend standing by his side, and the extended exhale *prāṇāyāma* we have been practicing.

The benefits of having a caregiver present during a videoconference session are apparent throughout the practice. This can be helpful due to the limited view-range using Zoom on a laptop. John is there to adjust Adam's alignment during tree pose (*vṛkṣāsana*), gently correcting his alignment of his lower leg. John also helps Adam get comfortable for guided relaxation and imagery, something that the yoga therapist would normally assist with when in-person. While the yoga therapist is normally able to observe the patient's breath rate, and other subtle, telling reflections of the patient's experience, these details can be difficult to pick up through videoconference sessions. Thankfully, the caregiver is available as a watchful extra set of eyes.

Toward the end of Adam's radiation treatment, more of the practice is done from the chair. Adam hasn't been eating or sleeping well, due to pain from radiation to the neck and mouth area. His energy is low, but he stays positive. There are days that I know he would cancel if our sessions involved him getting in the car, driving to our clinical space, and practicing yoga in-person. With the videoconference sessions, all Adam has to do is turn on the laptop and tell me what he feels able to do. Sometimes it's only a little gentle joint-loosening movements (*sūkṣmavyāyāma*) in the chair, and guided relaxation and imagery.

For Adam's last day of treatment, I drive to the proton therapy center to show support on his final day. The couple is elated to finally meet me in person (six feet away, with masks, due to COVID-19). Sadly, there are no hugs given, but there is still the feeling of *saṅgha* (community) and connection, created even through the veil of videoconferencing.

2.12 Oncology in-patient: delivering yoga at the hospital bedside

Background: In-patient yoga therapy

Johanne Lauktien, BA, RYT 500, C-IAYT and Leigh Leibel

Hospital admissions are part of the care trajectory of patients with cancer, often because of treatment complications such as neutropenia, thrombocytopenia, anemia,

infections, fever, mucositis, dehydration, and nausea and vomiting (Saxena et al. 2021). In fact, most older patients experience at least one hospitalization within 12 months of their cancer diagnosis, and the resulting prolonged bed rest can lead to unnecessary declines in function, muscle weakness and atrophy, pneumonia and other infections, and anxiety and depression (Halpern et al. 2020).

With medical permission, a wide variety of yogic techniques can be adapted for the hospital bedside and may be performed supine or seated, taking care with the IV (intravenous) pole, heart monitor, bags, and other devices and equipment. In the case of a critical illness requiring a stay in the intensive care unit (ICU), there are several research studies on the positive effects of early mobilization and rehabilitation. In 2017, a meta-analysis found that physical inactivity of patients in the ICU increases the risk for muscle weakness, delirium, and prolonged mechanical ventilation (Nydahl et al. 2017). These complications can lead to physical and cognitive impairments that can persist for years after discharge from the ICU.

Whether in the ICU or an in-patient oncology or specialty unit, yoga interventions at the bedside can mitigate many treatment side effects while safely increasing the level of physical activity through gentle movements and breathing tece weakness, and calming anxiety.

Patient story: Mario

Johanne Lauktien

Mario (he/his) is a 46-year-old Hispanic man diagnosed with hematologic cancer. His wife Carmen is in attendance as his caregiver.

Mario was diagnosed with non-Hodgkin lymphoma and had been admitted to the hospital for infusion chemotherapy, a grueling five consecutive-day regimen of multiple anti-cancer drugs. His wife Carmen is staying with him. They traveled from Colombia to receive treatment in Miami. They are far away from home. On day three,

I met Mario and Carmen in his new confined space – his room in the hospital – while they are watching the popular Telemundo show "Don Francisco Te Invita." Due to treatment, Mario is experiencing lack of sleep, pain and weakness, fatigue, nausea and vomiting, as well as lack of appetite. His emotional state is of constant anxiety, and he is angry with life.

Along with the news of a cancer diagnosis, a year ago he lost his company: "I am beginning to recognize the long-held sadness and anger accumulated inside me after losing my company"; then he says, "pain uncovers deep holdings within." Mario is ready to participate wholeheartedly in his discomforts and begin to release them. I explain how yoga, relaxation, breathing, and meditation can support his mind-body connection, and suggest we begin by paying close attention to discomfort through a "body sweeping" practice done in the spirit of discovery: turning toward the experience of the body with kindness, acceptance, compassion, and gratitude. I then guide him to gently engage the muscles of the lower and upper extremities while synchronizing the movement with breath to bring a meditative quality (Box 6.11). We practice with awareness of the breath, the physical movements, and the interaction between the various components of the body (bones, joints, ligaments, muscles). Mario and Carmen can do this together in the hospital several times a day.

> **BOX 6.11 A gentle sequence for the bedside**
>
> **Johanne Lauktien**
>
> Raise the head of the bed (Figure 6.10). When directing gentle movements, be sure to avoid direct compression of any lesion or tumor and do not strain a bone with metastasis. If there is a history of bone metastasis or osteoporosis, follow the accepted protocols for bone safety.
>
> - Lying stretch (fingers to toes)
>
> - Leg, ankle, and wrist rotation and bending
>
> *(continued)*

> *(continued)*
>
> - Hand clenching
>
> - Neck movements and shoulder roll
>
> - Lying gentle spinal twist
>
> - Guided meditation
>
> - Breathing guided practice: inhaling to count of 3, exhaling to count of 6 (with no breath holding in between)

2.13 Strength, step by step

Background: Exercise during cancer

Leigh Leibel

Strong epidemiologic evidence suggests that physical activity plays a critical role in improving the clinical and functional outcomes of many people with cancer (Mitgaard et al. 2015). Research also shows that physical activity can reduce the risk of cancer-specific and all-cause mortality for people diagnosed with early-stage breast, colorectal, and prostate cancers (Patel et al. 2019, Campbell et al. 2019, Schmitz et al. 2005). Given the data, physical activity has a strong evidence base to support its inclusion in most cancer care plans and can be recommended regardless of the type of cancer.

> People with cancer and survivors should always receive medical clearance before beginning any kind of physical activity program, including yoga.

Several organizations have issued recommendations and guidelines for exercise in cancer populations, including the National Comprehensive Cancer Network (NCCN), American Cancer Society (ACS), and the American College of Sports Medicine (ACSM). But not all people with cancer and survivors are able to engage in traditional aerobic and resistance training – for

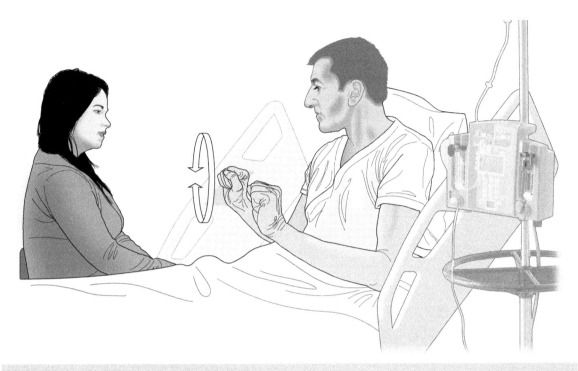

Figure 6.10
Bedside yoga

example, they may be too fatigued or ill to do so. There-fore, there is increased interest in exploring the safety and efficacy of different types of physical activity that fall outside of the exercise mainstream. With the increasing popularity of *Haṭha* yoga and other kinds of yoga in oncology, researchers are measuring the inten-sity of various yoga practices.

A 2016 systematic review of energy cost and meta-bolic equivalent of task (METs) of postural yoga practices suggests yoga is typically classified as a light-intensity physical activity. However, a few sequences and poses, including sun salutation (*sūryanamaskāra*), meet the criteria for moderate- to vigorous-intensity activity. The study concludes that in accordance with the NCCN, ACS, and ACSM recommendations for physical activity among people with cancer and survivors, the practice of *āsana* (posture) sequences with MET intensities higher than three (i.e., >10 min) can be accumulated through-out the day and count toward daily recommendations for moderate- or vigorous-intensity physical activity (Larsen-Meyer 2016).

Metabolic equivalent of task (MET)

A measure called the metabolic equivalent of task, or MET, is used to characterize the intensity of physi-cal activity. One MET is the rate of energy expended by a person sitting at rest. Light-intensity activities expend less than three METs, moderate-intensity activities expend three to six METs, and vigorous activi-ties expend six or more METs.

A customized yoga practice can address a patient's unique needs and can be titrated – *step by step* – to address cardiovascular fitness, muscular strength, and flexibility in a progressive manner, while balancing rest with increased activity. While more research is needed to understand the energy expenditure of yoga as a form of exercise, even if a yoga program does not reach the exercise goals recommended in the guidelines, it can promote required physical activity during cancer treatment, and help prepare the patient/client to engage in recommended types and levels of exercise over their lifetime.

> *Step by step,* a yoga practice can help people with cancer and survivors *strengthen* mind, body, and soul … *firm and steady, with gentleness and ease.*

Client story: Frances

Sharon Holly, E-RYT 500, RCYT, C-IAYT

Frances (she/her) is a 64-year-old White woman with a diagnosis of leiomyosarcoma, a rare and aggressive smooth muscle tumor.

Frances is a recently retired elementary school English teacher. She had been experiencing acid reflux which led her doctor to order a series of tests that led to the discovery of a 7-cm mass in her abdomen. Her specific kind of tumor typically has a five-year survival rate of

less than 50%. Her medical team recommended surgery and chemotherapy, followed by radiation.

Frances is referred to me by a mutual friend, and I meet her two weeks after her first chemotherapy treatment. She tells me she is experiencing a variety of symptoms including fatigue, difficulty with sleep, shortness of breath, nausea and constipation, and loss of appetite. She is also feeling lethargic, depressed, and anxious. In addition to dealing with the stress of this cancer diagnosis, she tells me she is caring for her ill father who was a Holocaust survivor, and that five years earlier, she lost her sister to breast cancer.

During our first session we discuss her goals. She says she is desperate to regain her quality of life, and maintaining strength during treatment is foremost on her list. Another big concern is being out of breath and not being able to take her beloved dog Shmoopy, a six-year-old Jack Russell terrier, for long walks. We decide to first address her stress and anxiety, and as she feels more balanced over the next weeks and months, we will begin introducing some gentle strengthening and active movement. I introduce her to various breathing practices (*prāṇāyāma*) and meditation to calm her nervous system. She especially likes cooling breath (*śītalī*)

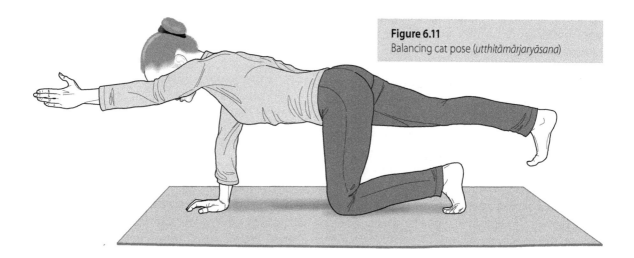

Figure 6.11
Balancing cat pose (*utthitāmārjaryāsana*)

and alternate nostril breathing (*nāḍīśodhana;* see Figure 6.2). I lead her through a guided *yoganidrā* (yogic sleep) meditation and provide a recording to help her with sleep.

In our next session, Frances tells me that she made good use of these breathing techniques when her anxiety began to rise at her last doctor's visit. When the nurse took her blood pressure after a brief breath practice, it was lower than it had been on previous visits. Since she is feeling a little stronger this session, I introduce her to an extended exhale breathing practice called *laṅghana* and combine it with gentle supine neck and shoulder stretches, as well as a gentle windshield wiper twist that she can do in bed.

Over the next several sessions, Frances reports that her sleep has improved. We continue *laṅghana* breath and integrate it with various gentle lower body poses such as knees to chest (*apanāsana*) and child's pose (*bālāsana*), moving on the exhale. Later, we add lying down pigeon (*suptakapotāsana*) and three-way hamstring stretch with a strap (i.e., central, external rotation, internal rotation of the hip). As we try these various poses, I invite her to check in with the felt sense in her body. I also check in with her in the days following our sessions to make sure we are moving in the right direction. She finds these practices are helping to ease the pain and the discomfort of constipation and sciatica.

Each session we have together is different. On days when Frances has a little more energy, we add gentle bridge pose (*setubandhasarvāṅgāsana*) and balancing cat pose (*utthitāmārjaryāsana;* Figure 6.11). On days she's fatigued, we do simple meditation and breathing. Sometimes it is one *krama-s* forward and two *krama* back.

One day she tells me her daughter is pregnant! This will be her first grandchild, a new motivation and purpose for living. Frances is dedicated, and

within another five months she is comfortably doing standing poses, such as dynamic warrior I and II (*vīrabhadrāsana I* and *vīrabhadrāsana II*) as well as warrior III (*vīrabhadrāsana III*) and tree (*vṛkṣāsana*). She is feeling more energized, sleeping better, and breathing more easefully. She has gradually increased her walks (with Shmoopy!) from ten minutes to forty minutes, and the walk often includes a small hill. With this newfound strength I can now introduce more active physical movement in our sessions to promote cardiovascular health. Energized, Frances flies off with her family to see her favorite band, Pearl Jam, in concert. She texts me, "I am so grateful. I am dancing and having the best time ever!"

Krama by *krama*

Vinyāsa (movement with breath) and *krama* (succession or steps) are fundamental yogic concepts that describe how a practice is constructed that is gradual and well thought-out, attaining a balance between *sthira* (firm and steady) and *sukha* (gentleness and ease). The first step or *krama* begins with *prāṇāyāma* (breath practice), then combined with *āsana* (dynamic movement) to warm up the muscles. The next *krama* is a static *āsana* (holding a posture) followed by breath extension or retention to build strength. At each session, progress is assessed, and together, yoga therapist and patient/client decide if they are ready to move to the next *krama*.

Section 2 references

Introduction

Danhauer, S.C., Addington, E.L., Cohen, L., et al., 2019. Yoga for symptom management in oncology: a review of the evidence base and future directions for research. *Cancer.* 125:1979–1989.

International Agency on Cancer Research (IARC), 2020. Latest global cancer data: cancer burden rises to 19.3 million new cases and 10.0 million cancer deaths in

2020. Available at: https://www.iarc.who.int/wp-content/uploads/2020/12/pr292_E.pdf.

Lin, P.J., Peppone, L.J., Janelsins, M.C., et al., 2018. Yoga for the management of cancer treatment-related toxicities. *Current Oncology Reports.* 20(1):5.

Milbury, K., Mallaiah, S., Mahajan, A., et al., 2018. Yoga program for high-grade glioma patients undergoing radiotherapy and their family caregivers. *Integr Cancer Ther.* 17:332–336.

Milbury, K., Liao, Z., Shannon, V., et al., 2019. Dyadic yoga program for patients undergoing thoracic radiotherapy and their family caregivers: results of a pilot randomized controlled trial. *Psychooncology.* 28:615–621.

Mustian, K.M., Sprod, L.K., Janelsins, M., et al., 2013. Multicenter, randomized controlled trial of yoga for sleep quality among cancer survivors. *J Clin Oncol.* 31:3233–3241.

National Cancer Institute (NCI), 2020. Cancer Statistics. Available at: https://www.cancer.gov/about-cancer/understanding/statistics.

Solzhenitsyn, Aleksandr, 1974. *Cancer Ward.* Farrar, Straus and Giroux; New York: p. 476.

2.1 Yoga in pediatric oncology – helping a child connect to his personal power

American Childhood Cancer Organization (ACCO), 2021. Childhood Cancer Statistics. Available at: https://www.acco.org/childhood-cancer-statistics/.

Kazak, A.E., Baxt, C., 2007. Families of infants and young children with cancer: a post-traumatic stress framework. *Pediatr Blood Cancer.* 49(7 Suppl):1109–1113.

Mu, P.F., Lee, M.Y., Sheng, C.C., et al., 2015. The experiences of family members in the year following the diagnosis of a child or adolescent with cancer: a qualitative systematic review. *JBI Database System Rev Implement Rep.* 13(5):293–329.

National Cancer Institute (NCI),2021. Childhood Cancers. Available at: https://www.cancer.gov/types/childhood-cancers.

Steliarova-Foucher, E., Colombet, M., Ries, L., et al., 2017. International incidence of childhood cancer, 2001–10: a population-based registry study. *Lancet Oncology.* 18(6):719–731.

2.2 Yoga for scan anxiety after a brain cancer diagnosis

Abreu, C., Grilo, A., Lucena, F., Carolino, E., 2017. Oncological patient anxiety in imaging studies: the PET/CT example. *Journal of Cancer Education.* 32(4), 820–826.

Bates, G.E., Mostel, J.L., Hesdorffer, M., 2017. Cancer-related anxiety. *JAMA Oncol.* 3(7):1007.

Deimling, G.T., Bowman, K.F., Sterns, S. et al., 2006. Cancer-related health worries and psychological distress among older adult, long-term cancer survivors. *Psychooncology.* 15: 306–320.

Feiler, B., 2011. Scanxiety. *Time.* Available at: http://content.time.com/time/specials/packages/article/0,28804,2075133_2075127_2075107,00.html.

Milbury, K., Li, J., Weathers, S.P., et al., 2019. Pilot randomized, controlled trial of a dyadic yoga program for glioma patients undergoing radiotherapy and their family caregivers. *Neuro oncol Pract.* 6(4):311–320.

Thompson, C.A., Charlson, M.E., Schenkein, E., et al., 2010. Surveillance CT scans are a source of anxiety and fear of recurrence in long-term lymphoma survivors. *Annals of Oncology.* 21: 2262–2266.

2.3 Titrating effort and ease for cancer fatigue

Bower, J.E., Garet, D., Sternlieb, B., et al., 2012. Yoga for persistent fatigue in breast cancer survivors: a randomized controlled trial. *Cancer.* 118(15): 3766–75.

Henry, D.H., Viswanathan, H.N., Elkin, E.P., et al., 2008. Symptoms and treatment burden associated with cancer treatment: results from a cross-sectional national survey in the U.S. *Support Care Cancer.* 16:791–801.

NCCN, 2022. NCCN Clinical Practice Guidelines in Oncology. Cancer Related-Fatigue. Available at: https://www.nccn.org/professionals/physician_gls/pdf/fatigue.pdf

Patel, A.V., Friedenreich, C.M., Moore, S.C., et al., 2019. American College of Sports Medicine Roundtable Report on Physical Activity, Sedentary Behavior, and Cancer Prevention and Control. *Med Sci Sports Exerc.* 51(11):2391–2402.

2.4 Embracing the challenges: axillary web syndrome – an underrecognized consequence of breast cancer surgery

Koehler, L.A., Blaes, A.H., Haddad, T.C., et al., 2015. Movement, function, pain, and postoperative edema in axillary web syndrome. *Physical Therapy.* 95(10), 1345–1353.

O'Toole, J., Miller, C.L., Specht, M.C., et al., 2013. Cording following treatment for breast cancer. *Breast Cancer Res Treat.* 140:105–111.

Torres Lacomba, M., Mayoral Del Moral, O., Coperias Zazo, J.L., et al., 2009. Axillary web syndrome after axillary dissection in breast cancer. *Breast Cancer Res Treat.* 117:625–630.

Yeung, W.M., McPhail, S.M., Kuys, S.S., 2014. A systematic review of axillary web syndrome. *J Cancer Surviv.* 9:576–598.

2.5 Cancer while Black – role of yoga in trauma stewardship and advocacy during breast cancer

Akinyemiju, T., Wilson, L.E., Deveaux, A., et al., 2020. Association of allostatic load with all-cause and cancer mortality by race and body mass index in the REGARDS Cohort. *Cancers.* 12(6):1695.

American Association of Cancer Research (AACR), 2021. Cancer Disparities Progress Report. Available at: https://cancerprogressreport.aacr.org/disparities/.

American Cancer Society (ACS), 2022. Cancer Disparities in the Black Community. Available at: https://www.cancer.org/about-us/what-we-do/health-equity/cancer-disparities-in-the-black-community.html

Cure Today, 2021. Cancer While Black: How Trauma, Fear, Generational Pain & Mistrust Impact Breast Cancer. Available at: https://www.curetoday.com/view/october-2020-cancer-while-black-how-trauma-fear-generational-pain-and-mistrust-impact-breast-cancer.

Ford, J.D., Courtois, C., 2020. *Treating Complex Traumatic Stress Disorders in Adults: Scientific Foundations and Therapeutic Models.* 2nd edition. Guilford Press.

National Cancer Institute (NCI), 2020. Cancer Disparities. Available at: https://www.cancer.gov/about-cancer/understanding/disparities.

Stephens, Mark, 2017. *Yoga Therapy Foundations, Methods and Practices for Common Ailments.* North Atlantic Books.

Van Der Kolk, B., 2015. *The Body Keeps the Score: Brain, Mind, and Body in the Healing of Trauma.* Viking.

Van Dernoot Lipsky, L., Burk, C., 2009. *Trauma Stewardship: An Everyday Guide to Caring for Self While Caring for Others.* Berrett-Koehler Publishers.

2.6 Yoga and lymphedema secondary to cancer treatment – the priority is *ahiṃsā* or "do no harm"

Aggithaya, M., Narahari, S., Ryan, T., 2015. Yoga for correction of lymphedema's impairment of gait as an adjunct to lymphatic drainage: a pilot observational study. *International Journal of Yoga.* 8:54–6.

Australasian Lymphology Association, 2019. ALA Position Statement on Early Detection of Breast Cancer-Related Lymphoedema. Available at: https://www.lymphoedema.org.au/about-lymphoedema/position-statements/.

Australasian Lymphology Association, 2020. About Lymphoedema. What is Lymphoedema? Available at: https://www.lymphoedema.org.au/about-lymphoedema/what-is-lymphoedema/.

Barbieux, R., Roman, M.M., Rivière, F., et al., 2019. Scintigraphic investigations of the deep and superficial lymphatic systems in the evaluation of lower limb oedema. *Science Reports.* 9(13691).

Baumann, F.T., Reike, A., Reimer, V., Schumann, M., Hallek, M., Taaffe, D.R., et al., 2018. Effects of physical exercise on breast cancer-related secondary lymphedema: a systematic review. *Breast Cancer Res Treat.* 170:1–3.

Fu, M.R., Ridner, S.H., Hu, S.H., et al., 2013. Psychosocial impact of lymphedema: a systematic review of literature from 2004 to 2011. *Psychooncology.* 22:1466–84.

International Society of Lymphology, 2016. The diagnosis and treatment of peripheral lymphoedema. Consensus document of the International Society of Lymphology. *Lymphology.* 49(4):170–184.

Loudon, A., Barnett, T., Piller, N., et al., 2014. Yoga management of breast cancer-related lymphoedema: a randomised controlled pilot-trial. *BMC Complementary and Alternative Medicine.* 14(214):1–13.

Loudon, A., Barnett, T., Piller, N., et al., 2016. The effects of yoga on shoulder and spinal actions for women with breast cancer related lymphoedema of the arm: a randomised controlled pilot study. *BMC Complementary and Alternative Medicine.* 16(343):1–15.

Loudon, A., Barnett, T., Williams, A., et al., 2017. Guidelines for teaching yoga to women with breast cancer-related lymphoedema: an evidence-based approach. *International Journal of Yoga Therapy.* 27(1):95–112.

Mazor, M., Lee, J.Q., Peled, A., et al., 2019. The effect of yoga on arm volume, strength, and range of motion in women at risk for breast cancer-related lymphedema. *Journal of Alternative and Complementary Medicine.* 24(2):154–160.

Olsson Möller, U., Beck, I., Rydén, L., Malmström, M.A., 2019. A comprehensive approach to rehabilitation interventions following breast cancer treatment – a systematic review of systematic reviews. *BMC Cancer.* 19(1):472.

Pasyar, N., Barshan Tashnizi, N., Mansouri, P., Tahmasebi, S., 2019. Effect of yoga exercise on the Quality of Life and upper extremity volume among women with breast cancer related lymphedema: a pilot study. *European Journal of Oncology Nursing.* 42:103–109.

Penny, J., Sturgeon, R., 2021. *An Integrative Approach to Cancer Care.* Handspring.

Saraswathi, V., Latha, S., Niraimathki, K. Vidhubala, E., 2021. Managing lymphedema, increasing range of motion and quality of life through yoga therapy among breast cancer survivors: a systematic review. *Int J Yoga.* 14:3–17.

Schmitz, K.H., Troxel, A.B., Cheville, A., Grant, L.L., Bryan, C.J., Gross, C.R., Lytle, L.A., Ahmed, R.L., 2009. Physical Activity and Lymphedema (the PAL trial): assessing the safety of progressive strength training in breast cancer survivors. *Contemporary Clinical Trials.* 30(3):233–245.

Singh, B., DiSipio, T., Peake, J., Hayes, S., 2016. Systematic review and meta-analysis of the effects of exercise for those with cancer-related lymphedema. *Archives of Physical Medicine and Rehabilitation.* 97(2): 302–315.

Suami, H., Scaglioni, M.F., 2018. Anatomy of the lymphatic system and the lymphosome concept with reference to lymphedema. *Seminars in Plastic Surgery.* 32(1):5–11.

Wanchai, A., Armer, J.M., 2020. The effects of yoga on breast cancer-related lymphedema: a systematic review. *Journal of Health Research.* 34(5):409–418.

2.7 Delivering yoga therapy in the chemotherapy infusion center – expanding the reach of mind-body therapies to patients in clinical settings

Sohl, S.J., Danhauer, S.C., Birdee, G.S., et al., 2016. A brief yoga intervention implemented during chemotherapy: a randomized controlled pilot study. *Complement Ther Med.* 25:139–42.

2.8 Coming of age with cancer – adolescents and young adults (AYAs)

American Cancer Society, 2020. Cancer Facts & Figures 2020. Cancer Statistics Center. Available at: http://cancerstatisticscenter.cancer.org.

Aubin, S., Rosberger, Z., Hafez, N., et al., 2019. Cancer!? I don't have time for that: impact of a psychosocial intervention for young adults with cancer. *Journal of Adolescent and Young Adult Oncology.* 8(2):172–189.

Cavallo, J., 2019. How cancer affects adolescents and young adults: a roundtable discussion with cancer survivors Lauren Ramer, Brian G. Smith, and Amanda Boser. *The ASCO Post.* Available at: https://www.ascopost.com/issues/may-25-2019/how-cancer-affects-adolescents-and-young-adults/.

Coccia, P.F., 2019. Overview of adolescent and young adult oncology. *Journal of Oncology Practice.* Available at: https://ascopubs.org/doi/abs/10.1200/JOP.19.00075.

Figueroa Gray, M., Ludman, E.J., Beatty, T., et al., 2018. Balancing hope and risk among adolescent and young adult cancer patients with late-stage cancer:

a qualitative interview study. *J Adolesc Young Adult Oncol.* 7(6):673–680.

Keegan, T.H., Ries, L.A., Barr, R.D. et al., 2016. Comparison of cancer survival trends in the United States of adolescents and young adults with those in children and older adults. *Cancer.* 122:1009–1016.

Knox, M., Hales, S., Nissim, R., et al., 2016. Lost and stranded: the experience of younger adults with advanced cancer. *Supportive Care in Cancer.* 25(2):399–407.

Lidington, E., Darlington, A.S., Din, A. et al., 2021. Describing unmet supportive care needs among young adults with cancer (25–39 years) and the relationship with health-related quality of life, psychological distress, and illness cognitions. *J Clin Med.* 10(19):4449.

Neff, K., 2019. Self Compassion. Available at: https://www.self-compassion.org.

Park, E.M., Rosenstein, D.L., 2015. Depression in adolescents and young adults with cancer. *Dialogues in Clinical Neuroscience.* 17(2):171–180.

Sanson-Daly, U.M, Wakefield, C.E., 2013. Distress and adjustment among adolescents and young adults with cancer: an empirical and conceptual review. *Translational Pediatrics.* 2(4):167–197.

Sender, A., Friedrich, M., Schmidt, R., Gueue, K., 2020. Cancer-specific distress, supportive care needs and satisfaction with psychosocial care in young adult cancer survivors. *European Journal of Oncology Nursing.* 44:101708.

Van der Gucht, K., Takano, K., Labarque, V. et al., 2017. Mindfulness-based intervention for adolescents and young adults after cancer treatment: effects on quality of life, emotional distress, and cognitive vulnerability. *J Adolesc Young Adult Oncol.* 6(2):307–317.

Zebrack, B., Bleyer, A., Albritton, K., et al., 2006. Assessing the health care needs of adolescent and young adult cancer patients and survivors. *Cancer.* 107(12):2915–2923.

Further reading

Cancer.Net, 2019. Coping with Changes to Your Body as a Young Adult. Available at: https://www.cancer.net/ navigating-cancer-care/young-adults-and-teenagers/ coping-with-changes-your-body-young-adult.

Chemocare, 2022. Depression and Chemotherapy. Available at: http://chemocare.com/chemotherapy/side-effects/ depression-and-chemotherapy.aspx.

Fardell, J.E., Patterson, P., Wakefield, C.E., et al., 2018. A narrative review of models of care for adolescents and young adults with cancer: barriers and recommendations. *Journal of Adolescent and Young Adult Oncology.* 7(2):148–152.

National Cancer Institute, 2020. Adolescents and Young Adults with Cancer. Available at: https://www.cancer.gov/ types/aya.

Muffly, L.S., Hlubocky, F.J., Khan, N., et al., 2016. Psychological morbidities in adolescent and young adult blood cancer patients during curative-intent therapy and early survivorship. *Cancer.* 2016 Mar 15;122(6):954–61.

2.9 Yoga to enhance caregiver connectedness during lung cancer treatment

Antoni, M.H., Dhabhar, F.S., 2019. Impact of psychosocial stress and stress management on immune responses in cancer patients. *Cancer.* 125(9):1417–1431.

Bevans, M., Sternberg, E.M., 2012. Caregiving burden, stress, and health effects among family caregivers of adult cancer patients. *JAMA.* 307(4), 398–403.

2.10 *Prāṇic* Energization Technique (PET) – can it improve symptoms associated with "chemo brain"?

Ahles, T.A., Saykin, A., Furstenberg, C.T., et al., 2002. Neuropsychologic impact of standard-dose systemic chemotherapy in long-term survivors of breast cancer and lymphoma. *J Clin Oncol.* 20:485–493.

Brezden, C.B., Phillips, K.A., Abdolell, M., et al., 2000. Cognitive function in breast cancer patients receiving adjuvant chemotherapy. *J Clin Oncol.* 18:2695–2701.

Cleeland, C.S., 2003. Are the symptoms of cancer and cancer treatment due to a shared biologic mechanism? A cytokine-immunologic model of cancer symptoms. *Cancer.* 97:2919–2925.

Jain, R.M., 2016. Effect of pranayama on cognitive functions of medical students. *Indian Journal of Basic and Applied Medical Research.* 6(1):471–476.

Jean-Pierre, P., 2010. Management of cancer-related cognitive dysfunction-conceptualization challenges and implications for clinical research and practice. *US Oncology.* 6:9–12.

Jerath, R., Edry, J.W., Barnes, V.A., Jerath, V., 2006. Physiology of long pranayamic breathing: neural respiratory elements may provide a mechanism that explains how slow deep breathing shifts the autonomic nervous system. *Medical Hypotheses.* 67(3):566–571.

Nagendra, H., 2005. *Pranic Energisation Technique (PET).* Swami Vivekananda Yoga Prakashana; Bangalore.

O'Shaughnessy, J.A., 2003. Chemotherapy-induced cognitive dysfunction: a clearer picture. *Clin Breast Cancer.* (Suppl. 2):S89–94.

Oswal, P., Nagarathna, R., Ebnezar, J., Nagendra, H.R., 2011. The effect of add-on yogic prana energization technique (YPET) on healing of fresh fractures: a randomized control study. *Journal of Alternative and Complementary Medicine.* 17:253–258.

Staat, K., Segatore, M., 2005. The phenomenon of chemobrain. *Clin J Oncol Nurs.* 9(6):713–721.

van Dam, F.S., Schagen, S.B., Muller, M.J., et al., 1998. Impairment of cognitive function in women receiving adjuvant treatment for high-risk breast cancer: high-dose versus standard-dose chemotherapy. *J Natl Cancer Inst.* 90:210–218.

Zauner, A., Daugherty, W.P., Bullock, M.R., Warner, D.S., 2002. Brain oxygenation and energy metabolism: part I-biological function and pathophysiology. *Neurosurgery.* 51(2):289–301; discussion 302.

Zelano, C.J., 2016. Nasal respiration entrains human limbic oscillations and modulates cognitive function. *Journal of Neuroscience.* 36(49):12448–12467.

2.12 Oncology in-patient – delivering yoga at the hospital bedside

Halpern, M.T., Zhang, F., Enewold, L., 2020. Hospitalizations following cancer diagnosis: national values for frequency, duration, and charges. *Journal of Clinical Oncology.* 38:15_suppl:12039.

Nydahl, P., Sricharoenchai, T., Chandra, S. et al., 2017. Safety of patient mobilization and rehabilitation in the intensive care unit. Systematic review with meta-analysis. *Ann Am Thorac Soc.* 14:766–777.

Saxena, A., Rubens, M., Ramamoorthy, V., et al., 2021. Hospitalization rates for complications due to systemic therapy in the United States. *Sci Rep.* 11:7385.

Further reading

Allen, C., Glasziou, P., Del Mar, C., 1999. Bed rest: a potentially harmful treatment needing more careful evaluation. *Lancet.* 354(9186):1229–1233.

Corcoran, P., 1991. Use it or lose it: the hazards of bed rest and inactivity. *West J Med.* 154(5):536–538.

Dittmer, D.K., Teasell, R., 1993. Complications of immobilization and bed rest, part 1: musculoskeletal and cardiovascular complications. *Can Fam Physician.* 39:1428–32, 1435–37.

Jairam, V., Lee, V., Park, H.S., et al., 2019. Treatment-related complications of systemic therapy and radiotherapy. *JAMA Oncol.* 5(7): 1028–1035.

2.13 Strength, step by step

Campbell, K.L., Winters-Stone, K.M., Wiskemann, J., et al., 2019. Exercise guidelines for cancer survivors: consensus statement from International Multidisciplinary Roundtable. *Medicine and Science in Sports and Exercise.* 51(11):2375–2390.

Larson-Meyer, D.E., 2016. A systematic review of the energy cost and metabolic intensity of yoga. *Med Sci Sports Exerc.* 48(8):1558–69.

Midtgaard, J., Hammer, N.M., Andersen, C., et al., 2015. Cancer survivors' experience of exercise-based cancer rehabilitation: a meta-synthesis of qualitative research. *Acta Oncol.* 54:609–617.

Patel, A.V., Friedenreich, C.M., Moore, S.C., et al., 2019. American College of Sports Medicine Roundtable Report on Physical Activity, Sedentary Behavior, and Cancer Prevention and Control. *Medicine and Science in Sports and Exercise.* 51(11):2391–2402.

Schmitz, K.H., Holtzman, J., Courneya, K.S., et al., 2005. Controlled physical activity trials in cancer survivors: a systematic review and meta-analysis. *Cancer Epidemiology, Biomarkers and Prevention.* 14(7):1588–1595.

Further reading

McTiernan, A., Friedenreich, C.M., Katzmarzyk, P.T., et al., 2019. Physical activity in cancer prevention and survival: a systematic review. *Medicine and Science in Sports and Exercise.* 51(6):1252–1261.

Rezende, L.F.M., Sá, T.H., Markozannes, G., et al., 2018. Physical activity and cancer: an umbrella review of the literature including 22 major anatomical sites and 770 000 cancer cases. *British Journal of Sports Medicine.* 52(13):826–833.

U.S. Department of Health and Human Services, 2018. 2018 Physical Activity Guidelines Advisory Committee Scientific Report. Available at: https://health.gov/sites/default/files/2019-09/PAG_Advisory_Committee_Report.pdf.

Section 3 Post treatment – cure, remission, or no evidence of disease (NED)

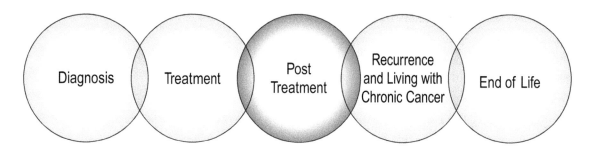

A bit of merry-making after long privation and powerlessness, the rejoicing of strength that is returning, of a reawakened faith in a tomorrow and the day after tomorrow, of a sudden sense and anticipation of a future, of impending adventures, of seas that are open again, of goals that are permitted again, believed again.

Friedrich Nietzsche,
The Gay Science

Introduction

Leigh Leibel

Post Treatment is the third of the five phases of the Yoga in the Cancer Care Continuum. In this phase of care, the primary or frontline treatment has been completed and the person with cancer is told they are cured, in remission, or have no evidence of disease (NED). *But for many, the end of cancer treatment doesn't mark the end of the cancer journey.*

While there are many cancer survivors who experience no physical after-effects of treatment and emerge with a renewed sense of life and purpose, many of the 32 million cancer survivors worldwide (Sung et al. 2021) will go on to face a host of unique medical, physical, functional, and psychosocial consequences of the disease and

its treatment for many months, years, or perhaps even the lifespan. To borrow a term coined during the global COVID-19 pandemic, they are cancer *long haulers*.

After months of harrowing and life-disruptive treatments, transitioning to a new way of life can be daunting for many survivors and their families as they adjust to new feelings, new and different medical problems, changes in support, financial impact of treatment, and different ways of looking at the world. Embedded within the construct of "survivorship" is also the ubiquitous need for routine medical surveillance to keep a watchful eye for cancer recurrence and/or signs and symptoms of adverse late effects of treatment. The byproduct is an anxiety-provoking landscape of physician check-ups, blood draws, and scans – for some, every three months,

What, exactly, is a cancer survivor?

The definition varies around the world: by country, by organization, and by individuals. In the United States, the National Institutes of Health/National Cancer Institute (NIH/NCI) and the American Cancer Society (ACS) describe a survivor as: "Everyone who's ever had cancer, from the time of diagnosis for the rest of their life." Family members are called "co-survivors."

continued

While this book follows the NIH/NCI definition of a cancer survivor, ultimately, it is up to each individual and their family to define what survivorship means to them personally.

for others, every six months. And as time passes without incident, many will graduate to yearly appointments and screenings, often for life. Because of this, the post treatment phase of cancer care marks the beginning of what is often called the *new normal* for this cohort of survivors.

The number of cancer survivors is growing. As mentioned in the introduction to this chapter, there are an estimated 32 million cancer survivors worldwide (IARC 2022), and as of January 2019, there were an estimated 16.9 million cancer survivors in the United States alone (NCI 2022). The U.S. number is projected to increase to 22.2 million by 2030 (NCI 2022); this is partly due to screening and early detection, improved therapies, and an aging population (Maule & Merletti 2012). The visibility of cancer survivors worldwide makes it increasingly clear that while many return to their pre-cancer routines and thrive, for many others, life after cancer treatment presents lasting challenges.

To better identify and address the unmet needs of cancer survivors, the National Coalition for Cancer Survivorship (NCCS) was established in 1985 in the United States to advocate for quality cancer care for all people touched by cancer. One of their early goals was to replace the words "cancer *victim*" with "cancer *survivor*" and create a different kind of cancer experience that embraced the full spectrum of survivorship and living well during treatment and beyond. In 2006, the Institute of Medicine (now the National Academy of Medicine[1]) issued a recommendation that every person with cancer in the United States should receive an individualized survivorship care plan with guidelines to monitor and maintain their health as they move beyond their treatment.

[1] National Academy of Medicine is a United States non-governmental agency that provides national and international advice on issues relating to health, medicine, health policy, and biomedical science.

The role of yoga in cancer survivorship

A successful transition from active cancer treatment to post-treatment care is critical to an individual's long-term health; today, in addition to regular visits to the oncologist, more and more cancer survivors worldwide are turning to integrative modalities that use holistic approaches to manage their ongoing concerns.

Given the popularity and widespread use of complementary therapies during and after cancer treatment, a growing number of randomized controlled trials and well-designed studies have begun to examine efficacy. Chief among these are mind-body interventions, defined by the National Center for Complementary and Integrative Health (NCCIH, the United States Federal Government's lead agency for scientific research on complementary and integrative approaches) as techniques designed to enhance the mind's capacity to affect bodily function and symptoms. Yoga is one such mind-body intervention that has been studied extensively in oncology populations. Evidence suggests yoga can improve overall health, quality of life, and physical function, as well as help reduce psychosocial distress, musculoskeletal symptoms, nausea, anxiety, depression, sleep disturbance, and fatigue – and it may have a positive effect on cognitive issues associated with treatment (Danhauer et al. 2019, Mustian et al. 2013, Chaoul et al. 2014, Narayanan et al. 2019).

Supported by solid research, in recent years clinical guidelines have begun including recommendations for nonpharmacologic therapies such as yoga and meditation to enhance quality of life among cancer survivors. In 2018, the Society for Integrative Oncology (SIO) issued evidence-based clinical practice guidelines the use of integrative therapies during and after cancer treatment. The guidelines were end the American Society for Clinical Oncolo The two organizations recommend yoga fo ety, as well as for improving quality of sive symptoms, fatigue, and sleep (

2022, SIO/ASCO issued guidelines for the use of Integrative Medicine for Pain Management in Adult Cancer Patients; yoga was included among the recommendations (Mao et al. 2022).

Society for Integrative Oncology (SIO)

According to its website, the Society for Integrative Oncology: "is a not-for-profit organization whose mission is to advance evidence-based, comprehensive, integrative healthcare to improve the lives of people affected by cancer. SIO encourages rigorous scientific evaluation of both pre-clinical and clinical science, while advocating for the transformation of oncology care to integrate evidence-based complementary approaches. The vision is to have research inform the true integration of complementary modalities into oncology care, so that evidence-based complementary care is accessible and part of standard cancer care for all patients across the cancer continuum. As an interdisciplinary and interprofessional society, SIO is uniquely poised to lead the 'bench to bedside' efforts in integrative cancer care. The Society brings together practitioners from multiple disciplines focused on the care of people with cancer and survivors" (SIO 2022). Society membership is open to anyone with an interest in integrative oncology, including yoga therapists and yoga professionals. SIO has an active Yoga Special Interest Group (SIG) with 50 members from US, Canada, UK, Australia, and India in 2022. Information: www.integrativeonc.org.

American Society of Clinical Oncology (ASCO)

The American Society of Clinical Oncology (ASCO), founded 1964, is the world's leading professional organization for physicians and oncology professionals caring for people with cancer. Information: www.asco.org

...milarly, the National Comprehensive Cancer Network (NCCN) *Survivorship Guidelines* recommend that ...nts "consider" yoga for improving distress, cog... functioning, menopausal symptoms, and pain

(Denlinger et al. 2018). Yoga is also listed in the NCCN *Clinical Practice Guidelines in Oncology* as an effective intervention for cancer-related fatigue and anticipatory nausea and vomiting (Berger et al. 2021, Ettinger et al. 2021). The guidelines suggest that when used in addition to conventional therapies, these interventions can help control symptoms and enhance patient well-being.

According to the 2017 National Health Interview Survey (NHIS) in the United States, the use of yoga among all populations increased (2012-2017) from 9.5% to 14.3%, and meditation from 4.1% to 14.2% (USDHHS 2018). However, a 2021 study (n=857) conducted by investigators at Memorial Sloan Kettering Cancer Center in New York City found that despite growing evidence supporting the benefits of yoga for cancer-related symptom management, yoga usage among cancer survivors is low (Desai et al. 2021). Investigators conclude patient preferences for yoga practice need to be adequately addressed in order to design effective yoga programs for people with cancer. We will discuss this in more detail in Chapter 7: Yoga Therapy in Oncologic Care - The Way Forward.

Those of us who practice yoga know through personal experience (the laboratory of our own bodies!) that it makes us feel good. But the reality is, it is solid research and scientific evidence that inform decision-making by healthcare professionals, health policymakers, and the public, regarding the integrated use of complementary health approaches in cancer care. The take-away for yoga professionals is:

1. Strong and growing evidence points to the benefits of yoga during cancer care and survivorship.

2. To design safe, effective, and inclusive yoga experiences for people who have experienced cancer and its treatment, their ongoing medical, physical, functional, psychosocial, as well as social determinants of health challenges must be considered.

3. We must ensure that yoga is available to all people, and we must train and mentor a more diverse yoga workforce.

As we have seen, the cancer journey doesn't always end with treatment.

On the following pages, twelve yoga professionals share stories of working with their patients and clients who are cancer survivors, all of whom experienced lingering symptoms and quality of life issues after completion of treatment. We'll see how incorporating yoga helped them live life more fully, robustly, and with joy. And in so doing, perhaps improved their overall health and well-being, and clinical outcomes.

3.1 Managing fear of cancer recurrence through efforts in "warrior-ness"

Background: Fear of cancer recurrence

Leigh Leibel

The fear of cancer recurrence (FCR) is a prevalent and widespread existential concern among cancer survivors, with nearly half reporting it provokes a moderate to high level of distress (Sharpe et al. 2018). FCR is defined as "fear or worry that cancer will return or progress" (Lebel et al. 2017). The often-consuming fear that cancer might eventually return is among a cancer survivor's most significant unmet needs (Simard et al. 2013). Mental health professionals understand this fear to be a situation-normal reaction to a cancer diagnosis and treatment, that can give rise to psychological sequelae (issues that arise following an initial event) such as intrusive thoughts about death and other post-traumatic symptoms. Examples include re-experiencing, avoidance, negative thoughts and feelings, and arousal or reactivity around cancer-related triggers or memories (Simonelli et al. 2017). While the intensity of fear may lessen over time, an individual may be triggered by many things, such as follow-up oncology visits, certain physical symptoms, the illness or death of a loved one, the anniversary date of the diagnosis, or even public health campaigns. Given the need for novel and effective treatments, multiple randomized controlled trials have examined the utility of mind-body approaches as an intervention to mitigate FCR's effect on survivors. According to a 2018 meta-analysis and systematic review by Daniel Hall, PhD and colleagues at Massachusetts General Hospital, Harvard Medical School, mind-body interventions (including yoga as meditative movement) are effective for reducing fear of cancer recurrence, with small-to-medium effect sizes persisting after the intervention ends (Hall et al. 2018).

Client Study: Simone

Teri Gandy-Richardson, RYT 500

Simone (she/her) is a 59-year-old Black woman diagnosed with triple negative breast cancer, who five years later received a diagnosis of myelodysplastic syndrome (MDS). This was likely caused by the first cancer treatment.

Simone is a strong, vibrant, tall, slender ex-athlete who is down to earth. She was referred to me over two years ago. We work together weekly. It's been 13 years since Simone was treated for triple-negative breast cancer, which was followed by a diagnosis of myelodysplastic syndrome (MDS) five years later. Long past treatment, Simone remains compromised by reduced upper body strength and range of motion in her arms and shoulders. She wants to build strength and reduce stress. My goal for Simone is to strategically employ yoga's blend of movement, stillness, and awareness to maximize her positive outlook, and to establish intelligent practices for longevity and graceful aging.

Before each session, I ask Simone how she's feeling. Today, Simone seems distracted with unusually low energy. "Are there any issues, pain or discomfort that require attention?," I ask. Simone shares that she's saddened by the passing of a colleague whose cancer had returned after many years. "I guess THAT possibility never completely goes away, huh?," she utters before revealing deeper concerns about recurrence apparently heightened by this difficult news. I relay that, "As survivors, while the fear of recurrence may never leave us, yoga is a tool that helps us connect to our bodies and builds our physical and emotional strength towards maintaining our health."

"It all begins with our breath," I say while placing two bolsters facing one another. I invite Simone to sit on one and position myself on the other. Once settled, I invite Simone to close her eyes. I guide her focus to the strength in her back…how engaged her muscles are to hold this posture while also supporting the lift of her chest. Next, I ask Simone to inhale and to experience the power of that. Her spine extends as breath fills her lungs.

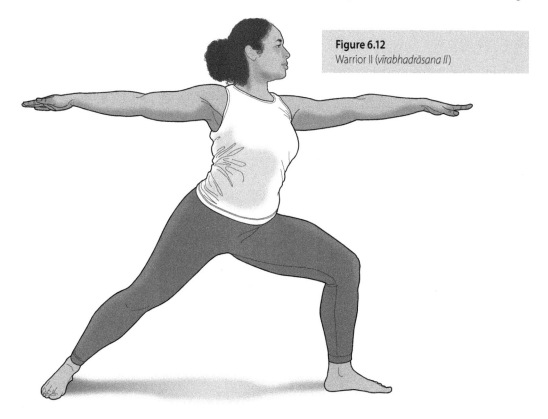

Figure 6.12
Warrior II (*vīrabhadrāsana II*)

Now, visibly more present, Simone is guided – on her exhale, to release, letting go of air and the holding on to anything that's possibly too much. We repeat this cycle a few more times. When we're done, Simone opens her eyes and appears lighter, steady, and ready to move on.

I wonder, "Simone, which of the yoga poses make you feel most strong?" She smiles and replies, "I feel strongest in warrior poses (*vīrabhadrāsana-s*). I also find that my balance is much better throughout the week after we practice and break down standing poses." To expand on that intelligence, I include a warrior I & II (*vīrabhadrāsana II & I*) *vinyāsa* (a sequence of moves). From warrior II (*vīrabhadrāsana II;* see Figure 6.12), I ask Simone to breathe into her lungs, expanding her ribcage and floating her arms out, and then up, while straightening her front leg. Then, we exhale and return to warrior II (*vīrabhadrāsana II*). Repeating this *vinyāsa*, together we revisit Simone's strength while acknowledging the ability in her back, arms, and legs required for this vigorous movement. Gradually, Simone embodies this pose. Through her own effort, body, and psyche, Simone collects the physical and emotional souvenirs of strength and autonomy. Having achieved this practice for herself, Simone now stands in "warrior-ness" towards managing her fears.

3.2 Tenderness and self-compassion: redefining strength after cancer

Background: Self-compassion

Leigh Leibel

Cancer can be a stressful and traumatic experience. In addition to the physical impact of cancer and its treatment, many survivors experience difficult thoughts, feelings, and memories during treatment and beyond. Today, many cancer centers and hospitals offer psychosocial oncology ("psycho-onc") services – a rising interdisciplinary cancer specialty that addresses the variety of psychological, behavioral, emotional, and social issues that arise for people affected by cancer.

Among oncology mental health professionals, there is increased focus on the importance of self-compassion, which is defined as a person's ability to turn love, understanding, and acceptance inward.

Research shows that high levels of self-compassion may have a positive impact on recovery from various life stressors including post-traumatic stress (Garcia et al. 2021), and that its practice can greatly enhance emotional well-being, boost happiness, reduce anxiety and depression, and can even help maintain healthy lifestyle habits such as diet and exercise (Kim & Ko 2018). Many cancer survivors who practice self-compassion find it to be a powerful tool to promote acceptance and emotional resilience. For some, the regular practice of self-compassion may be personally transformative.

Kristen Neff, PhD, widely recognized as one of the leading Western experts on mindful self-compassion, says being both mindful and compassionate leads to greater ease and well-being in daily life (Neff 2022a). Dr. Neff is the first to define the term academically, and describes the practice as having three elements:

Self-kindness: refraining from harsh criticism of the self.

Recognizing one's own humanity: the fact that all people are imperfect, and all people experience pain.

Mindfulness: maintaining a non-biased awareness of experiences, even those that are painful, rather than either ignoring or exaggerating their effect.

(Neff 2022a)

Through the expression of self-compassion, we offer ourselves the same kindness and care we'd extend to a good friend. Dr. Neff calls this "fierce self-compassion" (Neff 2022b). These types of practices – which are among the foundational principles of yoga – can be a source of strength and tenderness, a most welcome anchor to people with cancer and survivors in their journey to wellness.

Patient story: Mary Louise

Charlotte Nuessle, BSc, RYT 500, C-IAYT

Mary Louise (she/her) is a 54-year-old White woman diagnosed with DCIS (ductal carcinoma in situ), a non-invasive stage zero breast cancer of the milk duct.

Mary Louise is a biker and motorcycle enthusiast whose daily gym workouts have left her "buff and tough". Her siblings recognize her as the strong one in the family; the "go to" person for her nieces and nephews, all of whom admire her passion for her long career in healthcare. Yet even with her extensive medical background, she wasn't prepared for her own unexpected diagnosis of ductal carcinoma in situ (DCIS) breast cancer. Mary Louise underwent a lumpectomy, but just days later received a shock when the pathology report showed the outer margins of her surgical site weren't clean, meaning cancer cells remained. A second lumpectomy was repeated, this time showing more generalized disease. A mastectomy of the right breast was recommended. A new reality was unfolding as she faced a third surgery in just eight weeks. She set aside the "to do" list on her desk at work and took a medical leave of absence.

After healing from her mastectomy and reconstruction, her surgeons cleared her to exercise. Her nurse navigator referred her to me, and we met about eight times at the small hospital-based breast center where I work as part of the integrative healing team. Our program focuses on strengthening a patient's inner resources of well-being, such as learning to be kind to oneself. I incorporate a variety of experiential practices into my yoga therapy sessions to promote self-compassion and well-being, including gentle adaptive yoga and body-based movement, breath awareness, centering/meditation/visualization, discussion, journaling, and personal sharing.

Our center's yoga therapy sessions are semi-private and customized to each patient's special needs. Many of our patients with breast cancer have reported that one of the most important parts of the program was being in the company of other women on similar – yet unique – journeys. The shared experience evoked compassion for each other's suffering.

During our first yoga therapy session, Mary Louise told me she was experiencing chest tightness and was almost scared to move her right arm, so she wanted to work on her range of motion. I worked in tandem with her physical therapist to address imbalances compounded by the breast surgeries. We began gently with adaptive movements: an adapted gentle cat/cow (*mārjaryāsana*) in a chair, and explore supportive positions for her arms while supine in a comfortable resting pose. Mary Louise also said that before her surgery she had spent long hours at her desk, and I noted her posture and the medial rotation of the shoulders. This rotation was exacerbated by the breast surgeries that created scar tissue and further anterior myofascial shortness. To address this, we slowly incorporated the "superman stretch" performed in a warrior II (*vīrabhadrāsana II*) stance. Here, functional arm movements stretched the pectoralis minor and strengthened mid- and lower trapezius, both integral to functional shoulder movement.

Mary Louise said she drew strength from giving herself generous permission to be open to her body's experience. She enjoyed how her body *could move* instead of focusing on its current *limitations*. Experimenting with yoga poses, she found freedom to move in ways she hadn't been able to for several months. As she reconnected with her body, she touched into embodied memories of how, for her, exercise had been a source of vitality and identity. This helped her move forward into life with self-kindness, self-compassion, and a redefined self-image.

Mary Louise and I also practiced simple breathing awareness techniques to create more space and balance, physically and emotionally. Lying supine, a folded blanket under her head and with her lower legs at a 90-degree angle on a chair, she found her own natural fullness of breath and realized the extent to which her flow of breath had been constricted since her diagnosis.

As noted in the literature, compassionate exploration of one's breath has been shown to positively influence the nervous system toward a restorative state of safety (Conrad et al. 2007, Bernardi et al. 2000). It was through breath that she was able to extend acceptance and kindness to her body. This "compassionate breathing" was foundational in the gradual increase of physical range of motion on the right side. She continued this work in physical therapy.

Ultimately, Mary Louise recognized she'd been a private person in her life and instinctively knew it was essential for her healing to openly share her feelings; she couldn't do it alone. During treatment she had sought a safe connection with the nurse navigator whose warm, skillful presence contributed safe familiarity to the many women under her care. The special relationship that she cultivated with her nurse, coupled with our work together that named her physical tightness, gave her an embodied way to turn toward emotional tightness (the nervous system's guarded, protective response) and allow herself to soften.

Reflecting on her journey, Mary Louise remembered it had been impossible for her to speak without crying. For many long months her emotions were so close to the surface that she called herself a "basket case" and "teary." Yoga therapy gave her a way of compassionately partnering with herself to respect the suffering she'd felt, honoring with self-compassion and gratitude all her body *could* do.

3.3 Breathing into life

Background: Prāṇa, the breath of life – a parable

Leigh Leibel

To introduce this patient story, we draw inspiration from the wisdom of Yoga philosophy. In the *praśnopaniṣat* of the *artharvaveda* (an ancient Sanskrit text composed during the second half of the 1st millennium BCE), we are privy to a lively and provocative debate unfolding among the five faculties of the physical body as to which of them reigns supreme. Is it *prāṇa* (life-force or breath)? Mind? Speech? Hearing? Sight? As the group of five pontificates, a competition breaks out and each faculty races to leave the body to see which will be the most sorely missed:

First to go was speech; the body thrived, though mute.

Next to go were eyes; the body thrived, though blind.

Next to go were ears; the body thrived, though deaf.

Finally, the mind fled; yet still the body thrived, though unconscious.

But the moment prāṇa the breath of life, started to leave; the body began to die.

(Muller 1926)

Without the breath of life, how quickly the other faculties were losing their own life-force! Hurriedly, the four faculties gathered in a collective bow to *prāṇa* and admitted her supremacy, begging her to stay, exclaiming, "As a mother protects her children, O *prāṇa*, protect us and give us splendor and wisdom" (*Praśnopaniṣat* 2.13; Müller 1926). As this ancient parable illustrates, a steady and easeful breath is the very essence of life.

Patient story: Rachel

Kate Holcombe, MFA, E-RYT 500, C-IAYT

Rachel (she/her) is a 24-year-old White woman diagnosed with non-Hodgkin lymphoma

Rachel is a twenty-something medical student who moves with the fragility of someone much older. Her movement is slow, deliberate, and she speaks in a whisper. At our first session she shares her poignant story, an ordeal that first began with a misdiagnosis – a medical error that led to unnecessary surgery, chemotherapy, and chest radiation for a cancer she didn't have. Months later and still feeling ill, another medical team worked her up and made the correct diagnosis of non-Hodgkin lymphoma and she underwent a second, different chemotherapy protocol. The irony of Rachel's misdiagnosis is profound: her own medical colleagues were responsible for the misdiagnosis, and to make matters worse, they accidentally severed a nerve to her diaphragm while performing an unnecessary surgery. This caused left-side diaphragm paralysis and severely compromised her ability to breathe. With tears running down her cheeks Rachel says, "Yeah, I'm cured from my cancer, but because of a surgery I didn't actually need, I can barely breathe … I can barely move without triggering a coughing fit. I'm not sure I can go back to med school and be a doctor, or if I even want to. Everything I was working toward has been completely shattered."

Rachel has received medical clearance to work with me and I am excited to join her integrative healthcare team. During intake and assessment, she tells me she is scared to move and that even lying down triggers her cough; she must sleep slightly reclined in a chair. We decide together that our work will focus on that which is most difficult for her – *the breath*. As we sit facing each other, I note she continues to have chest pain and shortness of breath, and sudden moves elicit coughing bouts. If she shifts her position too quickly, or speaks too loudly or quickly, the coughing begins (and can last for several minutes), making her already labored breathing even more difficult. I note her inhale and exhale are rapid, barely lasting two seconds each. I invite her to soften her abdomen and join me in relaxed, diaphragmatic breathing. After a few minutes of gentle belly breathing, we practice a cooling breath called *śītalīprāṇāyāma*. As she draws air in through her curled tongue, I invite her to slightly raise her chin, as comfortable, with each inhale, and slowly lower her chin as she exhales through her nose. My hope is that this series will help address the tightness and stiffness in her neck from surgery and help to lengthen her breath.

"Oh," she says, "it feels so good to move and breathe," so we continue in rhythm and add gentle arm raises with lateral movement to help open her chest and stretch some of the muscles that have tightened post-surgery and radiation. She raises her elbows – first, one at a time, then, circling both elbows up and outward. She immediately asks for more! I invite her to stand and try a few simple movements facing the wall, hands placed firmly against it for support. On inhale, she gently arches and opens the chest. On exhale, she gently comes back to neutral (and if it feels comfortable) slightly rounding forward toward the wall. After our session I write out the practices and ask her to continue them at home each day.

A few sessions later, I introduce the use of sound with her movement, and she begins extending her exhale with a simple "*ahhh*" and "*mā*." Within weeks her breath capacity has increased enough to introduce her to the *kramaprāṇāyāma* technique. (The word *krama* comes from Sanskrit and means "step; part.") In *krama* breathing, the breath is divided into smaller parts within each inhale or exhale.) In a seated position, I invite her to inhale as she raises her arms up overhead beside her ears. On exhale, I invite her to lower her arms, pausing the arms at shoulder level as she simultaneously pauses the breath, then continuing to lower her arms back down to her sides as she completes the exhale. She then inhales freely as she raises her arms and repeats the "stepped" *krama* movement and breath on her exhale. After a few rounds, I ask her to reverse the process (on inhale, raise the arms to shoulder level, slightly pause, and then continue the inhale as the arms raise up beside the ears, followed by freely exhaling, as the arms lower down to the sides). This technique helps her establish a bit more control over her breath, and my hope is that it will help increase her breath capacity and stamina.

Over our weeks together, Rachel also practices each day at home, improves dramatically, and is no longer coughing. She is also walking every day. Soon we can introduce stronger *āsana*, including twists, supine and prone postures such as cobra pose (*bhujaṅgāsana*), modified bow pose (*dhanurāsana*), and sun salutation (*sūryanamaskāra*). Rachel tells me the sun salutations help her feel like her "old self," and that the *āsana* not only reconnect her to her body, but also help reduce the tightness and restriction in the thoracic area, and are helping with stamina, endurance, and strength. She is able to begin jogging, slowly, for very short distances – only a half-mile at first. After a few months, she is jogging three to four miles, and I can teach her stronger sequences.

Rachel is also working with a licensed mental health professional to unpack the emotional impact of her medical trauma. To supplement this work, Rachel says she wants to learn more about Yoga philosophy. At each session, we read passages from *Patañjali Yoga Sūtra-s* (PYS) and reflect on the concepts of *heyaṃ duḥkhaṃ anāgatam* (future suffering is to be avoided; PYS 2.16); *śraddhā* (inner strength, resilience, self-conviction; PYS 1.20); and *īśvara praṇidhāna* (do our very best in life but the results of our actions are out of our hands; PYS 2.1) (Desikachar 2003). These concepts give her insight toward forgiveness and most importantly, help her regain her sense of purpose. Rachel feels like she can continue her medical studies with clearer eyes and greater compassion for her patients, her colleagues, and herself.

3.4 Returning to work after cancer treatment: the "new" normal

Background: Post treatment – the "new" normal

Doreen Stein-Seroussi, MPA, MA, E-RYT, C-IAYT

Returning to work after cancer treatment is often seen as a sign of a return to normalcy (Isaksson et al. 2016), but for most cancer survivors, *normalcy* (at least the pre-cancer normalcy) does not exist (Henderson et al. 2019, Fitch et al. 2021). It is well described that a cancer experience can impact an individual both physically and emotionally, so it's no surprise that a return to the workplace environment can present unexpected hurdles (Fitch et al. 2021), especially if an individual is experiencing cognitive dysfunction because of chemotherapy. Unfortunately, these professional challenges occur at the same time well-intentioned family and friends believe the crisis is over and support is no longer needed. As a result, the cancer survivor can be left unmoored; drifting amid feelings of isolation and anxiety (Yarker et al. 2010). Yoga therapy can be an anchor during these difficult times.

Client story: Cheryl

Doreen Stein-Seroussi

Cheryl (she/her) is a 52-year-old Black woman diagnosed with colon cancer.

Cheryl is in treatment for colon cancer when we first meet. She is referred by her mental health therapist and her physical therapist. Throughout treatment she has been a regular yoga practitioner and has even shown up for group oncology yoga therapy classes on days that she felt ill, when she would remain lying down throughout the class. "It centered me to hear your voice and visualize the poses," she says. By the time Cheryl has returned to work, we have developed a solid therapeutic relationship. However, returning to work means she can't attend the yoga class, because it is in the middle of the day.

One day, Cheryl calls me from work in a panic. She's been back to work for three weeks and is facing difficulties. She tells me, "I can't concentrate and can't finish my work on time. I used to be a powerhouse and I was so efficient. I'm scared." As she talks, I can hear her breath becoming shallower and her voice rising with anxiety. I ask her to take a couple of deep, calm breaths and to ground herself by feeling her body in space. I know this is a technique that has worked for her in the past. I ask if she has time to meet me. She says she doesn't feel she can leave, or take a long lunch break, and after work she's exhausted. Because she's in a panic, we agree to talk on the phone. Before continuing, I make sure she's in a safe place where she can speak without fear of being overheard. She says she is.

I ask Cheryl to take a few more calming breaths, using the extended exhalation method to activate vagal nerve activity (see Chapter 2, section on "Cancer diagnosis through the lens of Polyvagal Theory"). She tells me, "This horrible chemo brain and insomnia is making concentration so difficult. I'm afraid I'll never be able to do the work again. Also, my colleagues, who were so supportive before now seem to think everything's better, but it isn't, and they're expecting me to carry the same workload. I'm so tired. I don't know if life will ever be normal again."

As we talk it becomes obvious that in the few weeks since returning to work, Cheryl's emotions have spiraled downward as she became overwhelmed and is now in a flight/fight/freeze situation. She is tired and her autonomic nervous system is overwhelmed by the many stresses. I explain that her stress hormones, such as cortisol, are likely elevated and that this can affect her ability to concentrate. That makes sense to her; she's noticed that her memory is worse when she is stressed or tired, but she can't help herself. Again, I hear her voice getting higher. Her words tell me that she's getting frustrated with herself and starting to blame herself for the situation. I want her to know it isn't her fault and I also want her to know that she can help herself, even if the problem cannot completely be resolved. A sense of control is important to Cheryl.

Cheryl is reluctant to use any movement practices at work, even simple ones, so we focus on meditation and breath-work. I ask her if there is an affirmation she would like to use. It takes a few minutes for her to settle on one, but she ultimately wants to focus on being calm. In her office, Cheryl puts a sign on her door not to be disturbed, puts me on speaker phone, and then gets into a comfortable position. She sits in her office chair near a wall so that she can rest her head. I begin to lead her through a guided meditation focusing on the breath. The meditation starts with body awareness, rotating awareness around the body, looking for tension and relaxation. I ask her not to judge how she is feeling, but to practice acceptance. I can hear Cheryl sigh as some tension naturally releases. I then ask Cheryl to notice emotions and mind chattering. I suggest this all can be done without judgment. The natural tendency is to judge ourselves, even our emotions, but we're practicing observing without judgment.

Then I ask her to focus her mind on her breath, noticing each breath in and each breath out. I guide her to say to herself the affirmation, "I am calm" with each exhalation. I remain quiet for a moment so she can breathe and focus. I can hear the calm rhythm of her breath. Slowly, she's guided to notice once again how she's feeling and to slowly bring herself back into the room. I ask her to open her eyes when she's ready. After a few moments of silence, she says, "Wow, that was amazing. I feel so much more relaxed. I can't believe how simple it was." We then practice the extended exhalation breath, something she knows, but forgets to use. Her voice lightens as she says, "I can use it in meetings when I'm feeling anxious." Cheryl also decides to use her online calendar to schedule breathing breaks during the day, one-minute check-ins for herself. "I forget how powerful the breath can be!" she comments.

We turn our attention to her workload and her colleagues' expectations. Cheryl knows she is going to have to talk to them, but says she isn't ready, yet. We discuss using visualization to help her through that meeting. It's something she wants to explore, but her lunch break is over. We arrange to talk in two days to see how she's feeling, adjust her routine, if needed, and to begin using visualization to help her prepare for the meeting.

3.5 Reframing caregiver distress
Background: Caregiver stress
Leigh Leibel

It can be devastating to a family when their primary caregiver is diagnosed with cancer. The newly diagnosed person must care not only for themselves during their own cancer treatments, but also for their loved one(s) at home who may be ill, disabled, dependent children or seniors, or otherwise accustomed to their support.

Caregiver burn-out is a national crisis in the United States. Today there are close to 53 million unpaid caregivers and the number is rising, according to statistics from the American Association of Retired Persons (AARP) and the National Alliance of Caregiving (NAC 2020). Caregivers are often overwhelmed by the emotional and physical responsibility of taking care of others. In fact, studies show that caregivers are much more likely than non-caregivers to suffer from health problems such as stress overload, depression, anxiety, and other issues (Inger 2022). According to an article in the journal of the American Academy of Family Physicians, many physicians are calling caregivers the "hidden patients" who may neglect their own medical and dental screenings and ignore new symptomatology (Roche 2009).

This is such a prevalent issue that there is a recognized condition called *caregiver stress syndrome* that is characterized by physical, mental, and emotional exhaustion. This syndrome typically occurs when a person neglects their own physical and emotional health because they are hyper-focused on caring for an ill, injured, or disabled loved one. Common feelings associated with this include being scared, sad, lonely, unappreciated, angry, frustrated, and guilty. To make matters worse, when caregivers are diagnosed with a serious medical condition, their pre-existing chronic stress is amplified, creating allostatic load, or accumulated "wear and tear on the body" that further impacts their health.

Caregiver stress syndrome

Caregiving has a substantial impact on the caregiver's physical health. According to data shared in the magazine *Today's Caregiver* (Inger 2022):

- "11% of caregivers state that their role has caused their physical health to decline.

- 45% of caregivers reported chronic conditions, including heart attacks, heart disease, cancer, diabetes, and arthritis.

- Caregivers have a 23% higher level of stress hormones and 15% lower level of antibody responses than non-caregivers.

- 10% of primary caregivers report that they are under physical stress from the demands of assisting their loved one physically.

- Women who spend 9 or more hours a week caring for a spouse increased their risk of heart disease by 100%.

- 72% of caregivers report that they had not gone to the doctor as often as they should have.

- 58% of caregivers state that their eating habits are worse than before they assumed this role.

- Caregivers between the ages of 66 and 96 have a 63% higher mortality rate than non-caregivers of the same age."

According to *Today's Caregiver*, "symptoms of caregiver stress syndrome may include changes in appetite, weight, or both; feeling blue, hopeless, irritable, or helpless; withdrawal from friends and family; changes in sleep patterns; getting sick more often; feelings of wanting to hurt yourself or the person for whom you are caring; loss of interest in activities previously enjoyed; emotional and physical exhaustion; and irritability" (Inger 2022).

Client story: Lizzie

Cheryl Fenner Brown, E-RYT 500, YACEP, C-IAYT

Lizzie (she/her) is a 76-year-old White woman diagnosed with DCIS (ductal carcinoma in situ), non-invasive stage zero breast cancer of milk ducts.

Lizzie is a 76-year-old woman with clinical depression. After three needle biopsies and a diagnosis of ductal carcinoma in situ (DCIS) breast cancer, her oncologist recommended a full mastectomy. Lizzie is in distress. To help her manage her extreme anxiety, her long-time psychiatrist prescribed anti-depressants and referred her to me for yoga therapy sessions. I began meeting with her two weeks prior to her scheduled surgery. She presented as severely fearful, exhausted, and anxious, and told me she was the primary caregiver for her 86-year-old husband who has advanced Parkinson's disease and severe dementia. Already incredibly stressed and depressed due to her role as his primary caregiver, her distress is now compounded by her own diagnosis. She says she chose not to tell her husband about her medical condition (fearing he would not understand nor remember) and thus does not have his support. She says she was completely blindsided by her diagnosis and is unable to fully process both her impending mastectomy and the fact that she does not have a family support system. Yet she must continue to care for her husband during her treatment. My goal is to support her, to help her take steps to protect her health and well-being with techniques for self-care. I share several yoga techniques with her, among them two simple practices – *saṅkalpa* (intention) and *mudrā* (symbolic hand gesture or body pose). My hope is that she can add them to her toolbox to redirect her distress and fearful thoughts and help her find a moment of calm strength, empowering her to take practical, conscious healing action in times of greatest need.

I guide Lizzie through a *saṅkalpa*-setting meditation to help her create an intention to use whenever she feels overwhelmed. Lizzie comes up with the *saṅkalpa* "I will survive." I suggest she rephrase it to "I am surviving." She agrees that the shift in language to the present tense helps her feel more capable and fully present in the moment.

We then turn our attention to the other simple yoga practice, *mudrā*. While there is not much research on *mudrā*, in the yogic tradition and in classic Indian dance it is said to be a powerful tool for stress-resilience and anxiety that is literally "in hand." Similar to reflexology, *mudrā* uses hand and finger positions that are thought to stimulate specific parts of the brain via energetic pathways. When pathways are activated, they elicit a response in the physical, mental/emotional, and energetic bodies. Specifically, I teach her *adhimudrā* (see Figure 6.3) which is achieved by holding the thumbs lightly inside of each fist and resting the hands (with backs of hands down) on the lap. It is believed this gesture can lengthen the exhalation and activate the parasympathetic nervous system which may help direct awareness inward and quiet the

mind (LePage et al. 2013). I suggest that she practices *adhimudrā* while simultaneously repeating her *saṅkalpa* "I am surviving" three times, whenever she feels she is getting caught up in negative thought patterns.

In the weeks following surgery, she reports that she has practiced *saṅkalpa* and *adhimudrā* several times a day and found calm and inner reserves of strength. She is able to reframe her distress into empowerment. I also encourage her to continue seeing her psychotherapist and physical therapist every week and to make time to do something for herself every day, for instance, taking a walk, going to a museum, or talking to a friend so that she would not feel isolated.

Since her surgery two years ago, Lizzie has no evidence of disease, and we continue to have weekly yoga therapy sessions. For many months after her surgery, she experienced an intense amount of stress as her husband's health deteriorated and she managed her own depression and fears around cancer recurrence without being able to rely on his support. Her husband passed away during this time, and Lizzie told me that the simple practice of *saṅkalpa* and *adhimudrā* allowed her to focus on survival in the midst of grief and sadness. It has been a privilege to stand beside her as she moved through the panic and disbelief of cancer diagnosis and treatment, to a place of understanding and gratitude of life with no evidence of disease.

Box 6.12 A *saṅkalpa*-setting meditation
Cheryl Fenner Brown

Setting an intention or *saṅkalpa* may help shift a client's mindset. When we focus on fear, anxiety, and negative self-talk, the mind can become trapped in a negative loop that erodes calm and reinforces helplessness. As we see in *Patañjali Yoga Sutra 2.33*, mentally repeating a positively stated intention

(continued)

Box 6.12 continued

can be a powerful tool for compassionate self-observation. It brings habitual negative thoughts to the surface of awareness, after which we can offer an opposing present-tense affirmation. In this way, negative mind states are gently re-framed in the moment to improve emotional self-regulation and promote stress resilience. *Saṅkalpa* is a powerful way for clients to manage their fear. *Saṅkalpa* comes from the heart – not the mind – and reshapes the circular nature of worry toward a peaceful connection to witness consciousness.

Example script

We begin with an intention-setting meditation that can be used to help calm the mind when you get stuck in a negative loop. Return to this meditation when you wake, before bed, and at any other time you need to. Repetition plants a seed for self-transformation deep within your mind, to assist you on your path towards self-compassion and well-being. Feel the breath gently directed into the chest, encouraging your deepest wish for self-transformation to arise. Bring to mind the current challenges that you are facing. Without dwelling on the details, recognize that all challenges are opportunities for personal growth and healing. Perhaps your current challenges have already set the stage for transformation in your life. Continue to visualize this challenging situation and hold it within the space of the heart, releasing any feelings of judgment or blame if they arise. Next, begin to visualize the best possible outcome for the challenges you are facing. If any thoughts of doubt begin to arise, redirect the mind towards receptivity and the positive resolution of your current situation. Whatever steps need to be taken, imagine taking them with self-confidence. Trust that you have the strength, courage, and ability to assist in bringing the imagined positive outcome into reality. Allow your intention to coalesce into a short, simple statement, phrased in the present tense beginning with the words "I am ...". State this silently three times. Trust that your *saṅkalpa* will manifest in the best possible way.

3.6 Ostomy and *āsana*

Backgound: Ostomy

Michelle Stortz, MFA, E-RYT 500, YACEP, C-IAYT and Leigh Leibel

An ostomy is a life-saving procedure that allows urine or stool to pass through a surgically created opening on the abdomen (a stoma) into a prosthetic device known as a pouch or ostomy bag worn on the outside of the body. The bag may be either permanent or placed temporarily to allow the affected organs to heal. An ostomy may be necessary due to colorectal, bladder, ovarian, and other cancers affecting the pelvis and abdomen, but it can also be a result of other medical conditions such as inflammatory bowel disease or diverticulitis. There are different kinds of ostomies, mostly located in the lower part of the abdomen, e.g., colostomy (lower left), ileostomy (lower right), and urostomy (lower area). There can also be a percutaneous endoscopic gastrostomy (PEG) tube placed in the abdomen for feeding. In Europe, approximately 700,000 people are living with a stoma, and in the United States, more than one million people have a stoma (Claessens et al. 2015).

The transition into life as an *ostomate* can be difficult. A 2016 systematic review of colorectal ostomates found that a stoma has a negative impact on a person's quality of life (Vonk-Klaassen et al. 2016). This is reinforced by a recent survey of ostomates that suggests almost half of those who responded perceive high levels of stigma around their ostomy (Jin et al. 2020). In practical terms, an ostomate must deal with many issues around emptying, cleaning, dressing, and supporting the pouch. Almost all report fear of leakage and smell; other common issues include sexual problems, depressive feelings, gas, constipation, dissatisfaction with appearance, change in clothing, travel difficulties, fatigue, and worry about noises – all of which can lead to low self-esteem (Vonk-Klaassen et al. 2016).

Another significant concern for ostomates is engaging in physical activity and exercise. Two recent surveys found that ostomates report a reduction in physical activity following their surgery (Beeken et al. 2019, Russell 2017). Many weren't active before their cancer diagnosis and are not inclined to develop new habits, while some are too fatigued to exercise (Russell 2017). Others say they don't exercise due to wounds from surgery, fear of/ or actual pouch leaks, feeling self-conscious, the need for professionals to better address specific stoma-related concerns, and concerns about risk of hernia (Saunders & Brunet 2019). Indeed, this population is at high risk for parastomal herniation, and preventative measures should be taken during physical activity (Box 6.13).

BOX 6.13 Parastomal herniation
Michelle Stortz

Parastomal herniation is a high-risk factor for ostomy patients and preventative measures should be taken. Parastomal hernia occurs when other abdominal contents protrude through the defect in the abdominal wall created for a stoma. Prevalence is estimated to be over 30% by 12 months, 40% by 2 years, and 50% or higher at long duration of follow-up. Studies highlight a trend toward inactivity after stoma formation surgery, with fear of hernia a major deterrent to being physically active. The hernia may happen when there's an increase in intra-abdominal pressure such as in sneezing, coughing, twisting, sudden moves, or lifting heavy objects. There are many strategies to prevent herniation such as wearing a support belt, not lifting anything heavy, and no quick, jerky movements. The best prevention is strengthening the abdominal wall – important not only for preventing herniation, but also for creating a better stomal grip.

(Association of Stoma Care Nurses [ASCN] 2016, Lowe et al. 2019, Saunders & Brunet 2019, Hubbard et al. 2020)

Another study suggests that ostomates aren't told about the importance of resuming an active lifestyle, or the vital role that physical activity and abdominal conditioning play in hernia prevention (Russell 2017). The irony is that it is well known that physical activity becomes even more important after a cancer diagnosis and treatment (Schmitz et al. 2010, Schwartz et al. 2017).

In fact, exercise contributes to reduced risk of cancer recurrence, reduced fatigue, and improved quality of life, physical function, and body composition (Schwartz et al. 2017). A statement from the Association of Stoma Care Nurses UK (ASCN UK) advises that ostomates return to all activities previously undertaken (Hubbard et al. 2017). (See gray box after client story for ASCN UK-endorsed core strengthening exercises). The American College of Sports Medicine concurs, adding that ostomates should progress slowly with strength building exercises and make modifications as necessary to avoid excessive intra-abdominal pressure (Campbell et al. 2019).

In sum, without activity, ostomates run the risk of deconditioning and weight gain which may lead to weakening of the abdominal wall (Russell 2017), and other metabolic and cardiovascular issues. They may also experience reduced quality of life. A yoga practice offers holistic healing – it can provide gentle abdominal conditioning and strength building, body awareness and self-regulating skills for calming and centering, and the opportunity to experience a therapeutic, holistic approach to well-being.

Points to remember

- The client should empty their bag before the yoga session. Ensure their privacy.

- Always clear exercises (*āsana*/movements) with the client's stoma nurse. Some ostomates may be advised not to do abdominal crunches or other moves per their individual circumstances.

- Avoid movement or positions that will put direct pressure on the stoma itself (prone postures may be OK if position is adjusted, perhaps with props, so there is no pressure on the stoma).

- The client may attend sessions wearing a belt, or tights for support (if directed by stoma nurse).

- For some people, as the bag fills it can make noise and/or there sometimes can be an odor.

(continued)

(continued)

- To help build abdominal strength, encourage daily home practice. Use mindset coaching to address obstacles, resistance, and strategies for the transition into yoga/exercise. Encourage baby steps, tiny habits, and make sure to celebrate the smallest wins.

Client story: Delia

Michelle Stortz

Delia (she/her) is a 67-year-old White woman diagnosed with bladder cancer who has a urostomy due to her disease and surgery.

Delia arrives at my yoga-for-cancer class and introduces herself. She is a survivor of bladder cancer. She wears a urostomy pouch and explains that even though her surgery was over a year ago, she's still afraid to move. She's afraid to bend over, lift even mildly heavy objects, or go down to the floor. She avoids any actions that involve her core lest she disrupt her stoma and pouch. Other than walking, Delia has no experience with exercise.

During intake, I explain that in our yoga therapy session we'll be going slowly and gently, and I will frequently ask her how movements are feeling. I assure her she doesn't have to go down to the floor. With that, I ask that she not hesitate to share what's happening and to not do anything she's uncomfortable with. She agrees. She wants to try to come regularly to yoga, so we talked about our plan going forward to help her build a stronger abdominal wall and how she can learn to sense its role in core support. I explain I want to help her understand sensations so that her confidence in movement can grow. I assured her that she will always dictate pacing and I will check in frequently about comfort. We agree that we will work with her stoma nurse to make sure all the practices are safe for her current condition.

We begin with breath awareness, drawing attention to its movement, then exploring a modest diaphragmatic

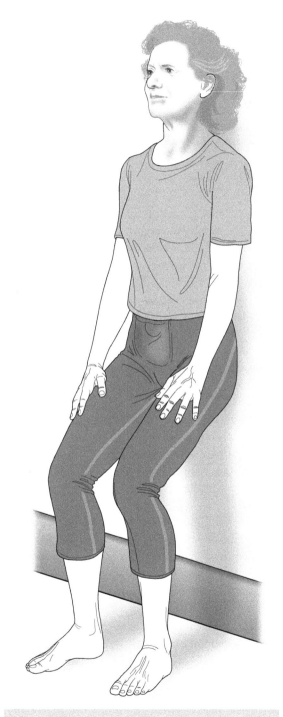

Figure 6.13
Engaging support at wall

breath with slight expansion in the belly on the inhale. We then move into a shallow spinal flexion/extension (cat/cow; *mārjaryāsana*) with no abdominal engagement. She says this feels great. We move into easy joint-opening movements, bringing awareness to these sensations. We periodically pause in neutral poses like seated or standing mountain pose (*tāḍāsana*) to simply feel the core area. We then mildly engage the abdominal muscles. When asked how it feels, she says, "It's OK," as she touches her belly and pouch. I ask often so she can confirm for herself and so I know that engagement is OK; there is no pain or unusual feeling in her abdomen or around the stoma. We progress to a stronger standing pose, warrior II (*vīrabhadrāsana II*). Here, I want her to feel the strength in her legs and to feel her belly's coordination with the activated legs. I don't ask her to engage abdominals. When checking in, she seems a little surprised that this is all just fine.

In our second class, Delia bravely ventures down to the floor. Using the chair for support as she makes her way down, then onto her back, all movements slow and mindful. Here we begin more intentional abdominal strengthening. With knees bent and feet flat on the floor, I ask her to simply engage her abdominals on her exhalations. Next, windshield wipers, knees falling to one side, then the other. She says that this movement feels good. We add a posterior pelvic tilt with active abdominal engagement.

In the third class, lying on her back, we add bridge pose (*setubandhasarvāṅgāsana*) which requires more core activation. We follow this with "hugging knees into chest" (*apāsana*), which can be disconcerting for many ostomates because it will put pressure on the bag. She found she could gauge her level of flexion to suit her moment-to-moment condition. She approaches all these challenges slowly and mindfully. In subsequent sessions we add stronger abdominal engagement, pressing belly toward spine.

Many more core-strengthening *āsana-s* were explored throughout many months, and now years, of working together. She has become comfortable and confident with core engagement and continues to build overall strength.

Four core strengthening exercises for ostomates endorsed by the Association of Stoma Care Nurses (ASCN 2016)

These are general guidelines, and all exercise should be cleared by the patient's personal stoma nurse or surgeon.

- Lying supine, knees bent, engage abdominals, hold for 3 seconds.

- Posterior pelvic tuck with abdominal engagement, hold for 3 seconds.

- Knee rolling (windshield wipers) with abdominal muscles engaged, lower knees to one side as far as is comfortable. Return to center. Other side.

- Standing at a wall (see Figure 6.13), engage abdominals, pulling low back to the wall, hold for 3 seconds.

3.7 Guided yogic meditation for anxiety during cancer remission: MSRT and PET techniques

Background: MSRT and PET yogic meditation techniques – current research

Leigh Leibel

Cancer survivors often experience mental health concerns after completion of their cancer treatment that can include subclinical or clinical depression and anxiety. These conditions can have a significant impact on their well-being, quality of life, and clinical outcomes. Nonpharmacologic mind-body interventions such as yoga are increasingly being explored as important and effective adjuncts to psychotherapy with licensed mental health professionals.

A 2021 systematic review and meta-analysis conducted in Australia evaluated the effect of yoga-based interventions on self-reported depression and anxiety symptoms in people with cancer. The review included 42 studies that were designed as randomized controlled trials: 26 for depressive symptoms and 16 for anxiety symptoms. Investigators found evidence that in people with cancer, yoga-based interventions are associated with improved depression and anxiety symptoms, suggesting the types of yoga practices included in the studies are a promising therapeutic modality for their management (Gonzalez et al. 2021).

Mind Sound Resonance Technique (MSRT)

There are other novel yogic-based mindfulness and relaxation techniques that warrant study in cancer populations for the management of mood concerns and quality of life. One is called Mind Sound Resonance Technique (MSRT; Box 6.14). This technique uses *mantra* to induce deep relaxation for mind and body and has been studied in India in both clinical (hypertension, general anxiety disorder) and nonclinical (high schoolers, schoolteachers, IT professionals) populations for anxiety and depressive symptoms. It shows promising results in these populations. Below, we describe three MSRT studies – two are randomized controlled trials in nonclinical populations and the other is a pilot study in hypertension.

- A 2021 randomized controlled trial looking at MSRT's efficacy as an extracurricular activity on the psychological state and cognitive function in high school students (n=60) showed the practice led to enhanced psychological functions and improved cognition in teenagers (14–16 years of age) facing high levels of stress, anxiety, and depression arising from peer pressure (Anusuya et al. 2021).

- A 2017 randomized controlled trial looking at the effects of MSRT on psychological states, sleep quality, and cognitive functions in female teachers (n=60) working in primary schools in India showed a reduction in their levels of stress, anxiety, fatigue, and psychological distress, and enhanced levels of self-esteem and quality of sleep (Rao et al. 2017).

- A 2018 pilot study to assess the acute effect of MSRT intervention on blood pressure, heart rate, and state anxiety in Indian patients (n=30) with essential hyper-

tension demonstrated the usefulness of a single session of MSRT in reducing blood pressure, heart rate, and state anxiety among individuals with hypertension as compared to supine rest, the control group (Wang et al. 2018).

BOX 6.14 Mind Sound Resonance Technique (MSRT)

Satyam Tripathi, Bhavani Munamarty, and Kiran Shenoy

MSRT is an advanced meditation practice developed in India (Nagendra 2001). It systematically takes patients to a deeper layer of silence. It starts with systematic proper intonation which produces resonance within. Spoken first out loud, and then silently in the mind, the patient is asked to produce three sounds, *AAA, UUU, MMM* in low, medium, and high pitch and is guided to feel the subtle vibrations. Audible *AUM* sound is produced to feel the vibration in the entire body. With practice, repeating this three times with deep sensitivity and calmness helps to reach a subtle layer of consciousness. *AUM* sound represents the primal vibrations which are repeated with effort nine times silently in the mind, allowing us to disconnect from the various thoughts that come to the mind. The patient repeats *AUM* silently in the mind, and is guided to focus on the intervals of silence. This focusing leaves the patient experiencing deep inner peace for a few minutes. This is followed by a resolve that strengthens the will and the immune defense.

Prāṇic Energization Technique (PET)

Another novel yogic-based relaxation technique developed in India is *Prāṇic (life-force)* Energization Technique (PET; see Box 6.10). This technique involves breath regulation (*prāṇāyāma*), chanting, and visualization. The belief is that this practice may revitalize the tissues by activating the subtle energies (*prāṇa*) within the body; *prāṇa* is a fundamental concept in the traditional teaching of yoga. In a randomized controlled study looking at the effect of add-on PET on healing of fresh bone fractures (n=30), investigators concluded that PET practiced twice a day (30 minutes/session) for three weeks using taped audio instructions (after learning under supervision for one week) accelerates fracture healing, as compared to controls (Oswal et al. 2011).

As seen in the 2021 systematic review (Gonzalez et al. 2021) that we described earlier, various yoga-based relaxation techniques have shown promise for the management of depression and anxiety in cancer populations. The novel MSRT and PET mindfulness and relaxation techniques are recognized in India as having a positive influence on physical and psychological health. Both warrant study in cancer populations for management of mood, stress, and quality of life.

Patient story: Lu

Satyam Tripathi, BAMS, MD (Yoga & Rehab), E-RYT 500, C-IAYT
Bhavani Munamarty, MSc, CYT 500, YIC 200
Kiran Shenoy, E-RYT 200, CYT 500, RYT 200

Lu (she/her) is a 33-year-old woman of Chinese descent diagnosed with diffuse large B-cell lymphoma.

Patient Lu is an anesthesiologist in Singapore who has a good understanding of health, in a scientific way. She has gone through a bone marrow transplant after rounds of chemotherapy. Initially diagnosed with diffuse large B cell lymphoma, she underwent chemotherapy and was in complete remission, but the cancer recurred a year later. Lu came to our Integrative Center looking for complementary and integrative therapy to deal with anxiety and low energy levels. I greet Lu and try to make small talk, but she seems lost and withdrawn from the surroundings. Lu says, "I feel weak, breathless, and I just can't stop the constant looping of thoughts. This makes me very anxious. I want to try yoga to help me relax." During our intake and assessment, Lu says she is ambitious, result-oriented, and highly competitive – as such, her stress levels are high, and she has struggled to cope with an ever-demanding lifestyle (both mentally and physically) after remission. She also shares that she has trouble sleeping and wakes up often in a light sweat

in the middle of night. Being on the quieter side, she is uncomfortable expressing emotions openly.

I invite Lu to lie down on the yoga mat, close her eyes if she'd like to, and observe the breath and thoughts: "Try to make your exhalations longer than your inhalations and with every breath you exhale, try to first acknowledge and then gently remove whatever thought comes to your mind." I observe that after a couple of rounds, Lu is breathing smoothly. I continue, "If the mind begins to drift away, don't worry. It's the nature of the mind. Use your breath as an anchor to bring your mind to the present and connect it to your body." After a few rounds, I observe that Lu's breath has deepened, and the shoulders relaxed. I ask Lu to observe the body and mind and pay attention to the subtle changes taking place. Afterward, she says she is willing to try other advanced meditation and relaxation techniques.

During the next few weeks, we work on two meditations, Mind Sound Resonance Technique (MSRT) and *Prāṇic* Energization Technique (PET) to help her relax. Both are advanced yoga techniques developed at S-VYASA Yoga University in Bengaluru, India, to induce a deeply rested state of body. If we can change the response of the perceiving system, then we can achieve mastery over the stress response of the mind-body.

We begin with Mind Sound Resonance Technique (MRST; see Box 6.14). I place a bolster under the knees to make the patient more comfortable and encourage the patient to take a few easy breaths. With legs stretched, arms by the side and eyes closed, I ask Lu to take a deep breath and make the sound "A" (*A-kāra*). Lu hesitates a little and makes a very soft sound. I explain the importance of the sounds produced and lead towards the next round. The chanting in the next round is louder and Lu seems to be loosening up. We complete two more rounds of *A-kāra* and continue with three rounds of sound "U" (*U-kāra*), "M" (*M-kāra*), and "AUM" (*AUM-kāra*). Beautiful vibrations of the chanting fill the room with positive, healing energy. I could see its effect on Lu, and the patient is slipping into a restful state. Lu opens her eyes gently and gives a smile, "I feel relaxed." I ask her to stay in silence (a thoughtless wakeful state) for a few minutes. Before we end the session, I ask Lu to think of a resolve (a short positive statement) and repeat it mentally. I say, "When repeating the resolve, mean and say each word like it is really happening in the body." Lu repeats "I am strong and full of energy" mentally, nine times.

At our next appointment, the second advanced meditation we practice is PET in which we observe the flow of energy or *prāṇa* through the body (see Box 6.10). This can help energize the body by allowing the mind to concentrate and move the energy inside our body in a guided manner. This helps us to feel the forces as the energy moves around. Beginning in a seated position, the patient is guided to balance breath by alternate nostril breathing (*nāḍīśodhana*; see Figure 6.2). The patient feels the air flowing in and out of the respiratory system by following mindfully the path of breath. The nerve impulses traveling from between index finger and thumb to brain are guided to be felt, for 4–5 minutes. The patient then lies down, brings their palms close to each other, and rubs the palms together, feeling the energy generated between the palms. Recognizing the force i.e., *vyānaprāṇa* (subtle energy) between the palms can lead to recognize and feel the subtle energy in other parts of the body. The patient is then led to scan and move this *prāṇa* to each side of the body, and then the entire body and each organ, observing the feeling for a few minutes, while keeping all thoughts at bay and emotions subsided to reach the deep state of rest; then a resolve is made.

After a few sessions using these techniques on alternate days, Lu's breath has become slower and deeper, the mind calmer. After more than six months into the therapy, her physician says her blood work shows promising results. Lu visits the yoga center regularly, enjoying sessions, and making slow, but steady progress. She says, "I look forward to these sessions as I feel a deeper sense of relaxation in both body and mind. My mind is calmer,

and my anxiety has reduced. I feel this sense of relaxation has had a positive impact on my sleep and I am able to deal with stress better." Lu understands that yoga is a journey, not a destination. It will be a long journey on the path of healing and self-discovery. Lu has made good progress and we are happy to be walking alongside her and help her get back on track.

3.8 Yogic management of chemotherapy-induced peripheral neuropathy (CIPN)

Background: Chemotherapy-induced peripheral neuropathy

Robyn Tiger, MD, C-IAYT and Leigh Leibel

Several common chemotherapy agents are known to be toxic to the peripheral nerves that carry sensation, control movements of the arms and legs, and control the bladder and bowel (Brown et al. 2019). When chemotherapy damages these nerves it causes peripheral neuropathy, more accurately called chemotherapy-induced peripheral neuropathy (CIPN). Common therapies that contribute to this condition include the platinum drugs, taxanes, vinca alkaloids, and bortezomib. Risk of nerve damage is thought to be dose dependent and made worse when multiple drugs are given at the same time, or when additional cycles of chemotherapy are administered.

CIPN is a painful condition that can significantly impact quality of life, for example, affecting the ability to button a shirt, or even to walk without assistance. Symptoms are usually symmetrical and begin in the fingers and toes, progressing inwards. Symptoms present immediately, or weeks to months later. They include:

- Tingling or pins-and-needles sensation
- Pain, burning, numbness
- Sensitivity to hot or cold

The effects of CIPN may persist for years or last indefinitely. In one study of over 500 cancer survivors, nearly half experienced persistent neuropathy up to six years following completion of their chemotherapy treatment (Winters-Stone et al. 2017). In another study, almost 50% of breast cancer survivors experienced CIPN symptoms for years after treatment (Wildes et al. 2016).

In addition to pain and discomfort, functional deficits caused by CIPN include fundamental motor skills and manual dexterity (Naumann et al. 2015), as well as deficits in distal sensation, balance, and strength and mobility (Ness et al. 2012). This can lead to an increased fall risk which is a hazard in an aging population, especially if there is co-existing bone fragility. Osteoporosis and other conditions such as obesity and psychosocial health may be part of a complex interaction that limits physical activity and exercise. This can lead to further health concerns and metabolic and cardiovascular risk factors.

Several recent studies have looked at the role of yoga in CIPN management. Two recent pilot studies evaluated the effectiveness and impact of a somatic-based *Haṭha* yoga and meditation protocol in individuals with CIPN. Both demonstrated promising results including decreased fear of falling, as well as improvement in flexibility, balance, and quality of life (Galantino et al. 2019, 2020). Another study by Bao et al. at Memorial Sloan Kettering Cancer Center in New York City found that among breast and gynecological cancer survivors with moderate-to-severe CIPN, yoga was safe and showed promising efficacy in improving symptoms (Bao et al. 2020).

There is no cure for CIPN, and pharmaceuticals have limited impact and carry side effects. These three yoga studies suggest a role for an interventional yoga program as an adjunct nonpharmacologic treatment for cancer survivors experiencing CIPN. Further research is warranted.

Client story: group yoga therapy to address CIPN

Robyn Tiger

Ten cancer survivors (median age 64 years) with CIPN participated in a group class as part of a research study on the effect of yoga on CIPN symptoms. Participants had previously completed treatment for ovarian, breast, colon, uterine, and bladder cancers and were continuing to experience CIPN symptoms months to years after completion of treatment.

As the lead yoga therapist for a research study (Galantino et al. 2020) on chemotherapy-induced peripheral neuropathy (CIPN), I observe carefully as ten courageous individuals walk into our classroom in an outpatient rehabilitation center – some without difficulty, others with the aid of canes and walkers – to join our eight-week yoga and meditation pilot study. The heaviness in the room is palpable. The participants had previously completed chemotherapy treatment for ovarian, breast, colon, uterine, and bladder cancers and were continuing to experience life-impacting neuropathy symptoms. I explain there will be a total of 16 classes (twice a week for eight weeks) with home assignments, and each session will follow the same format: verbal check-in; baseline breath and body scan; somatic movements; iRest *yoganidrā* (yogic sleep); *śavasāna* (corpse pose); a post practice check-in; and closing affirmation that incorporates grounding *mudrā-s* (hand gestures). The program is designed to decrease the symptoms of CIPN, including pain, numbness, and tingling in the extremities, with the objective of improving flexibility, pain, proprioception, agility, balance, and kinesthetic sense.

As we begin our first session together, students choose whether to use floor mats or chairs. Once everyone is settled, we focus on mindset, immediately addressing CIPN, "the elephant in the room," and many eyes that were previously gazing downward look up to meet mine. I acknowledge and validate their CIPN symptoms and listen closely to their stories. The heaviness in the room begins to lift. I extend the invitation to "meet yourself exactly where you are" and assure everyone that it is their choice to rest at any time. The heaviness in the room lifts even more.

We begin our practice with the three-part check-in of the mind, breath, and body. As we begin to breathe together, I can see that most participants are "stress breathing" in their chest. Today, and in each of our 16 sessions, I teach diaphragmatic (belly) breathing and other types of breath that activate the parasympathetic nervous system. This includes beak (*kākī*) breath either on inhale (cooling) or exhale (calming); cleansing breath; breath of the bee (*bhramarī*); and alternate nostril breathing (*nāḍīśodhana*) using index fingers instead of the whole hand *mudrā* due to neuropathy symptoms.

After we complete our breathing practices, we begin our somatic-based movements. (See Box 6.15 for more about the research study.) As I give instructions for each pose, I first describe the poses verbally to create a motor map in the mind prior to beginning the movement. This can make the moves easier to learn. I also emphasize the importance of connecting movement with the breath. This can lead to improvement in flexibility, strength, stability, and balance, all of which are frequently negatively affected with cancer treatment.

Upon completion of our body-based movement, we transition to our relaxation - iRest *yoganidrā*, a very effective somatic-based trauma-informed meditation with decades of documented research. I guide students to either lie down or find a seated position for this phase of practice. After relaxation, we complete our session with *maṇḍalamudrā* (gesture of the circle; see Figure 6.3) and an affirmation for wholeness that we repeat together either quietly or aloud: "I am complete and whole exactly as I am."

Our first class went very well, and we continue to meet for 15 more sessions, always following the same yoga protocol but modifying and customizing for the students' evolving needs. On the final day of our program one student shares with the group, "After practice, I am not focused on the numbness or pain, my mind is elsewhere." Another student tells us, "Concentration on the belly breathing has cooled some of the sensation of fire in my feet – lasting a little longer after each breathing session. I am very grateful for the relief I experience for long periods after practice and whenever I breathe through my nose." After we say our goodbyes, I share the last elevator ride with a student who tells me yoga "saved his life." I respond, "Thank yourself for saving your own life!" And as I turn to walk to my car, I begin to sob tears of gratitude for having gained the knowledge and opportunity to teach those with CIPN how to help themselves through yoga therapy.

BOX 6.15 Details of the research protocol (Galantino et al. 2020)
Robyn Tiger

Attentive listening

Individuals with CIPN frequently feel frustrated and unheard, and may feel that the progress of their cancer treatment is given priority over their distressing symptoms. They may feel disheartened and at times depressed, having found no relief from medications. For this reason, it is important that the yoga therapist commence the therapist-client relationship with an initial focus on mindset prior to initiating any practice, by acknowledging and validating clients' symptoms with attentive listening skills, and in turn begin to develop their trust and confidence.

Cooling breath

It is best to teach clients with CIPN calming and cooling, as opposed to energizing and heating breath practices that can activate the sympathetic nervous system and exacerbate their underlying symptoms.

(continued)

BOX 6.15 continued

As the weeks pass, I see that for some students it takes several sessions for them to soften into belly breath. For others, *kākīprāṇāyāma* breath on the exhale (breathing through pursed lips that resemble that of a crow's beak) is easier to learn and is calming as well. Overall, they are amazed how much calmer they feel when they are finally able to belly breathe.

I also emphasize that these breathing practices can help to improve sleep. Many people with CIPN experience sleep difficulties because the touch of sheets and blankets on their feet can cause pain and discomfort. Often, they must sleep without covers which can make them feel unsafe and exposed.

Somatic-based movement

Since CIPN symptoms fall under the umbrella of disembodiment, in this research study we address symptoms through a somatic-based yoga therapy approach designed to enhance cognitive awareness and body reintegration. While there are many types of somatic movement, our study uses a particular methodology that has a foundation in *Haṭha* yoga that was developed by Thomas Hanna of Hanna Somatics (Hanna 1979; 1988) and Eleanor Criswell of Somatic Yoga (Criswell 1987). It is based on their research that includes biofeedback.

By mindful interoceptive pandiculation (involuntary stretching of soft tissue), muscles are voluntarily contracted and eccentrically (slowly) de-contracted while focusing on the sensation of each movement. In this first-person approach, the resting lengths of chronically tense muscles are increased over time by engaging the brain, creating more space and comfort in the body. This methodology is unlike traditional yoga in which muscles are passively stretched and reflexively re-contracted at the level of the spinal cord. In addition, by its meditative nature, somatic movement decreases the stress response and increases the relaxation response. A chronic stress response causes chronic muscular contraction and inflammation which may compress and irritate nerves. Upregulation of the parasympathetic nervous system with somatic movement

(continued)

(continued)

enhances muscle relaxation and decreases inflammation (Galantino et al. 2019).

iRest

These meditations, developed by Richard Miller, PhD (Miller 2010), are trauma-informed and evidence-based, and support healing, personal growth, and well-being over a broad range of populations, including individuals with cancer. It was chosen for this protocol because this type of meditation has been shown to decrease the stress hormone cortisol, which drives the upregulation of the sympathetic nervous system. In 2010, iRest was endorsed by the United States Army Surgeon General and Defense Centers of Excellence as treatment for chronic pain (Miller 2015).

Mudrā (see Figure 6.3)

As with movement and breath, I teach clients calming and cooling *mudrā-s* that are said to enhance *apānavāyu* (downward moving energy) for grounding, stability, and security, as well as those that are said to enhance immune function (LePage & LePage 2013). I carefully choose *mudrā-s* to include simple hand positioning accessible to individuals with neuropathy symptoms so that they feel at ease during the practice. These may include:

- *adhimudrā* (gesture of primordial stillness)
- *cinmudrā* (gesture of consciousness)
- *bhūmudrā* (gesture of the Earth)
- *bhramaramudrā* (gesture of the bee)
- *hṛdayamudrā* (gesture of the spiritual heart)
- *kuberamudrā* (gesture of the Lord of Wealth)
- *apānamudrā* (gesture of downward current of purifying energy)
- *hākinīmudrā* (gesture of the Goddess Hākinī)
- *padmamudrā* (gesture of the lotus)
- *maṇḍalamudrā* (gesture of the circle)

The overall experience may be enhanced by teaching affirmations with the *mudrā* practice, with the invitation to repeat the affirmations quietly or aloud.

3.9 Yoga for bone health in a leukemia patient

Background: Bone health during cancer treatment

Leigh Leibel

Cancer survivors are at high risk for local or generalized bone loss, bone fragility, and bone fractures due to the deleterious impact of metastases and disease on the skeleton and its structure, as well as the toxic effect of anticancer therapies on bone cells (Drake 2013). Treatments that contribute to this include chemotherapy, radiotherapy, glucocorticoids, aromatase inhibitors, and androgen deprivation therapy, among others. Bone loss caused by the various cancer therapies occurs at a faster and more severe rate than that caused by normal aging – reported to be seven times higher (Guise et al. 2006, Dalton 2019). Given this, osteoporosis in cancer populations is a prevalent and debilitating disease that contributes to impaired health-related quality of life, disability, and death.

In 2019, the American Society for Clinical Oncology (ASCO) issued *Clinical Practice Guidelines for the Management of Osteoporosis in Cancer Survivors.* In their recommendation, the panel says, "Clinicians should actively encourage patients to engage in a combination of exercise types, including balance training, flexibility or stretching exercises, endurance exercise, and resistance and/or progressive strengthening exercises, to reduce the risk of fractures caused by falls" (Shapiro et al. 2019). While ASCO guidelines acknowledge that there is conflicting data as to whether exercise preserves bone density mass in cancer populations (as compared to healthy populations), they nonetheless recommend exercise in this population as a nonpharmacologic management intervention due to its known benefits to overall health, including improved sleep, mood, fitness, and a reduction in the risk of cancer recurrence and/or certain new cancers (Shapiro et al. 2019).

Weight-bearing and muscle-strengthening exercises are also recommended in the *Clinician's Guide to Prevention and Treatment of Osteoporosis* developed by multispecialty medical experts at the Bone Health and Osteoporosis Foundation (BHOF) (known as the National Osteoporosis Society [NOS] until October, 2021). In their recommendations they name yoga, pilates, and tai chi as exercises to improve agility, strength, posture, and balance to reduce the risk of falls (Cosman et al. 2014).

As the importance of exercise on skeletal health in at-risk cancer populations is increasingly recognized by oncologists, more research on the impact of exercise (including postural yoga) on bone density in cancer survivors is warranted. Today, there is still not enough research data to identify the most beneficial yoga poses for cancer survivors who are at risk for reduced bone density due to anticancer therapies, or to identify which yoga postures present the least risk for fracture or injury in this population. Research and literature on this subject exist (Sfeir et al. 2018, Smith & Boser 2013, Lu et al. 2016), but their findings are not mutually conclusive. Standardization of future research and broad inclusive discussions are needed.

However, widespread agreement does exist that movements emphasizing flexion of the thoracic spine and extreme thoracic twists are contraindicated for those people with, or at risk for osteoporosis, whether due to aging or disease. There is also agreement that moderate weight-bearing activities are beneficial to strengthen the muscles supporting the spinal column, promote balance, improve posture, reduce risk of falls, and enhance quality of life (Chan et al. 2003, Papaioannou et al. 2010, Sinaki 2012a & b, Sinaki & Mikkelsen 1984). This is endorsed by the BHOF in their public-facing patient information (see Box 6.16). Well-designed empirical studies are needed to further the understanding of which yoga poses are of greatest benefit and present the least risk to people with cancer and survivors who have bone health issues.

Given the above, yoga therapists and yoga professionals must exercise caution when working with people with cancer and survivors who are confirmed to have osteoporosis or are known to be at risk of developing it. Yoga programs should be designed to address each patient/client's current bone health status and comorbid conditions. There are many benefits of a yoga practice in cancer populations, including improved posture, balance, gait, coordination, strength, and range of motion, as well as reduced anxiety – all of which contribute to the health and well-being of people with cancer and survivors (Galantino et al. 2012, Järvinen et al. 2008, Smith & Boser 2013, Prado et al. 2014, Salem et al. 2013, Payne & Crane-Godreau 2013, DiBenedetto et al. 2005).

BOX 6.16 Bone Health and Osteoporosis Foundation website advice (BHOF 2022)

According to their website, "If you have osteoporosis, you should avoid any movements that require you to bend forward from the waist, such as doing a toe touch. When you bend forward from the waist, your shoulders and back become rounded. This is also known as spine flexion and can increase the risk of a spine fracture. If you have osteoporosis or are otherwise at risk of breaking bones in your spine, you should avoid twisting to a point of strain.

- Do not bend forward from the waist.

- Do not twist and bend at the torso (trunk) to an extreme.

- Do not lift/carry heavy objects.

- Do not bend forward when coughing and sneezing.

- Do not reach for objects on a high shelf.

- Do not do toe-touches, sit-ups, or abdominal crunches."

Client story: Bryan

Tari Prinster, RYT 200, C-IAYT

Bryan (he/his) is a 54-year-old White man diagnosed with acute lymphoblastic leukemia (ALL) and post-transplant graft-versus-host disease (GVHD).

Bryan is an acclaimed orthopedic surgeon who has led research on osteoporosis. He was diagnosed with acute lymphoblastic leukemia (ALL) after he was taken to the emergency room complaining of a rapid heart rate, shortness of breath, and a severe pounding headache. At time of diagnosis, he was physically fit, a life-long sports enthusiast, a proud father, and head surgeon at a local orthopedic center.

Upon diagnosis of ALL, Bryan immediately began a grueling six-month treatment protocol to prepare him for an allogeneic (donor) stem cell transplant. The induction phase consisted of six cycles of chemotherapy, including significant doses of glucocorticoids, and a strong dose of radiation therapy. Once his disease was controlled, he received a pre-transplant dose of chemotherapy designed to eradicate any residual disease including his bone marrow stem cells. He then received an infusion of stem cells from a donor.

Four months after his transplant, Bryan began losing weight, and experienced gastrointestinal distress and musculoskeletal pain. Movement was extremely difficult, "I felt like the Tin Man, grunting and moaning with the simplest movements." These symptoms led to the diagnosis of chronic graft-versus-host disease (GVHD), a syndrome commonly associated with allogeneic stem cell transplant, which is characterized by inflammation of various body organs. GVHD happens when the donated tissue (graft) recognizes the recipient (host) as foreign and the donor's white blood cells in the transplanted tissue attack cells of the recipient's body.

As a result of GVHD, Bryan underwent ten months of treatment and was bed-ridden for weeks at a time. He consequently lost body mass and strength. During this time, he lost over 35 pounds or 23% of his total body weight and he struggled to engage in any type of physical activity. As an orthopedic surgeon, Bryan knew the long-term risks caused by his cancer treatments and his increased risk of developing glucocorticoid-induced osteoporosis. He also knew exercise supports bone health. But how could he exercise with his fragile physical circumstances? A friend suggested yoga.

Bryan was referred to me for yoga therapy by a mutual friend, and I worked with him over a six-week period.

Each weekly yoga therapy session was 90 minutes. At our first session together, we thoroughly discuss his current health condition. He said his medical team had not ordered a DEXA scan (dual-energy X-ray absorptiometry) which is a measurement of bone density, even knowing his high risk of treatment-induced osteoporosis. Bryan and I prioritized safety and were extremely careful to protect his spine by selecting yoga poses that avoid stress on the spine which would increase the likelihood of breaking a bone.

With these precautions in mind, we designed a yoga program to include no forward bends, no gazing to ceiling in spinal extension, and no extreme twisting. The program had an emphasis on weight-bearing movement between poses, resistance holding poses to build bone and muscle strength, and movements to improve the strength and flexibility of the spine. A body weight metric was taken for each session. This is an overview of Bryan's program based on clinical notes:

- Supine with blanket neck adjustment, a belt was used for extension and flexion of knee to chest (*apāsana*) and lateral abduction and adduction of legs to the side. This helped support the lower spine and initiated connection with synchronized breathing.

- Other supine spine movements included: elongation, flexion (knees to chest; *apāsana*), and extension (modified bridge; *setubandhasarvāṅgāsana*) all with synchronized breathing.

- From a comfortable seated position or hero pose (*vajrāsana*), a centering breath and warm up arm *vinyāsa*, moving the spine in five directions taking all safety precautions and with proper breath was sequenced.

- From hands and knee sequences, moving the spine in five directions with all safety precautions with proper breath was completed.

- Seated with "legs-extended, forward folding" with straight back using a belt, followed by seated half cob-

bler pose (*ardhabaddhakoṇāsana*), both poses careful to keep spine elongated and properly aligned.

- Steps back to standing poses: lunge (*utthitāśvasañcalāsana*), modified sun salutation (*sūryanamaskāra*), and warrior I (*vīrabhadrāsana I*) using blocks, flowing with properly synchronized breath, created standing sequences.

- A modified kickstand tree (*vṛkṣāsana*) with heel resting to ankle and using the wall for balance was timed each session and included a breath awareness exercise.

- Legs-up-the-wall (*viparītakaraṇi*) at a >60 degrees each session.

In each weekly session the yoga intervention was similar, but the intensity was increased. We added movement sequences between standing poses and increased durations in standing/balancing poses. Additionally, an at-home, self-led practice was constructed for mid-week use.

- Session 1: Bryan was curious and, despite his weakness, eager. The first session included all sequences, except standing poses. Bryan struggled with the breath synchronization and tired easily. Weight 120 lbs.

- Session 2: Bryan maintained a daily self-directed practice of 30 minutes and extended legs-up-wall (*viparītakaraṇi*). He reported improved appetite. The second session included a simple step back to knee down for modified sun salutations (*sūryanamaskāra*) with spinal safety precautions, high lunge (*aṣṭacandrāsana*), and a 30-second tree pose (*vṛkṣāsana*). Weight 125 lbs.

- Session 3: Medication adjustment lead to spurred energy resulting in lengthened self-practice. Bryan was eager to learn more demanding standing poses. Weight 130 lbs.

- Session 4: Bryan continued to gain weight, strength, and confidence. He was curious about breathing practices in standing poses because this seemed

173

to increase his focus to hold poses longer. He was excited to see the increased time he could hold tree pose (*vṛkṣāsana*) without significant wobble. His professional experience and knowledge helped his appreciation of this pose, not only to meet his personal goals, but as a future appropriate intervention for his patients. Weight 134 lbs.

- Session 5: Recently, Bryan had a flare up of his GVHD that included muscle and fascial pain, skin changes, and GI irritability. A return to a higher dose of steroids was recommended by his doctors. However, Bryan continued self-practice, and he enjoyed modest weight gain and gained confidence in his strength and steadiness. Regardless of the treatment setback and anxiety about a poor prognosis, Bryan was increasingly enthusiastic about yoga as a tool to manage his future. Weight 136 lbs.

- Session 6: Session six gave witness to a one-minute tree pose (*vṛkṣāsana*) which was not only easy for him but accomplished without wobbling. Both results indicated increased muscle strength. He was inspired. Weight 140 lbs.

During the six weeks of yoga therapy sessions, Bryan also started light biking and hiking on his "good" days. He credited the yoga sessions with enabling this increased activity. He was impressed at how much body awareness yoga afforded him, "connecting top and bottom" as he described, "rather than speed and effort, and yet providing core work."

Three months later, Bryan came back for another yoga therapy session. He had continued to gain weight, build muscle mass, remain active with snowboarding, and had continued yoga three to four times a week. Additionally, he had introduced weight training and mountain biking. Corticosteroid dosage continued, so his challenges and risk of osteoporosis remained. In the meantime, he maintains his musculoskeletal fitness and bone strength with daily yoga, snowboarding, and biking. Weight after three months: 155 lbs.

Bryan credits yoga for giving him a way to come back to his beloved other sports. He said, "Yoga became a vital adjunct in my recovery, with multiple sessions per week over several months, and my strength and mobility improved. Yoga had a profound effect on my well-being, ability to concentrate and find confidence to get back to snowboarding without fear of fracture. Yoga will be an integral part of my future to mitigate the stiffness that occurs with aging and post-transplant challenges I will face the rest of my life."

3.10 Grief interrupted: finding a path forward

Background: Prolonged grief disorder (PGD)

Leigh Leibel

Grief is a natural and unavoidable reaction to loss – whether the death of a loved one, the news of a terminal medical diagnosis, or other life-impacting event such as job loss or divorce. Grief is unique to the individual and may be profound, eliciting a succession of feelings including sadness, anger, denial, guilt, bitterness, or shock. For most, these feelings will gradually diminish, usually within six months to a year (Royal College of Psychiatrists 2020). But for some, the normal grief reaction lingers and can be debilitating, especially if there is a second traumatic experience that "interrupts" the grieving process (Prigerson et al. 2009). When grief interferes with daily living, it is known as complicated grief or prolonged grief disorder (PGD); this disorder puts people at higher risk for medical problems (cancer, high blood pressure, heart and immunological issues) and warrants intervention by bereavement specialists and psychotherapists (Prigerson et al. 2009).

In late 2021, the American Psychiatric Association announced that PGD would be added to the newest version of the *Diagnostic and Statistical Manual of Mental Disorders* (DSM-5-TR) — the main guide for diagnosing mental health problems (American Psychiatric Association 2022).

Additional resources on PGD may be found on the website of the Center for Prolonged Grief at Columbia University (www.prolongedgrief.columbia.edu)

See also:

https://www.psychiatry.org/newsroom/news-releases/apa-offers-tips-for-understanding-prolonged-grief-disorder

https://complicatedgrief.columbia.edu/for-the-public/complicated-grief-public/overview/

The tools of yoga can help support the bereaved through their journey of heartbreak and loss, gently guiding them through darkness to light. In the book *Yoga for Grief and Loss*, Karla Helbert (licensed professional counselor and certified yoga therapist) writes, "The practice of yoga addresses self-care, helps to integrate the experience of loss, and supports feelings of connection and relationship with loved ones who have died" (Helbert 2016). Yoga therapists and yoga professionals can accompany bereaved patients/clients through compassionate communication and a created sense of safety, providing sacred space for them not only to explore their painful life events, but also to hold and carry their grief.

Client story: Teresa

Karen Apostolina, E-RYT 500

Teresa (she/her) is a 58-year-old Italian American woman diagnosed with stage II breast cancer.

Teresa's diagnosis, surgery, and first round of chemotherapy occurred when she was moving her husband to hospice care after a recurrence of untreatable stage IV germ cell cancer. Her second round of chemotherapy took place while planning his funeral. Suddenly a single mother, she was charged with running her husband's business investments during her continuing cancer treatment and she felt grief would have to wait. In ongoing survival mode, she relegated her sadness to the dark spaces occupied by earlier losses: her father when she was 28 and her brother from bone cancer when she was 19.

During our first session, Teresa tells me she has spent the last two years stuffing down all thoughts of her husband and hasn't cried in a year. She also recently began working with a mental health professional to help her process her lingering grief. She says she is stressed, has difficulty concentrating, and honestly doesn't know "who she is anymore." She tells me she's irritable and tired, yet in the next breath says she is thinking of remodeling her house! I let all of this sit for a moment, then I ask, "Where do you feel tightness in your body?" She places her hands over her heart and throat. Suddenly the weight of her sadness fills the room, and she says that a family member accused her of causing her husband's cancer by not contributing more financially to the marriage. We sit silently while these painful words hang in the air. "I know it's not my fault," she says. Tears well up.

I ask her to keep her hands over her heart, and sitting on my rug, we practice belly breathing. Once her breath calms, I show her "reclining bound angle" pose (*suptabaddhakoṇāsana*) over a bolster. As she lies back, she sighs deeply. Next, I suggest supported child's pose (*sālambabālāsana*) with her belly resting on the bolster. We finish with a simple body-scanning *yoganidrā* (yogic sleep), recording it so she can practice at home.

Next session, Teresa still feels anxious, but she reports an increase in well-being and calmer breath. She says a few days ago, while ironing a tablecloth and listening to the soundtrack of *Wicked*, she suddenly began to cry. Grief can erupt at any moment. We discuss how focusing on humble work such as ironing, cooking, and mending can be very much like meditation, so I encourage her to pursue this method of stilling her mind. Teresa loves music but doesn't feel comfortable chanting, so we discuss singing as a means of sound therapy; it turns out, music is a powerful release valve for her. In addition, we add simple core-strengthening *āsana* (posture) to her home practice to increase feelings of stability and confidence, and cobra poses (*bhujangāsana*) to bring awareness to the heart (*anāhata cakra*). In child's pose (*balāsana*), I add the weight of multiple blankets on her back to ease anxiety. For another version of *yoganidrā* (yogic sleep) I guide her in reclining bound angle pose (*suptabaddhakoṇāsana*), and suggest retrieving some peaceful images from her past. She remembers falling asleep in her father's lap as a child. This, and another beautiful image of rocking her own baby to sleep, evoke feelings of peace and provide an inner sanctuary, guiding her focus away from some of the disturbing thoughts she's been experiencing.

In the following weeks, Teresa reports her pain, fatigue, throat tightness, and anxiety have all decreased. Her release of emotion and the cultivation of positive images from her pre-loss life seem to correlate with an uptick in well-being. I ask her to describe more images – she shares memories of summers in Italy, sleeping as a child on her uncle's boat, and napping in the afternoon with her husband and kids while on family vacations at the desert or the beach. These common themes of sun-drenched slumber evoke happiness. Again, I cover her with multiple blankets before our *yoganidrā*. She says the blankets feel like a "warm hug," as opposed to grief, which "feels like a cold stone." Here she experiences the warmth she's been craving and is now learning to access this ease and relaxation on her own. Teresa smiles and says, "I think it's time to plan a trip to the beach and make some new memories." In that moment, Teresa seems radiant, a woman in full possession of her past and present, peacefully looking toward the future.

Section 3 references

Introduction

Berger, A.M., Mooney, K., Aranha, O., et al., 2021. NCCN Clinical Practice Guidelines in Oncology: Cancer-Related Fatigue. Version 1.2021. Available at: https://www.nccn.org/professionals/physician_gls/pdf/fatigue.pdf.

Chaoul, A., Milbury, K., Sood, A.K., et al., 2014. Mind-body practices in cancer care. *Curr Oncol Rep.* 16:417.

Danhauer, S.C., Addington, E.L., Cohen, L., et al., 2019. Yoga for symptom management in oncology: a review of the evidence base and future directions for research. *Cancer.* 125:1979–1989.

Denlinger, C.S., Sanft, T., Baker, K.S., et al., 2018. NCCN Clinical Practice Guidelines in Oncology: Survivorship. Version 3.2018. Available at: https://www.nccn.org/professionals/physician_gls/pdf/survivorship.pdf.

Desai, K., Bao, T., Li, Q.S., et al., 2021. Understanding interest, barriers, and preferences related to yoga practice among cancer survivors. *Support Care Cancer.* 29(9):5313–5321.

Ettinger, D.S., Berger, M.J., Arnand, S., et al., 2021. NCCN Clinical Practice Guidelines in Oncology: Antiemesis. Version 1.2021. Available at: https://www.nccn.org/professionals/physician_gls/pdf/antiemesis.pdf.

IARC, 2022. Global Cancer Observatory. International Agency for Research on Cancer. World Health Organization. Available at: https://gco.iarc.fr/.

Lyman, G.H., Greenlee, H., Bohlke, K., et al., 2018. Integrative therapies during and after breast cancer treatment: ASCO endorsement of the SIO clinical practice guideline. *J Clin Oncol.* 36:2647–2655.

Mao, J., et al., 2022. Integrative Medicine for Pain Management in Oncology: Society for Integrative Oncology–ASCO Guideline. *J Clin Oncol. 2022 Sep 19:JCO2201357.*

Maule, M., Merletti, F., 2012. Cancer transition and priorities for cancer control. *Lancet Oncol.* 13:745–746.

Mustian, K.M., Sprod, L.K., Janelsins, M., et al., 2013. Multicenter, randomized controlled trial of yoga for sleep quality among cancer survivors. *J Clin Oncol.* 31:3233–3241.

Narayanan, S., Francisco, R., Lopez, G., et al., 2019. Role of yoga across the cancer care continuum: from diagnosis through survivorship. *J Clin Outcomes Manag.* 26:219–228.

National Cancer Institute (NCI), 2020. Cancer Statistics. Available at: https://www.cancer.gov/about-cancer/understanding/statistics/.

Nietzsche, F., 1886. *The Gay Science.*

Society for Integrative Oncology, 2022. Available at: www.integrativeonc.org.

Sung, H., Ferlay, J., Siegel, R.L., et al., 2021. Global Cancer Statistics 2020: GLOBOCAN Estimates of Incidence and

Mortality Worldwide for 36 Cancers in 185 Countries. *CA Cancer J Clin.* 71(3):209–249.

U.S. Department of Health and Human Services (USDHHS), 2018. Use of yoga, meditation, and chiropractors among U.S. adults aged 18 and over. Available at: https://www.cdc.gov/nchs/data/databriefs/db325-h.pdf.

3.1 Managing fear of cancer recurrence through efforts in "warrior-ness"

Hall, D.L., Luberto, C.M., Philpotts, L.L., et al., 2018. Mind-body interventions for fear of cancer recurrence: a systematic review and meta-analysis. *Psychooncology.* 27(11):2546–2558.

Lebel, S., Ozakinci, G., Humphris, G., et al., 2017. Current state and future prospects of research on fear of cancer recurrence. *Psychooncology.* 26:424–427.

Sharpe, L., Curran, L., Butow, P., Thewes, B., 2018. Fear of cancer recurrence and death anxiety. *Psychooncology.* 27(11):2559–2565.

Simard, S., Thewes, B., Humphris, G., et al., 2013. Fear of cancer recurrence in adult cancer survivors: a systematic review of quantitative studies. *J Cancer Surviv.* 7(3):300–322.

Simonelli, L.E., Siegel, S.D., Duffy, N.M., 2017. Fear of cancer recurrence: a theoretical review and its relevance for clinical presentation and management. *Psychooncology.* 26(10):1444–1454.

3.2 Tenderness and self-compassion – redefining strength after cancer

Bernardi, L., Wdowczyk-Szulc, J., Valenti, C., et al., 2000. Effects of controlled breathing, mental activity and mental stress with or without verbalization on heart rate variability. *J Am Coll Cardiol.* 35(6):1462–1469.

Conrad, A., Müller, A., Doberenz, S., et al., 2007. Psychophysiological effects of breathing instructions for stress management. *Appl Psychophysiol Biofeedback.* 32(2):89–98.

Garcia, A.C.M., Camargos Junior, J.B., Sarto, K.K., et al., 2021. Quality of life, self-compassion and mindfulness in cancer patients undergoing chemotherapy: a cross-sectional study. *Eur J Oncol Nurs.* 51:101924.

Kim, C., Ko, H., 2018. The impact of self-compassion on mental health, sleep, quality of life and life satisfaction among older adults. *Geriatr Nurs.* 39(6):623–628.

Neff, K., 2022a. Definition of Self-Compassion. Available at: https://self-compassion.org/the-three-elements-of-self-compassion-2/.

Neff, K., 2022b. Fierce Self-Compassion. Available at: https://self-compassion.org/fierce-self-compassion/.

Taimni, I.K., 2014. *The Science of Yoga: The Yoga Sutras of Patanjali in Sanskrit.* Theosophical Publishing House; Wheaton, IL.

3.3 Breathing into life

Desikachar, T.K.V., 2003. *Reflections on Yogasūtra-s of Patañjali.* Krishnamacharya Yoga Mandiram.

Müller, F.M., 1926. Prasna Upanishad, Second Question Verse 2.1. In: *The Upanishads*, *Part 2.* Oxford University Press, pp. 274–275. Available at: https://archive.org/details/upanishads02ml/page/274/mode/2up?view=theater.

3.4 Returning to work after cancer treatment – the "new" normal

Fitch, M.I., Nicoll, I., Lockwood, G., 2021. Exploring the impact of physical, emotional, and practical changes following treatment on the daily lives of cancer survivors. *J Psychosoc Oncol.* 39(2):219–234.

Henderson, F.M., Cross, A.J., Baraniak, A.R., 2019. 'A new normal with chemobrain': experiences of the impact of chemotherapy-related cognitive deficits in long-term breast cancer survivors. *Health Psychology Open.* 6(1):2055102919832234.

Isaksson, J., Wilms, T., Laurell, G., et al., 2016. Meaning of work and the process of returning after head and neck cancer. *Support Care Cancer.* 24(1):205–213.

Yarker, J., Munir, F., Bains, M., et al., 2010. The role of communication and support in return to work following cancer-related absence. *Psychooncology.* 19(10):1078–1085.

3.5 Reframing caregiver distress

Inger, R., 2022. Caregiver Stress Sydrome. *Today's Caregiver.* Available at: https://caregiver.com/articles/caregiver-stress-syndrome/.

LePage, J., 2013. *Mudras for Healing and Transformation*. Integrative Yoga Therapy.

National Alliance for Caregiving (NAC), 2020. Caregiving in the U.S. 2020. Available at: https://www.caregiving.org/caregiving-in-the-us-2020/.

Roche V., 2009. The hidden patient: addressing the caregiver. *Am J Med Sci*. 337(3):199–204.

Taimni, I.K., 2014. *The Science of Yoga: The Yoga Sutras of Patanjali in Sanskrit*. Theosophical Publishing House; Wheaton, IL.

3.6 Ostomy and *āsana*

Association of Stoma Care Nurses UK (ASCN), 2016. ASCN Stoma Care National Clinical Guidelines. Available at: https://www.sath.nhs.uk/wp-content/uploads/2017/11/Stoma-Care-Guidelines.pdf.

Beeken, R.J., Haviland, J.S., Taylor, C., et al., 2019. Smoking, alcohol consumption, diet and physical activity following stoma formation surgery, stoma-related concerns, and desire for lifestyle advice: a United Kingdom survey. *BMC Public Health*. 19(1):574.

Campbell, K.L., Winters-Stone, K.M., Wiskemann, J., et al., 2019. Exercise guidelines for cancer survivors: consensus statement from international multidisciplinary roundtable. *Medicine & Science in Sports & Exercise*. 51(11):2375–2390.

Claessens, I.P.R., Tielemans, C., Steen, A., et al., 2015. The ostomy life study: the everyday challenges faced by people living with a stoma in a snapshot. *Gastrointest Nurs*. 13(5):18–25.

Hubbard, G., Beeken R., Taylor C., et al., 2017. Physical activity programme for people recovering from bowel cancer surgery with a stoma: manual. University of the Highlands and Islands, Inverness.

Hubbard, G., Taylor, C., Watson, A., et al., 2020. A physical activity intervention to improve the quality of life of patients with a stoma: a feasibility study. *Pilot and Feasibility Studies*. 6, 12.

Jin, Y., Ma, H., Jiménez-Herrera, M., 2020. Self-disgust and stigma both mediate the relationship between stoma acceptance and stoma care self-efficacy. *J Adv Nurs*. 76(10):2547–2558.

Lowe, B., Alsaleh, E., Blake, H., 2019. Assessing physical activity levels in people living with a stoma. *Nurs Stand*. 35(1):70–77.

Russell, S., 2017. Physical activity and exercise after stoma surgery: overcoming the barriers. *British Journal of Nursing*. 26(5):S20-S26.

Saunders, S., Brunet, J., 2019. A qualitative study exploring what it takes to be physically active with a stoma after surgery for rectal cancer. *Support Care Cancer*. 27(4):1481–1489.

Schmitz, K.H., Courneya, K.S., Matthews, C., et al., 2010. American College of Sports Medicine roundtable on exercise guidelines for cancer survivors. *Medicine & Science in Sports & Exercise*. 42(7):1409–1426.

Schwartz, A., de Heer, H.D., Bea, J.W., 2017. Initiating exercise interventions to promote wellness in cancer patients and survivors. *Oncology (Williston Park, NY)*. 31(10):711.

Vonk-Klaassen, S.M., de Vocht, H.M., den Ouden, M.E., et al., 2016. Ostomy-related problems and their impact on quality of life of colorectal cancer ostomates: a systematic review. *Qual Life Res*. 25(1):125–133.

3.7 Guided yogic meditation for anxiety during cancer remission – MSRT and PET techniques

Anusuya, U.S., Mohanty, S., Saoji, A.A., 2021. Effect of Mind Sound Resonance Technique (MSRT - a yoga-based relaxation technique) on psychological variables and cognition in school children: a randomized controlled trial. *Complement Ther Med*. 56:102606.

Gonzalez, M., Pascoe, M.C., Yang, G., et al., 2021. Yoga for depression and anxiety symptoms in people with cancer: a systematic review and meta-analysis. *Psycho-Oncology*. 30(8):1196–1208.

Nagendra, H.R., 2001. *Mind Sound Resonance Technique (MSRT)*. Swami Vivekananda Yoga Prakashana; Bangalore: p. 51.

Oswal, P., Nagarathna, R., Ebnezar, J., Nagendra, H.R., 2011. The effect of add-on yogic prana energization technique (YPET) on healing of fresh fractures: a randomized control study. *J Altern Complement Med*. 17(3):253–258.

Rao, M., Metri, K.G., Raghuram, N., Hongasandra, N.R., 2017. Effects of Mind Sound Resonance Technique (yogic relaxation) on psychological states, sleep quality, and cognitive functions in female teachers: a randomized, controlled trial. *Adv Mind Body Med.* 31(1):4–9.

Wang, Y., Metri, K., Singh, A., Raghuram, N., 2020. Immediate effect of mind sound resonance technique (MSRT – a yoga-based relaxation technique) on blood pressure, heart rate, and state anxiety in individuals with hypertension: a pilot study. *Journal of Complementary and Integrative Medicine.* 17(2):20170177.

3.8 Yogic management of chemotherapy-induced peripheral neuropathy (CIPN)

Bao, T., Zhi, I., Baser, R., 2020. Yoga for chemotherapy-induced peripheral neuropathy and fall risk: a randomized controlled trial. *JNCI Cancer Spectr.* 4(6):pkaa048.

Brown, T.J., Sedhom, R., Gupta, A., 2019. Chemotherapy-induced peripheral neuropathy. *JAMA Oncol.* 5(5):750.

Criswell, E., 1987. *How Yoga Works: An Introduction to Somatic Yoga.* Novato, CA; Freeperson Press.

Galantino, M.L., Tiger, R., Brooks, J., et al., 2019. Impact of somatic yoga and meditation on fall risk, function, and quality of life for chemotherapy-induced peripheral neuropathy syndrome in cancer survivors. *Integr Cancer Ther.* 18:1534735419850627.

Galantino, M.L., Brooks, J., Tiger, R., et al., 2020. Effectiveness of somatic yoga and meditation: a pilot study in a multicultural cancer survivor population with chemotherapy-induced peripheral neuropathy. *International Journal of Yoga Therapy.* 30(1):49–61.

Hanna, T., 1979. *The Body of Life: Creating New Pathways for Sensory Awareness and Fluid Movement.* Rochester, VT; Healing Arts Press.

Hanna, T., 1988. *Somatics: Reawakening the Mind's Control of Movement, Flexibility, and Health.* Boston, MA; Da Capo Press.

Le Page, J., Le Page, L., 2013. *Mudras for Healing and Transformation.* Sebastopol, CA; Integrative Yoga Therapy.

Miller, R., 2010. *Yoga Nidra: A Meditative Practice for Deep Relaxation and Healing.* Boulder, CO; Sounds True, Inc.

Miller, R., 2015. *The iRest Program for Healing PTSD.* Oakland, CA; New Harbinger Publications.

Naumann, F.L., Hunt, M., Ali, D., et al., 2015. Assessment of fundamental movement skills in childhood cancer patients [published correction appears in *Pediatr Blood Cancer.* 2016;63(3):574]. *Pediatr Blood Cancer.* 62(12):2211–2215.

Ness, K.K., Hudson, M.M., Pui, C.H., et al., 2012. Neuromuscular impairments in adult survivors of childhood acute lymphoblastic leukemia: associations with physical performance and chemotherapy doses. *Cancer.* 118(3):828–838.

Wildes, T.M., Depp, B., Colditz, G., Stark, S., 2016. Fall-risk prediction in older adults with cancer: an unmet need. *Support Care Cancer.* 24:3681–3684.

Winters-Stone, K.M., Horak, F., Jacobs, P.G., et al., 2017. Falls, functioning, and disability among women with persistent symptoms of chemotherapy-induced peripheral neuropathy. *J Clin Oncol.* 35(23):2604–2612.

3.9 Yoga for bone health in a leukemia patient

Bone Health and Osteoporosis Foundation (BHOF), 2022. Frequently asked questions. Available at: https://www.bonehealthandosteoporosis.org/patients/patient-support/faq/.

Chan, M.C., Anderson, M., Lau, E.M.C., 2003. Exercise interventions: defusing the world's osteoporosis time bomb. *Bulletin of the World Health Organization.* 81(11):827–830.

Cosman, F., de Beur, S.J., LeBoff, M.S., et al., 2014. Clinician's Guide to Prevention and Treatment of Osteoporosis. *Osteoporosis International.* 25(10), 2359–2381.

Dalton, M., 2019. ASCO Provides Guidance on Managing Osteoporosis in Cancer Survivors. *The ASCO Post.* Available at: https://ascopost.com/issues/november-25-2019/asco-provides-guidance-on-managing-osteoporosis-in-cancer-survivors/.

DiBenedetto, M., Innes, K.E., Taylor, A.G., et al., 2005. Effect of a gentle Iyengar yoga program on gait in the elderly: an exploratory study. *Arch Phys Med Rehabil.* 86:1830–1837.

Drake, M.T., 2013. Osteoporosis and cancer. *Current Osteoporosis Reports.* 11(3):163–170.

Galantino, M.L., Green, L., Decesari, J.A., et al., 2012. Safety and feasibility of modified chair-yoga on functional outcome among elderly at risk for falls. *Int J Yoga.* 5(2):146–150.

Guise, T.A., 2006. Bone loss and fracture risk associated with cancer therapy. *Oncologist*. 11:1121–1131.

Järvinen, T.L.N., Sievänen, H., Khan, K.M., et al., 2008. Shifting the focus in fracture prevention from osteoporosis to falls. *BMJ*. 336:124.

Lu, Y-H., Rosner, B., Chang, G., et al., 2016. Twelve-minute daily yoga regimen reverses osteoporotic bone loss. *Topics in Geriatric Rehabilitation*. 32(2)81–87.

Papaioannou, A., Morin, S., Cheung, A., et al., 2010. 2010 clinical practice guidelines for the diagnosis and management of osteoporosis in Canada: summary. *Canadian Medical Association Journal*. 182(17):1864–1873.

Prado, E.T., Raso, V., Scharlach, R.C., Kasse, C.A., 2014. Hatha yoga on body balance. *Int J Yoga*. 7(2):133–137.

Salem, G.J., Yu, S.S., Wang, M.Y., et al., 2013. Physical demand profiles of hatha yoga postures performed by older adults. *Evid Based Complement Alternat Med*. 2013:165763.

Sfeir, J.G., Drake, M.T., Sonawane, V.J., Sinaki, M., 2018. Vertebral compression fractures associated with yoga: a case series. *Eur J Phys Rehabil Med*. 54(6):947–951.

Shapiro, C.L., Van Poznak, C., Lacchetti, C., et al., 2019. Management of osteoporosis in survivors of adult cancers with non-metastatic disease: ASCO Clinical Practice Guideline. *J Clin Oncol*. 37:2916–2946.

Sinaki, M., 2012a. Exercise for patients with osteoporosis: management of vertebral compression fractures and trunk strengthening for fall prevention. *PM&R*. 4(11):882–888.

Sinaki, M., 2012b. Yoga spinal flexion positions and vertebral compression fracture in osteopenia or osteoporosis of spine: case series. *Pain Practice*. 13(1):68–75.

Sinaki, M., Mikkelsen, B.A., 1984. Postmenopausal spinal osteoporosis: flexion versus extension exercises. *Arch Phys Med Rehabil*. 65(10):593–596.

Smith, E.N., Boser, A., 2013. Yoga, vertebral fractures and osteoporosis: research and recommendations. *Int J Yoga Therap*. 23(1):17–23.

3.10 Grief interrupted – finding a path forward

American Psychiatric Association, 2022. *Diagnostic and Statistical Manual of Mental Disorders: DSM-5-TR*. 5th edition. Text revision. American Psychiatric Association Publishing; Washington, D.C.

Helbert, K., 2016. *Yoga for Grief and Loss*. Philadelphia, PA; Singing Dragon.

Prigerson, H.G., Horowitz, M.J., Jacobs, S.C., et al., 2009. Prolonged grief disorder: psychometric validation of criteria proposed for DSM-V and ICD-11. *PLoS Med*. 6(8):e1000121.

Royal College of Psychiatrists, 2020. Bereavement. Available at: https://www.rcpsych.ac.uk/mental-health/problems-disorders/bereavement.

Section 4 Recurrence and living with chronic cancer

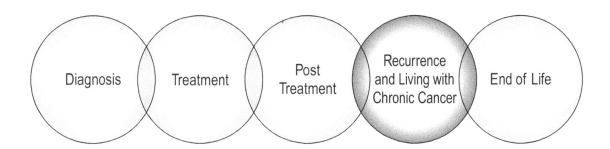

What if this mixture do not work at all?

Romeo and Juliet, Act 4: Scene 3

Introduction

Leigh Leibel

Recurrence and Living with Chronic Cancer is the fourth of the five phases of the Yoga in the Cancer Care Continuum. In this phase of care, the cancer has returned after treatment, and after a period of the patient having no clinical evidence of disease (typically, at least 12 months). The cancer may return to its original location, to nearby lymph nodes, or to other parts of the body. Some cancers may recur several times. A cancer recurrence is confirmed through imaging, lab tests, and biopsy. Each malignancy is unique. The intent of treatment for a cancer recurrence may be cure/remission, disease stabilization, or palliation. (See Chapter 4: Understanding Cancer and its Treatment.)

Recurrence is often described as one of the most stressful phases of the Cancer Care Continuum. A re-diagnosis can evoke strong emotions that may be more intense than those of the initial diagnosis. A 2010 Spanish study looking at the psychosocial impact of recurrence on survivors of cancer and their family members found that learning the cancer had recurred a second time was more devastating than the initial diagnosis (Vivar et al. 2010). All the participants in the study used the term *again* to describe recurrence of the disease. They identified the shock of recurrence and interruption of family life as a cause of great psychological distress.

A cancer recurrence tends to be harder to treat and control. However, for many survivors, improved and different anti-cancer therapies are transforming a cancer recurrence from a rapidly progressing condition to a chronic illness that people can manage and live with for many years or decades. In the exquisitely poignant memoir *When Breath Becomes Air*, Paul Kalanithi, a 36-year-old neurosurgeon, and new father diagnosed with stage IV metastatic lung cancer writes:

Until I actually die, I am still living.

Kalanithi (2016)

On the following pages, four yoga therapists share stories of working with their patients and clients whose cancer returned. We'll see how a yoga practice supported them through the emotional impact of a re-diagnosis and the management of treatment side effects – and helped them adjust to a new prognosis, an uncertain future, and regain a sense of agency in their lives. Not just being alive...*living.*

Recurrence, second cancers, and progression

According to the National Cancer Institute (NCI), "Recurrence rates can vary widely among cancer types, and within cancer types according to stage, histology, genetic factors, patient-related factors, and treatments. Some cancers are difficult to treat and have high rates of recurrence, while others, particularly when treated in earlier stages, have low recurrence rates. A *recurrence* is different from a *second* cancer that develops in another type of cell, and *progression* of cancer is different from a recurrence. Recurrence is cancer that goes away and comes back, while progression is cancer that worsens or spreads. Cancer that seems to return quickly may have become resistant to treatment, so it is considered progression, not recurrence." (NCI, 2020)

It is important for yoga professionals to remember that patients/clients who experience recurrence and/ or progression must be assessed for new and changing medical conditions before each yoga/yoga therapy session so that appropriate modifications may be made to ensure their safety during yoga.

Contributing authors to Section 4*

*Patient/client names have been changed and the stories edited to assure confidentiality. Each contributor has chosen whether to use the term "patient" or "client."

4.1 Full catastrophe living wake – coping with metastatic breast cancer

Background: Metastatic breast cancer

Chandrika Gibson, PhD, ND, PhD, MWell, E-RYT 500, C-IAYT and Leigh Leibel

Breast cancer remains the most common cancer in women[1] worldwide (World Cancer Research Fund 2020). Despite pink ribbon awareness campaigns and robust international advocacy, in 2020, more than 2.3 million women globally were newly diagnosed with breast cancer. This means that one in eight women will be diagnosed with breast cancer at some point in their lives (Siegel et al. 2017). Tragically, despite calls for early detection, risk reduction, and the development of new and different kinds of cancer therapies, breast cancer remains the leading cause of cancer-related death in women in both developed and undeveloped countries (World Health Organization 2020).

> Yoga therapists and advanced practice yoga teachers need to know that all people can develop breast cancer, and that breast cancers aren't the same: each is a different disease. Their respective treatments will have differing side effects and impacts on a yoga practice.

Within the breast cancer population, there is a subset of patients who have advanced or late-stage disease, meaning cancerous cells have been found in distant visceral organs such as lungs, liver, or in brain or bones. They are described as having stage IV metastatic breast cancer (MBC). Some present at diagnosis with end-stage disease, while some are diagnosed early-stage and their disease has progressed.

In 2017, it was estimated that about 155,000 women in the United States were living with MBC (Mariotto et al. 2017); the global estimates are not well described.

[1]Men and non-binary people may also develop breast cancer; in the United States, men represent approximately 1% of all newly diagnosed cases (American Cancer Society 2020).

For many, the diagnosis of MBC can be life-limiting, and/or the cancer must be actively managed as a chronic disease for the rest of their lives. This is particularly true if the cancer is classified as "triple-negative breast cancer" (TNBC), which is a complex disease well known for its aggressive behavior. It is a difficult type of cancer to treat. While TNBC accounts for just 10% to 20% of the worldwide breast cancer burden (Perou 2011), it disproportionately affects Black and Hispanic populations. Several large-scale population-based studies (Bauer et al. 2007) show that:

- TNBC is up to three times more likely to occur among premenopausal women of African American/Black descent.

- Younger, non-Hispanic Black and Hispanic women diagnosed with TNBC had more aggressive tumors and poorer survival regardless of stage of disease.

- Non-Hispanic Black women with late stage TNBC had the poorest survival rate of any comparable group.

TNBC also tends to affect younger White premenopausal women, as well as women of any age who have BRCA 1 or 2 or Li-Fraumeni Syndrome gene mutations.

MBC is a grossly underrepresented disease in cancer care, and in fact, cancer registries don't even track metastatic recurrences. Advocates call for MBC's increased inclusion in clinical trials and to prioritize the development of new lifesaving and life-extending drugs (Thrift-Perry et al. 2018).

Understandably, patients with advanced breast cancer and their families have complex needs that if not addressed, can result in severe distress. Disease and treatment-related symptoms can negatively impact quality of life, causing psychological distress, anxiety, depression, sleep disturbance, fatigue, and pain (Irvin et al. 2011, Ganz & Stanton 2015). This can have a significant impact on social, occupational, and emotional functioning, particularly when the person has a family with young children. While experiences of parents/mothers with metastatic cancer vary,

a theme running through much of the literature is that the tragedy of MBC is compounded for those who have dependent children (Bell & Ristovski-Slijepcevic 2011). The biographical disruption (changes in parent/child relationships) is made even more complex when the life of the primary caregiver is likely to be shortened due to disease (Bury 1982). The whole family ecosystem is impacted by the unknown timeline for treatment, the possibility of remission, and the likelihood of death.

Given this, a meticulous multidisciplinary approach to care is needed to support the well-being of MBC patients and their families, and especially their children. Ideally, the integrative team includes yoga therapists who are skilled at stress management and creating therapeutic relationships, and who are committed to continuity of care. Today, the focus of clinical care is shifting not only to increasing *quantity* of life, but also *quality* of life. This is especially true among women living with MBC. The symptom burden is high, yet survival rates are improving as new drugs come into play.

MBC Resource: "Project Life" is a free membership-based virtual wellness house for those living with metastatic breast cancer and their loved ones: https://www.projectlifembc.com.

Client story: Michelle

Chandrika Gibson

Michelle (she/her) is a 42-year-old White woman diagnosed with metastatic stage IV triple-negative breast cancer that has spread to the spinal cord and brain.

Michelle is a vivacious woman with four young children. Seven years ago, she was diagnosed with stage II triple-negative breast cancer (TNBC) and underwent a double mastectomy with reconstruction and chemotherapy. Three years later the cancer recurred, and she was told she now has incurable metastatic disease. At the time of recurrence, she was aged 39 and the youngest of her four children was just 16 months old.

During this second cancer go-round, her oncology team advised five months of intense chemotherapy, plus the addition of a newly approved immunotherapy drug to treat triple-negative breast cancer. She immediately started treatment and managed side effects such as headaches and nausea with medication. It was during this phase of care that she began attending community yoga-for-cancer classes. She found support being with other women with a shared cancer experience. For example, when the drugs caused her hair to start falling out in clumps, she invited yoga friends over to shave her head. Her husband and eldest son joined them. Difficult weeks ensued and her friends stood by in support. As with many cancer patients, her veins "collapsed" (veins may become scarred after multiple needle sticks), and she needed a port placed in her chest to receive chemotherapy. Her body rejected multiple ports, she had infections around the port site, and needed repeated surgeries to replace ports.

In the three years since her metastatic diagnosis, through ups and downs, she has been a regular at group yoga. Michelle's determined mindset and outgoing personality have drawn people to her. Along the way she has shared openly on social media, made vlogs while in hospital, and encouraged her friends to use the life-embracing language she prefers:

I want to continue walking and staying fit and I want to break down those misconceptions about metastatic breast cancer. I'd love for people to use the term "chronic disease" instead of "terminal disease or stage IV disease." I hate those words so don't use them around me.

She has also made deep friendships through a metastatic breast cancer support group, has reconnected with old school friends, reached out to her local community, engaged in fundraising events for cancer charities, and gathered her community – her *sangha* – at every opportunity. However, her attachments to others going through a similar experience with metastatic disease have ended in heartbreak numerous times, bringing to the front of her mind the reality of her life-limiting diagnosis. With each loss she forges on, determined to live her dharma or "right way of living" without attachment to the outcome. Each time a friend from support group dies, Michelle mourns for their families left behind, while strengthening her own resolve to live well:

As sad as this is, life does go on. It deepens my resolve to enjoy my life and take every opportunity to squeeze every drop of love, laughter, joy, and hope out of what time I have left! Don't worry, I'll be bugging you all for a good time yet! So, expect nothing different, plenty of adventures, social gatherings, holidays, and big birthdays (even if they aren't big ones).

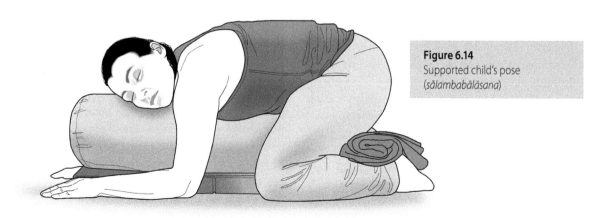

Figure 6.14
Supported child's pose
(*sālambabālāsana*)

Unfortunately, when Michelle's brain tumor began to affect her ability to drive, she was no longer able to attend classes, so she turned to me for one-on-one yoga therapy in her home (Box 6.17). During one of our sessions, she told me she wanted to throw herself a living wake. We enjoyed planning it! She invited her boarding school friends to drink, eat, cry, recount their school day memories of her, and cozy up together in pajamas for an emotional sleepover. She gave a speech about her life, her impending death, and what she wants when she's gone. It is her wish for everyone to do what matters for them without hesitation. Emotions ran high at this event, with the specter of Michelle's mortality contrasting with her effervescent hostess style. While alcohol flowed freely, this was not a *tamasic* (melancholic) environment, rather one of joyous celebration of this cherished woman's life and laughter.

Michelle holds onto hope that she will be among the few who defy this diagnosis. She wants to see her children reach adulthood, maybe even hold a grandchild or two – yet she maintains a pragmatic approach, knowing her death could come sooner rather than later. When that day comes, it will be a poignant close to a remarkable life, one that has inspired, educated, and prompted all people around her to live fully and with the undeniable knowledge of death.

BOX 6.17 Considerations when working with metastatic breast cancer

Chandrika Gibson

Key issues identified during intake and assessment: low back pain and concerns about mortality

Each session began with a check-in and ongoing assessment, particularly around pain, fatigue, lymphedema, breast reconstruction, port infection, and leg strength. Michelle's goals for yoga therapy were staying well enough to walk her children to and from school, manage back pain related to spinal metastases without needing high doses of pain medi-

(continued)

(continued)

cation, and having a space to discuss death with someone outside the family unit.

In the first two sessions, she talked at length about facing her fear of death, her desire to leave a meaningful legacy for her children and community, and her burgeoning spiritual perspective including dreams of a deceased friend welcoming her to a peaceful afterlife. In later sessions this theme recurred when friends in her metastatic cancer support group died.

Yoga therapy goals

Psycho-spiritual well-being through focus on *vijñānamayakośa* (sheath of wisdom), an intention to balance *pitta* (an *Āyurvedic* quality based on fire) (especially when skin irritation/infection was flared up), and support to maintain a *sāttvic* (quality of purity/goodness; one of the three *guṇa-s* from *Saṅkhyā* philosophy) inner and outer environment (see Chapter 2, *Yoga philosophy*).

The initial assessment occurred at a time when Michelle had been suffering sleep disturbance, was undergoing 12 weeks of chemotherapy, had back pain rated at 7/10, and was generally very fatigued, rating her energy at 3/10. This meant that initial yoga therapy practices involved bolsters and cushions to provide comfort in moderate-long held restorative poses such as *suptabaddhakoṇāsana* (reclining bound cobbler pose), *jānuśīrṣāsana* (head-to-knee pose), *viparītakaraṇī* (legs-up-the-wall pose), *sālambabālāsana* (supported child's pose, see Figure 6.14) and supported *śavāsana* (corpse pose). During each pose, a mindful breath awareness, and body scanning helped manage pain. A *yoganidrā* (yogic sleep) recording was provided for home practice.

Checking-in before each session

At the start of each yoga therapy session, a brief check-in showed that Michelle's needs were different each week, depending on treatment, sleep, and emotional fluctuations. When she had more energy, the practice included standing postures, flowing arm movement, *utkaṭāsana* (chair pose) and *vīrabhadrāsana* (warrior pose) to rebuild leg strength. Her goals to stay active and engaged with her family didn't waiver, no matter how uncomfortable she felt.

(continued)

185

BOX 6.17 continued

Managing lymphedema

This meant avoiding overheating by resting between active postures, while bringing rhythmic movement to arms intended to move stagnant lymphatic fluid. Active practices included rotating wrists, circling shoulders, and moving from *vīrabhadrāsana I* (warrior I) to *vīrabhadrāsana II* (warrior II). To avoid worsening lymphedema, there was minimal time spent weight-bearing through arms. Seated cat/cow and hamstring stretches such as *paścimottānāsana* (seated forward bend) fulfilled some of the same goals as "kneeling" cat/cow (*mārjaryāsana*) and *adhomukhaśvānāsana* (downward-facing dog), and an attitude of exploration was encouraged.

Navigating her port

Michelle's port produced blood clots within the region and as a result her right arm swelled up, causing a limited range of motion in her neck and right shoulder. The doctor who was treating the clots with an anti-coagulant cleared her for movement. Cues included reminders to move within pain-free range. Despite having a port in her chest, Michelle found restorative postures such as *sālambabālāsana* (restorative child's pose; see Figure 6.14) over a bolster very comfortable, and this position in particular gave relief to her lower back pain.

Bone metastases

Triple-negative breast cancers are more likely to spread to "visceral organs" such as the brain, liver, and lungs, and unlike estrogen-positive tumors, are less likely to spread to bones. Unfortunately, bony metastases were found in Michelle's mid-low back around T5 and her right ileum bone. The risk of fractures became a consideration when planning all movement, and even when she had energy for standing postures, the couch was always within arm's reach to lower the risk of a fall.

Practices on difficult days

With a staph infection causing itchy skin that bled and scabbed, tightness in her chest and back from multiple surgeries, pain radiating from her lower back, and discomfort in her elbow when lymphedema flared

(continued)

(continued)

up, it was not surprising to hear her express frustration. On those days we used more mindfulness-based approaches, very gentle limbering movements, slow, steady, diaphragmatic breathing, moving awareness through the body without judgment, and the cultivation of self-observation, allowing the thoughts and feelings of grief and frustration to be present without entering into battle with them.

Mindful yoga intervention for MBC: results of a randomized controlled trial (RCT)

Women with metastatic breast cancer (MBC) may experience pain, fatigue, sleep disturbance, and mental health issues. In an RCT study of women with MBC (n=64), "higher mindfulness" was associated with lower symptom levels including lower pain severity, pain interference, fatigue, anxiety, depression, and sleep disturbance. The study investigators concluded that mindfulness – and in particular "nonreactivity, nonjudging, and describing" – may help women cope with their disease (Zimmaro et al. 2020).

In the investigators' words: "For women with MBC, nonreactivity may be particularly useful for noticing and stepping back from – as opposed to getting overtaken by – distressing thoughts and feelings. Women high in nonreactivity may be able to redirect their attention to the present moment more effectively, while letting any thoughts or feelings that may cause significant distress to exist in the background. Such nonreactivity may promote a more balanced and calm mental response to typically distressing stimuli, thus lowering sympathetic nervous system arousal, hypothalamic-pituitary-adrenal (HPA) axis dysregulation, and downstream immune dysregulation. Such physiological processes are thought to be mechanisms by which meditation interventions produce beneficial outcomes."

(Zimmaro et al. 2020)

L.L.

4.2 Making meaning after recurrence

Background: Meaning-making and existential distress

Tina Paul, MS, E-RYT 500, C-IAYT and Leigh Leibel

For many people with cancer, being diagnosed with a life-threatening illness can evoke existential distress and trigger a desire to search for greater meaning and purpose in their lives (Greisinger et al. 1997, Kissane 2000). While many in the medical community recognize that patient-centered care means attending to the *whole* person (including their existential concerns), the reality is that for many people with cancer and survivors, their spiritual health and well-being continues to be an unmet psychosocial need (Piderman et al. 2015, Greisinger et al. 1997).

In the seminal Holocaust survival memoir *Man's Search for Meaning*, Victor Frankl, MD, an Austrian psychiatrist, writes that man's primary motivation in life is the desire to find meaning.

Elaborating on Friedrich Nietzsche's wisdom in the book *Twilight of the Idols*, Dr. Frankl quotes Nietzsche: *"If we have our own 'why' in life, we shall get along with almost any 'how.'"* Dr Frankl believed that finding a purpose in life is *"a tangible way to decrease suffering"* (Frankl 1998), and that *meaning* can be born in each moment and cherished…even during times of suffering:

For the meaning of life differs from man to man, from day to day and from hour to hour. What matters, therefore, is not the meaning of life in general but rather the specific meaning of a person's life at a given moment.

Victor Frankl, *Man's Search for Meaning*

A sense of purpose is, of course, personal – and unique to everyone. But researchers have identified some universal themes. In a 2013 focus group study of cancer survivors (n=23) in the Netherlands, Dutch investigators found that the most frequently mentioned themes around "meaning-making in cancer" were relationships and experiences. In general, study participants experienced enhanced meaning during cancer through five areas: relationships, experiences, resilience, goal-orientation, and leaving a legacy. Paradoxically, however, some participants said they (also) experienced a loss of meaning in their lives through experiences, social roles, relationships, and uncertainties about the future (van der Spek et al. 2013). At the time, this was the first study that used patient focus groups to look at meaning-making in cancer survivors. Today, it continues to inform meaning-based interventions in oncology.

In another study, Livestrong (a cancer charity in the United States) asked 429 lymphoma survivors to explore the themes of meaning, cancer worry, security, identity, grief, and guilt, and their impact on their lives post-treatment. Most (73–86%) endorsed existential concerns, with 30–39% also reporting related perceived functional impairment. Not surprisingly, the study found existential challenges impacted their lives for years after diagnosis (Posluszny et al. 2016).

These studies provide important feedback for developing successful interventions to better support cancer populations. Since we know that being able to sustain meaning during cancer treatment can buffer against hopelessness, despair, and suicide ideation (Breitbart et al. 2018), it makes sense that raising awareness and helping patients reconnect to a source of meaning can help them cope with overwhelming emotions and existential concerns. Given this, yoga therapy, as a spiritual practice, can help guide patients in their quest to rewrite their own narratives in the face of protracted illness, and support them as they strive to form a new self-identity. For some, purpose may be a life raft in a sea of uncertainty.

Patient story: Anu

Tina Paul

Anu (she/her) is a 54-year-old woman of South Asian descent who has been diagnosed with recurrent epithelial ovarian cancer.

Anu arrives and sits down. She is focused, yet seems anxious. Her petite, slender frame is retracted in the seat. Three years ago, she was treated for stage III ovarian cancer. Her end-of-therapy PET scan (positron emission tomography) showed she had no evidence of disease (NED), yet in the back of her mind she knows that her type of cancer has a statistically high incidence of recurrence. She has been doing well in the years since she completed treatment, but she has lingering effects of neuropathy from the cisplatin chemotherapy treatment, presenting mainly as numbness in her fingers and toes.

In the last few months, she has been experiencing fatigue, bloating, abdominal pain, and a sense of "fullness" after eating a few bites of food – signs and symptoms that the ovarian cancer may have returned. She is worried. She has been in touch with her oncologist, and in addition to medical tests, he has referred her to me for help managing anxiety and insomnia. In our last yoga therapy session, she was waiting for the results of her CA-125 serum blood test and CT scan. Today, she shares that the fear and worry she spoke of in our last session have spilled into a new understanding that the ovarian cancer is back. She is preparing for another round of chemotherapy and immunotherapy that is to start in a few weeks. She is scared, and her wish is to counteract symptoms as much as she possibly can and not be a burden on her family. "I'm mostly worried about my family and how they are handling things. Neither of my children has expressed much, but there's this heaviness between us," she states softly, with teary eyes. We sit quietly.

She tells me she has asked her oncology team for a referral to a licensed mental health professional who specializes in anxiety and family grief. I assure her that I will work alongside her psychologist to reinforce her goals of care and help her with relaxation techniques to better manage anxiety.

I ask her how she feels. She says she is experiencing some abdominal discomfort and chronic numbness from neuropathy, as well as a tightness in her chest (like she can't take a full breath in), and her mind is racing. I ask what she wants to gain from the session, and she says to support her despair, calm her mind, and to find something that might help the numbness in her feet. I ask about some of her favorite places that draw forth a sense of meaning, purpose, and joy. She mentions long walks, birdwatching in her quiet yard, the ocean, spending time with her family, and stillness.

We begin our practice on the floor in a constructive rest pose (*śavāsana* variation with bent knees; see Box 6.18), with her legs over stacked blocks and a bolster, and a small blanket tucked underneath her head. Soft singing bowl sounds play in the background. I invite Anu to slowly notice how her body is making contact with the floor, how her clothes are making contact with the body, and to notice the sounds in the room, near and far. She gently rocks her head from side to side. I invite her to place both hands on her collarbone, with the elbows softly on the floor, and notice any movement underneath her hands. Once she's comfortable, I ask if there's a word or image – perhaps a favorite place at the ocean's edge – that brings joy: "in your mind's eye, bring forth a word, image, place, person, pet – anything that brings you a feeling of equanimity, peace, and calm." She nods and says, "my family cottage." I continue, "Allow this place to fill your senses on the inhale. Allow the sensation to permeate throughout the space underneath your hands on the exhale."

Using this breath visualization, I slowly guide her through her body, from the area of the ribcage to her low belly. I notice that Anu's face becomes soft and more relaxed, and I see her breath begin to ebb and flow in her chest, ribs, and belly. While in constructive rest pose I invite Anu to point and flex her toes, synching with the inhale and exhale, and slowly rotate her feet in one direction, and then the other, in a joint-freeing (*pavanamuktāsana*) series. She laughs, "I can feel my numb feet, if only a little. It's not painful."

We remove the bolster from underneath her knees, and with Anu still on her back, explore gentle knee to chest (*apānāsana*) movements. We draw the right knee into the chest and pause for several breaths while she visualizes birdwatching with her family. I invite her to release the right leg to the floor and notice both sides (legs). "The right side feels heavier, closer to the ground, and more relaxed," she says. We continue to the left side, drawing the knee gently toward the chest, pausing on this side. As she relaxes and breathes slowly in and out, she imagines the ocean and her children playing in the waves. She releases the left side slowly to the floor and says, "I feel closer to the ground and more relaxed, the tightness in my chest has melted. Actually, it sounds crazy, but it feels like my heart is warm and full." We complete the practice with a guided relaxation, a soft blanket covering her whole body for warmth.

Anu notes that her presence has shifted. She reports feeling lighter, calm, and more "in her body." We revisit the concept of meaning and purpose, and ways of incorporating what is most meaningful to her in her day-to-day life. "After today, all I want to do is spend more time with my family, be in nature, and rest in stillness." Anu's eyes brighten as she anticipates visiting her family cottage where she can enjoy stillness and birdwatching before our next session together.

BOX 6.18 Yoga therapy and meaning-making

Tina Paul

Yoga therapy offers a safe container for "meaning-making" in the present moment. An integrated practice of movement, breathing, meditation, and meaning-centered inquiry offers a practice that meets the patient right where they are, and helps support self-regulatory skills, emotional regulation, and re-appraisal of life situations (Sullivan et al. 2018). Meditative breathing techniques draw awareness back to the present moment and cultivate calm. It is this practiced calm – and a reliable ability to return

(continued)

(continued)

to it – that allows a patient to choose their mindset, and to identify and engage with activities and ideas that hold profound meaning.

Three-part breath and gentle movement

Utilizing three-part breath (*dīrghaprāṇāyāma*) in constructive rest pose (*śavāsana* variation with bent knees) we bring our focus to grounding and awareness, directing it to different parts of the body that are clenching in fear. This practice brings somatic awareness to the belly, ribcage, and upper chest, and anchors the patient to the present moment while witnessing movement and expansion in the body. The patient is encouraged to notice movement at the collarbones, expansion in the ribcage, and sense the rise and fall of the abdomen. The patient is led through a series of yoga postures including knee to chest (*apānāsana*), with a guided reminder of infusing each shape with a connection to an idea that holds meaning for the patient.

4.3 Addressing hyperkyphosis

Background: Hyperkyphosis

Marianne Woods Cirone, MS, MFA, CYT 500

Hyperkyphosis is the exaggerated anterior curvature in the thoracic spine, sometimes referred to as a "hunchback." Though typically associated with aging, people with cancer and survivors can be at increased risk for hyperkyphosis because of bone loss, protective posturing, muscle weakness, pain, as well as the effects of surgeries, radiotherapy, and medications. Some of the common medications with deleterious effects on bone health include (Panday et al. 2014):

- Glucocorticoids

- Proton pump inhibitors

- Selective serotonin reuptake inhibitors

- Thiazolidinediones

- Anticonvulsants

- Medroxyprogesterone acetate

- Hormonal therapies: aromatase inhibitors and androgen deprivation

- Heparin

- Calcineurin inhibitors

- Some chemotherapies

People with cancer often receive combinations of these medications, potentially compounding their harmful effects. Other important facts about hyperkyphosis include:

- The condition correlates with osteoporosis (bone loss) and is also an independent risk factor for other health problems (Roghani et al. 2017), including impaired mobility, increased risk of falls and fractures, restricted breathing, the impairment of organ functioning, and lymphatic flow (Tominaga 2016, Sinaki et al. 2005).

- It can lead to negative psychological effects by affecting the vagus nerve and the autonomic nervous system (van der Jagt-Willems et al. 2015), and even lead to an increased risk of mortality (Kado 2009).

- It can also have a "snowball" effect, predisposing those with the condition to spinal compression fractures, leading to more hyperkyphosis.

Although postural abnormalities can be debilitating and tend to be progressive, they are often overlooked by the medical establishment. Fortunately, hyperkyphosis and osteoporotic bone loss can both potentially be prevented or limited with intervention (Jang et al. 2019), and through the use of appropriate yoga therapies (Lu et al. 2016, Norlyk Smith & Boser 2013, Fishman 2010).

Client story: Arlene

Marianne Woods Cirone

Arlene (she/her) is a 64-year-old White woman with a recurrence of breast cancer occurring ten years after her primary diagnosis and treatment.

Arlene has recently undergone a double mastectomy without reconstruction or chemotherapy. Because of her type 1 diabetes, Arlene wears an insulin pump on her front body and cannot lie in a prone position. She's also had axillary lymph node dissection and is at risk for lymphedema, although she hasn't developed symptoms. After treatment, her physician ordered a DEXA (dual-energy X-ray absorptiometry) scan which is an imaging test that measures bone density or strength. It shows she has osteoporosis secondary to several risk factors (age, thin body type, genetics, and a history of bone-weakening medications). Her end-of-therapy CT scan showed no evidence of bone metastases. Unfortunately, Arlene's surgeon did not give her any exercises to do after surgery and she has developed hyperkyphosis and a reduced range of motion in her upper body, although she does not have adhesive capsulitis, or so-called "frozen shoulder."

> Diabetes is a common comorbidity in people with cancer. In addition to observing current best practices in yoga in cancer, yoga therapists and yoga professionals should observe all precautions and best practices for yoga in diabetic populations.
>
> L.L.

When Arlene is medically cleared, we schedule a session and I ask questions to determine the modifications she'll need. She's a bubbly person with curly red hair, a quick talker with a bright smile. From an *Āyurvedic* perspective, osteoporosis and the related hyperkyphosis are associated with an imbalance of *vātadoṣa* (an *Āyurvedic* mind-body element associated with air and space). In addition, both cancer and osteoporosis are primarily found in those aged 60 and over, corresponding to the *vāta* stage of life. In *Āyurvedic* medicine, type 1 diabetes is typically considered an imbalance of *vātadoṣa*. In addition to her physical conditions, Arlene experiences severe anxiety, also associated with a *vāta* imbalance. To pacify *vātadoṣa*, we'll do gentle, warming movements, combined with restorative poses, slow breathing, body awareness, *mudrā-s* (hand gestures), and *yoganidrā* (yogic sleep). We will also include a thoracic spine-focused backbend to build spinal strength and improve her posture.

We start with a reclining chest opener. A folded blanket is positioned along and under the spine encouraging chest opening, spinal length, and alignment. A second blanket is placed under the head, with the edge rolled under, supporting the neck. We are cautious about adding elevation beneath the thoracic spine (as often seen in standard reclining chest openers) since lying flat can feel like a backbend for a person with hyperkyphosis. Here, Arlene takes slow, full breaths, focusing on the exhalation to help calm her nervous system.

Hyperkyphosis is often associated with shortened hamstrings and hip flexors, so I guide Arlene through "reclining hand to big toe" pose (*suptapādāṅguṣṭhāsana*) I, II, and III. *Suptapādāṅguṣṭhāsana* is the safest way to lengthen hamstrings for people with bone loss in the spine, there being no risk of spinal rounding, as exists in seated and standing forward bends. To work on upper- and mid-body mobility, we include:

- Raised hands pose (*ūrdhvahastāsana*): reclining dynamic and static versions, using a block between the hands.

- Upward facing dog pose (*ūrdhavamukhaśvānāsana*) against the wall (to reduce lymphedema risk).

- Reclined Lord of the Fishes pose (*suptamatsyendrāsana*) and seated Lord of the Fishes pose (*matsyendrāsana*).

To increase spinal mobility and to elongate the psoas muscles, we include supported bridge pose (*setubandhasarvāṅgāsana*) with one leg extended, and reclining postures to increase hip mobility. Next, we practice *pavanamuktāsana* series, a joint-freeing series (Stiles 2000), seated in a chair so as not to risk rounding the spine. Arlene pauses here to do the *daṇḍasvāsthyamudrā* for spinal health ("spinal column established in well-being" *mudrā* [hand gesture]): in this, the thumb, middle, and pinky fingers of the right hand will touch each other, while the thumb of the left hand will press on the second phalange of the folded index finger (Arora 2015; see Figure 6.3).

We then practice a thoracic extension technique (see Box 6.19), starting seated in a chair and building up to versions in chair pose (*utkaṭāsana*) and warrior I (*vīrabhadrāsana I*) in future sessions. Arlene feels fatigue in her mid-back, an area not accustomed to strength-building, and we stop before she overworks the area. We end with *yoganidrā* (yogic sleep) in a restorative pose, and a silent *śavāsana* (corpse pose) to still the mind and integrate the *koṣa-s* (in yogic philosophy, the five sheaths of existence; see *Yoga philosophy* in Chapter 2). As we conclude, Arlene smiles with a calm expression I haven't seen in her before.

After months of working together and with everyday home study, Arlene returns to a full range of shoulder movement and improved posture. Her mental and physical recovery is very good, and her surgeon tells her that she's "done better than his other patients." The degree of her hyperkyphosis appears decreased (this is our observation – we haven't measured pre-post), and her posture appears more upright. She can freely lift and open her chest and the mobility in her shoulders has significantly increased. Arlene continues to use yoga to help with her anxiety, to keep her posture aligned, and to help her to stay mobile, yet grounded. She lives each day with joy, often babysitting for her young granddaughters and spending time in her garden.

BOX 6.19 Thoracic extentsion technique for hyperkyphosis

Marianne Woods Cirone

To improve posture and counter the effects of gravity, bone loss, muscular weakness, and other issues contributing to hyperkyphosis, the sequence presented below focuses on a specific back bend technique. An older, but pivotal study (Sinaki & Mikkelsen 1984), clearly demonstrates the protective benefits of backbends for women with osteoporosis. This landmark research implicated forward bends, finding an 89% correlation between a practice of forward bends and the appearance of new spinal fractures. As it is unethical to do a similar study after such compelling evidence of risk, we still rely on this older study to guide us, although more recent case studies also show the damaging effects of flexion (Sinaki 2012). The safest and most effective practice for spinal health for those with bone loss includes appropriate back bends and excludes rounding the spine, which increases the risk for spinal fractures and hyperkyphosis.

Additionally, this sequence incorporates modifications often needed by people with cancer to address commonly co-occurring conditions such as osteoporosis, lymphedema, and joint pain. Championed by Dr. Gill Solberg, an Israeli kinesiologist and yoga therapist, and the author of *Postural Disorders and Musculoskeletal Dysfunction: Diagnosis, Prevention and Treatment*, the movements isolate extension in the thoracic spine, an area often unaddressed in "global" backbend poses due to compensatory hyperextension in the cervical and lumbar spine (Solberg 2008). Without isolating the extension in the thoracic spine, improvements will not be optimal. While many common chest openers, backbends, and extensor strengthening poses are done in a prone position, this can be uncomfortable or contraindicated for some cancer patients. Fortunately, this extension technique can be done in other positions, including in standing poses such as chair pose *(utkaṭāsana)* and warrior I *(vīrabhadrāsana I)* as well as seated in a chair, or even while kneeling.

(continued)

(continued)

Isolated spinal extension

- Clients start from a position (standing, seated, or kneeling) where the angle between the spine and the thighs is less than 90 degrees. For example, in a seated position, done most easily seated on a chair, the client sits tall with the spine long and a slight anterior tilt of the pelvis. The client leans forward with spine pitched at an angle of approximately 45 degrees. Holding the arms out wide at shoulder height, thumbs facing downward, helps to isolate the movement in the thoracic spine.

- From the starting position, the client externally rotates the arms, thumbs turning upward, while coming into a slight backbend that starts at the lower thoracic spine. The movement is subtle, but it focuses the effects on the mid-thoracic spine. Because of the angle of the spine, there is little possibility of a compensatory extension occurring in the cervical and/or lumbar spine, and the maximum extension occurs in the mid-thoracic spine. This focus of the movement in the thoracic spine gives it the greatest chance of reducing the hyperkyphosis, or excessive curve in the spine.

4.4 Imagine that!

Background: Spiritual care

Leigh Leibel

Spiritual care is increasingly recognized by healthcare providers as an essential part of caring for people with cancer. In fact, spiritual *distress* – including existential distress, hopelessness, despair, and anger at a higher power (however each of us defines that) – is acknowledged as a possible source of severe pain for people with cancer that can result in poorer health outcomes across physical, social, and emotional domains, as well as contribute to a reduced quality of life (Puchalski et al. 2019, Breitbart 2002).

The American Society of Clinical Oncology (ASCO) recommends that clinicians address a patient's spiritual needs, and in 2018, this was included in their *Guidelines for Palliative Care* (Osman et al. 2018). Further, in a joint statement with the American Academy of Hospice and Palliative Medicine (AAHPM), these two organizations identified spiritual and cultural care as one of the nine components of high-quality palliative care in oncology (Bickel et al. 2016). This sentiment is mirrored in Europe in the European Association for Palliative Care (EAPC) 2014 *Guidelines* (EAPC 2015) that also advocate for patients' spiritual needs to be addressed.

While many definitions of spirituality exist in the literature, consensus conferences in both the USA and Europe have defined spirituality in patient care as a "broad construct that is inclusive of both religious and non-religious forms" (Puchalski et al. 2009; 2014, NICE 2011). Spiritual care in oncology, including the incorporation of patient religious beliefs when appropriate, is an important step toward good patient care. A recent systematic review that looked at hospital in-patient spiritual distress showed their levels of distress ranged from 16% to 63%, with 96% of patients experiencing spiritual pain that they characterized as "deep in the being that is not physical" (des Ordens et al. 2018). But ironically, an earlier 2012 study found that among patients surveyed, most had never received any form of spiritual care from their oncology nurses (87%) or physicians (94%) (Balboni et al. 2013). This is discordant, as many studies have shown that most patients would like to have their spiritual concerns addressed (Balboni et al. 2007).

Given the data around the importance of spirituality in cancer care, healthcare providers should strive to make it a cornerstone of supportive oncology care. Integrative practices should include yoga, which at its roots is a spiritual practice. Not surprisingly, a systematic review of the literature looking at the relationship between yoga and spirituality shows that a yoga practice is positively associated with various aspects of spirituality, including spiritual aspiration, a search for insight and wisdom, integrated worldview, and a sense of

meaning, peace, faith, hope, compassion, and inner happiness (Csala et al. 2021).

In the presence of a compassionate listener, a patient's voice can be amplified, and their suffering witnessed and validated, perhaps leading to an increased sense of coherence, healing, and hope. Creating safe, nonjudgmental space is among the guiding principles of yoga therapy.

Client story: Elizabeth

Nischala Joy Devi, C-IAYT

Elizabeth (she/her) is a 65-year-old White woman who is diagnosed with a recurrence of breast cancer metastatic to the lung.

Elizabeth is a very loving and proper woman who follows a fundamental Christian religion. Her devotion to the sacred heart of Jesus is her strength and power. At the referral of her doctor, she came to see me at a time when her breast cancer had recurred and metastasized to her lung. It seemed that with her present state of health and her religious openness, imagery would be a good modality for her (see Box 6.20). At each yoga therapy session, we practiced relaxation and she was a willing student. When we included imagery with the relaxation, she had some apprehension in choosing her image. What comes to her suddenly is her favorite picture of Lord Jesus in long flowing white robes, holding the sacred heart. Since we were meeting just once a week, Elizabeth continued to practice her relaxation and imagery every day on her own at home. Soon, she was feeling less pain and anxiety and experienced a sense of peace.

A few weeks after beginning the imagery, Elizabeth arrived on time for her appointment. She reported that her imagery and relaxation sessions had been proceeding nicely, but reported: "Last night, instead of just imagining Lord Jesus, he really appeared and then turned into pure white light. I could feel the light enter my body right here." She points to the third eye center, between her eyebrows. "I felt the light travel all through my body and a profound feeling of peace, love, and joy permeated my whole body and mind. I've never felt anything like this."

We speak together about her unexpected experience of passive imagery, this feeling of having received a profound felt sense of loving kindness. Elizabeth's eyes are sparkling, and she says she feels effervescent and calm at the same time. She leaves the session, radiant, with the promise to return in one week.

When she did not arrive for her next appointment, I phoned hoping to reach Elizabeth directly. She answered and hesitantly told me, "I told my pastor. He yelled and screamed and said 'It is the work of the devil. Not only do you have cancer of the body, now you have cancer of the soul! Never do anything like that again or you will go to hell for sure!' So, I am afraid to do it again."

I listen with great empathy. I want to find a way, if she is willing, to help her continue her inner work within her religious frame of reference. "If you decide to come back, be sure to bring your Bible." Not surprisingly, Elizabeth arrived at her next session with Bible in hand. I began cautiously, "Do you know the part where it says, 'When thine eye becomes single'?" "Yes," she replied, "... 'the whole body fills with light.'"

"This," I pointed to the middle of my forehead, "is called the third eye. When the two eyes draw inward from the worldly sights to the heavenly realm, they form a third eye. This eye opens to allow heavenly light to enter and then the whole body fills with light. Perhaps the light, Elizabeth, was a gift from Lord Jesus."

"Oh my, then maybe the healing light *is* from Lord Jesus after all. Perhaps this *is* a religious and spiritual experience." She is brightening by the second. "Maybe I *am* filled with healing light."

Elizabeth continues her imagery work, in addition to many gentle practices of *prāṇāyāma* (breath-work), often receiving unexpected feelings of calm and bliss.

Instead of separating her from her religious beliefs, her practice has strengthened them. She returns to the safe haven of her church with an inner smile, knowing she was filled with Jesus's light.

BOX 6.20 Active and passive imagery

Nischala Joy Devi

Imagery, an ancient and subtle practice in yoga, is widely used today. In cancer care, it is a practice accessible to all, especially when a client feels particularly unwell, or their suffering is more in the realm of spiritual disconnection or lack of hope. Imagery can be done in an active or passive form. Each can be used according to one's own temperament, or one form can follow the other.

Active imagery

Active imagery is a practice wherein we formulate an action to work directly on an area in need of healing. Working with concentration through the lens of the *manomayakośa* (mind sheath), we project that image to do the task (see Chapter 2, *Yoga philosophy*). It is often helpful to choose images clients are familiar with and use in everyday life. For example: a delete button to purge unwanted emotions; a sponge to soak up debris; a broom to sweep away pain; a vacuum cleaner to open vessels; soap that wipes away tumors; a paint brush to change a hot spot to a cool spot. When transmitting the image to a particular part of the body or mind, it is important to be relaxed, focused, and directed, allowing the body to soften, open, and accept the image. Do not try to use force; instead, allow the body to accept the healing.

Passive imagery

Passive imagery is quite different (more in the realm of *vijñānamayakośa* [wisdom sheath] or *ānand-amayakośa* [bliss sheath]; see Chapter 2, *Yoga philosophy*) and can happen spontaneously, sometimes as a surprising expansion of an active imagery practice. It is received instead of being self-generated, and often creates profound feelings of "goodness" and

(continued)

spiritual connection. When we cultivate an openness, this practice allows us to go beyond day-to-day consciousness and connect with the divine.

Points to remember

Person-centered care builds on the therapeutic relationship between the clinician and patient/client and acknowledges the person's serious illness. Inherent in this aspect of spiritual care is the practice of compassionate presence, characterized as "being fully present with another person as a witness to their own experience." Healing may occur through finding meaning, hope, or a sense of coherence during illness.

A few reminders:

- Spirituality is unique to everyone. Some people may not be interested in yoga philosophy, and a patient/client's values and beliefs may be quite different – or even at odds – with those of a yoga therapist, or of yoga or Hindu philosophy. Good spiritual care involves understanding and accepting this diversity.

- If the patient so desires, their individual religious beliefs can be incorporated into their yoga practice. Yoga therapists can be attentive to what they observe in the environment as potential resources, for example, sacred texts, spiritual music, spiritual symbols in the room, or what the patient is wearing.

- Yoga therapists may work in partnership with chaplains and/or they may refer to trained chaplains who are experts in spiritual care.

L.L.

Section 4 references

Introduction

Kalanithi, P., 2016. *When Breath Becomes Air*. Random House.

Shakespeare, W., 1913. Act 4, Scene 3. In: *Romeo and Juliet*. J.B. Lippincott; Philadelphia, PA: p. 229.

Vivar, C.G., Whyte, D.A., McQueen, A., 2010. 'Again': the impact of recurrence on survivors of cancer and family members. *J Clin Nurs*. 19(13–14):2048–2056.

4.1 Full catastrophe living wake – coping with metastatic breast cancer

American Cancer Society (ACS), 2020. Male Breast Cancer. Available at: https://www.cancer.org/cancer/breast-cancer-in-men.html.

American Cancer Society (ACS), 2011–12 Breast Cancer Facts. Available at: https://www.cancer.org/content/dam/cancer-org/research/cancer-facts-and-statistics/breast-cancer-facts-and-figures/breast-cancer-facts-and-figures-2019-2020.pdf.

Bauer, K., Brown, M., Cress, R., Parise, C.A., Caggiano, V., 2007. Descriptive analysis of estrogen receptor (ER)-negative, progesterone receptor (PR)-negative, and HER2-negative invasive breast cancer, the so-called triple-negative phenotype: a population-based study from the California Cancer Registry. *Cancer*. 109:1721–1728.

Bell, K., Ristovski-Slijepcevic, S., 2011. Metastatic cancer and mothering: being a mother in the face of a contracted future. *Medical Anthropology*. 30(6):629–649.

Bury, M., 1982. Chronic illness as biographical disruption. *Sociology of Health and Illness*. 4(2):167–182.

Ganz, P.A., Stanton, A.L., 2015. Living with metastatic breast cancer. In *Improving Outcomes for Breast Cancer Survivors*. Springer, pp. 243–254.

Irvin, W. Jr., Muss, H.B., Mayer, D.K., 2011. Symptom management in metastatic breast cancer. *Oncologist*. 16(9):1203–1214.

Mariotto, A.B., Etzioni, R., Hurlbert, M., Penberthy, L., Mayer, M., 2017. Estimation of the number of women living with metastatic breast cancer in the United States. *Cancer Epidemiol Biomarkers Prev*. 26(6):809815.

Perou, C.M., 2011. Molecular stratification of triple-negative breast cancers. *Oncologist*. 16(Suppl 1):61–70.

Siegel, R.L., Miller, K.D., Jemal, A., 2017. Cancer statistics, 2017. *CA: A Cancer Journal for Clinicians*. 67(1):7–30.

Thrift-Perry, M., Cabanes, A., Cardoso, F., Hunt, K.M., Cruz, T.A., Faircloth, K., 2018. Global analysis of metastatic breast cancer policy gaps and advocacy efforts across the patient journey. *Breast*. 41:93–106.

World Cancer Research Fund, 2020. Available at: https://www.wcrf.org/dietandcancer/cancer-trends/breast-cancer-statistics.

World Health Organization, 2020. Available at: https://www.who.int/news-room/fact-sheets/detail/breast-cancer.

Zimmaro, L.A., Carson, J.W., Olsen, M.K., Sanders, L.L., Keefe, F.J., Porter, L.S., 2020. Greater mindfulness associated with lower pain, fatigue, and psychological distress in women with metastatic breast cancer. *Psychooncology*. 29(2):263–270.

4.2 Making meaning after recurrence

Breitbart, W., Pessin, H., Rosenfeld, B., et al., 2018. Individual meaning-centered psychotherapy for the treatment of psychological and existential distress: a randomized controlled trial in patients with advanced cancer. *Cancer*. 124(15): 3231–3239.

Fishman, L., Saltonstall, E., 2010. *Yoga for Osteoporosis: The Complete Guide*. WW Norton and Company.

Frankl, V., 1998. *Man's Search for Meaning: An Introduction to Logotherapy*. Random House; London, UK.

Greisinger, A.J., Lorimor, R.J., Aday, L.A., et al., 1997. Terminally ill cancer patients. Their most important concerns. *Cancer Practice*. 53(3):147–154.

Kissane, D.W., 2000. Psychospiritual and existential distress. The challenge for palliative care. *Aust Fam Physician*. 29(11):1022–102.

Piderman, K.M., Kung, S., Jenkins, S.M., 2015. Respecting the spiritual side of advanced cancer care: a systematic review. *Curr Oncol Rep*. 17(2):6.

Posluszny, D.M., Dew, M.A., Beckjord, E., et al., 2016. Existential challenges experienced by lymphoma survivors: results from the 2010 LIVESTRONG Survey. *J Health Psychol*. 21(10):2357–2366.

Sinaki, M., Brey, R.H., Hughes, C.A., et al., 2005. Balance disorder and increased risk of falls in osteoporosis and kyphosis: significance of kyphotic posture and muscle strength. *Osteoporos Int*. 16:1004–1010.

Sullivan, M.B., Erb, M., Schmalzl, L., et al., 2018. Yoga therapy and polyvagal theory: the convergence of

traditional wisdom and contemporary neuroscience for self-regulation and resilience. *Front Hum Neurosci*. 12:67.

Tominaga, R., Fukuma, S., Yamazaki, S., et al., 2016. Relationship between kyphotic posture and falls in community-dwelling men and women: The Locomotive Syndrome and Health Outcome in Aizu Cohort Study. *Spine (Phila Pa 1976)*. 41(15):1232–1238.

van der Spek, N., Vos, J., van Uden-Kraan, C.F., et al., 2013. Meaning making in cancer survivors: a focus group study. *PLoS One*. 26;8(9):e76089.

4.3 Addressing hyperkyphosis

Arora, I., 2015. *Mudrā: The Sacred Secret*. Yogsadhna; Downers Grove, IL.

Jang, H-J., Hughes, L.C., Oh, D-W., Kim, S-Y., 2019. Effects of corrective exercise for thoracic hyperkyphosis on posture, balance, and well-being in older women. *Journal of Geriatric Physical Therapy*. 42(3):E17–E27.

Kado, D.M., 2009. Hyperkyphosis predicts mortality independent of vertebral osteoporosis in older women. *Annals of Internal Medicine*. 150(10):681.

Lu, Y-H., Rosner, B., Chang, G., Fishman, L.M., 2016. Twelve-minute daily yoga regimen reverses osteoporotic bone loss. *Topics in Geriatric Rehabilitation*. 32(2):81–87.

Norlyk Smith, E., Boser, A., 2013. Yoga, vertebral fractures, and osteoporosis: research and recommendations. *International Journal of Yoga Therapy*. 23(1):17–23.

Panday, K., Gona, A., Humphrey, M.B., 2014. Medication-induced osteoporosis: screening and treatment strategies. *Therapeutic Advances in Musculoskeletal Disease*. 6(5):185–202.

Roghani, T., Zavieh, M.K., Manshadi, F.D., et al., 2017. Age-related hyperkyphosis: update of its potential causes and clinical impacts—narrative review. *Aging Clinical and Experimental Research*. 29(4):567–577.

Sinaki, M., Mikkelsen, B., 1984. Postmenopausal spinal osteoporosis: flexion versus extension exercises. *Arch Phys Med Rehabil*. 65:593–596.

Sinaki, M., 2012. Yoga spinal flexion positions and vertebral compression fracture in osteopenia or osteoporosis of spine: case series. *Pain Practice*. 13(1):68–75.

Solberg, G., 2008. *Postural Disorders and Musculoskeletal Dysfunction.* 1st ed. Churchill Livingstone Elsevier; Edinburgh, UK.

Stiles, M., 2000. *Structural Yoga Therapy: Adapting to the Individual.* Weiser Books; York Beach, ME.

van der Jagt-Willems, H.C., de Groot, M.H., van Campen, J.P., et al., 2015. Associations between vertebral fractures, increased thoracic kyphosis, a flexed posture and falls in older adults: a prospective cohort study. *BMC Geriatrics.* 15:34.

4.4 Imagine that!

Balboni, T.A., Vanderwerker, L.C., Block, S.D., 2007. Religiousness and spiritual support among advanced cancer patients and associations with end-of-life treatment preferences and quality of life. *J Clin Oncol.* 25(5):555–60.

Balboni, M.J., Sullivan, A., Amobi, A., et al., 2013. Why is spiritual care infrequent at the end of life? Spiritual care perceptions among patients, nurses, and physicians and the role of training. *J Clin Oncol.* 31:461–7.

Bickel, K.E., McNiff, K., Buss, M.K., et al., 2016. Defining high-quality palliative care in oncology practice: an American Society of Clinical Oncology/American Academy of Hospice and Palliative Medicine Guidance Statement. *J Oncol Pract.* 12:e828–38.

Breitbart, W., 2002. Spirituality and meaning in supportive care: spirituality- and meaning-centered group psychotherapy interventions in advanced cancer. *Support Care Cancer.*10:272–280.

Csala, B., Springinsfeld, C.M., Köteles, F., 2021. The relationship between yoga and spirituality: a systematic review of empirical research. *Front Psychol.* 12:695939.

des Ordons, A., Sinuff, T., Stelfox, H., et al., 2018. Spiritual distress within inpatient settings—a scoping review of patient and family experiences. *J Pain Symptom Manage.* 156:122–145.

EAPC, 2022. EAPC Reference Group on Spiritual Care. Available at: https://www.eapcnet.eu/eapc-groups/reference/spiritual-care/.

National Institute for Health and Care Excellence (NICE), 2011. Quality Standard [QS13]: End of Life Care for Adults. Available at: https://www.nice.org.uk/guidance/QS13.

Osman, H., Shrestha, S., Temin, S., 2018. Palliative care in the global setting: ASCO Resource-Stratified practice guideline. *J Glob Oncol.* 4:1–24.

Puchalski, C., Ferrell, B., Virani, R., et al., 2009. Improving the quality of spiritual care as a dimension of palliative care: the report of the consensus conference. *J Palliat Med.* 12:885–904.

Puchalski, C.M., Vitillo, R., Hull, S.K., et al., 2014. Improving the spiritual dimension of whole person care: reaching national and international consensus. *J Palliat Med.* 17:642–656.

Puchalski, C.M., Sbrana, A., Ferrell, B., et al., 2019. Interprofessional spiritual care in oncology: a literature review. *ESMO Open.* 4:e000465.

Taimni, I.K., 2014. *The Science of Yoga: The Yoga Sutras of Patanjali in Sanskrit.* Theosophical Publishing House; Wheaton, IL: 1.9.

Section 5 End of life

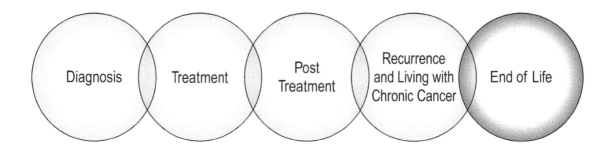

Death is not extinguishing the light; it is only putting out the lamp because the dawn has come.

Rabindranath Tagore (1861–1941)[1]

Introduction
Leigh Leibel

In the first four sections of this chapter, we have accompanied yoga therapists and yoga professionals and their patients/clients with cancer on dynamic journeys through cancer diagnosis, treatment, post treatment, and recurrence. And now, we arrive at the fifth phase of the Yoga in the Cancer Care Continuum, *End of Life*. To best frame our eight yoga therapy contributor stories presented in this chapter, we define end-of-life care in accordance with the National Hospice and Palliative Care Organization (NHPCO) in the United States. The NHPCO characterizes end of life as the last six months of a patient's estimated lifespan; the estimate is determined by two physicians who base it on a patient's current health status according to the ECOG (Eastern Cooperative Oncology Group) Performance Status (ECOG 2022) and the usual or expected trajectory of their specific cancer (NHPCO 2022).

---

[1]Rabindranath Tagore, an Indian, was the first non-European to receive a Nobel Prize in Literature (1913). Throughout India, this quotation is widely attributed to Tagore, though no original source is found.

Palliative care vs. hospice care: definitions

There is often confusion about the role of these two systems of care, when in fact they are very different. Palliative care is a medical discipline, much like cardiac care is a medical discipline, whereas hospice is a care model for end of life. Here are the definitions recognized in the United States (definitions vary by country):

Definition of palliative care

The Center to Advance Palliative Care (CAPC) in the United States offers the most structured definition:

Palliative care, and the medical subspecialty of palliative medicine is specialized medical care for people living with serious illness. It focuses on providing relief from the symptoms and stress of a serious illness. The goal is to improve the quality of life for both the patient and the family. Palliative care is provided by a team of palliative care doctors, nurses, social workers, and others who work together with a patient's other doctors to provide an extra layer of support. It is appropriate at any age and any stage in a serious illness and can be provided along with curative treatment.

CAPC (2022)

It is important to reiterate that palliative care is not just for the terminally ill. It is available for any patient undergoing cancer treatment – including treatments with

(continued)

(continued)
curative intent – to help manage difficult symptoms. Palliative care aims to treat holistically, taking into consideration factors beyond merely the patient's diagnosis.

Definition of hospice care

The Centers for Disease Control and Prevention (CDC) in the United States offers this definition:

Hospice is a special model of care for patients who are in the late phase of an incurable illness and wish to receive end-of-life care at home or in a specialized care setting.

CDC (2022)

According to the CDC, "A major priority of hospice is to incorporate the principles of palliative care to minimize pain and discomfort in the face of advanced or terminal disease. The essential components of hospice are:

- Ongoing communication among patients, families, and providers.

- Aggressive pain control and management of symptoms such as nausea, fatigue, anxiety, shortness of breath, and tissue breakdown.

- Medication monitoring and maintenance.

- Assistance with limited activities of daily living such as bathing.

- Advance care planning, although this is not as important as in other situations.

- Psychosocial and spiritual care.

- Grief and bereavement counseling for the patient and family."

CDC (2022)

As we saw in Chapter 4: Understanding Cancer and its Treatment, and in this chapter's previous section 4 on *Cancer recurrence and living with chronic cancer*, many people with non-curable cancer can, and do, live well for many months, many years, or for some, decades, while managing cancer as a chronic disease. But eventually, for most, there comes a point when they make the difficult decision to transition to end-of-life care.

Perhaps their treatments have stopped working and cancer and comorbidities have progressed, or perhaps they have become too frail to continue with arduous and toxic therapies. Either scenario triggers tough decisions around next steps:

- Should the patient continue aggressive treatment in the hopes of prolonging life for an indeterminate period, without regard to quality of life?

- Or should they turn toward comfort care (hospice) that focuses on the palliation of pain and symptoms, and attends to emotional and spiritual well-being during the remaining days, weeks, months?

This is a very personal patient decision made with support of family and their oncology team, and in many countries with guidance from the American Society of Clinical Oncology (ASCO) end-of-life care guidelines (Prigerson et al. 2015). Whatever the patient's choice, it is to be respected.

Important cultural considerations

Yoga therapists must be aware that in many cultures it is not appropriate to discuss impending death. Always respect the beliefs of patients/clients and their families.

However, not all people with cancer have the option of choosing how to die. Some of our most vulnerable populations across rural or segregated areas of the United States and other developed countries, as well as those in under-resourced and low-and-middle income countries (LMICs) don't have access to a broad range of cancer therapies, clinical trials, lifesaving treatments, palliative and pain medications, or even supportive care for mental health and symptom management (see *Cancer health disparity* in Chapter 4). Disparity in healthcare – and indeed, disparity in death – is among the world's biggest social injustices. A position statement of the World Health Organization (WHO) affirms that it is the ethical duty of all stakeholders in our global healthcare community to respect a person's dignity in illness and to relieve their suffering (WHO 2020).

In the thought-provoking book *The Lost Art of Dying: Reviving Forgotten Wisdom*, Lydia Dugdale, MD, director of Columbia University's Center for Clinical Medical Ethics, advocates for a new global paradigm in end-of-life care that provides all patients and their families with comfort, peace, and dignity during their most vulnerable moments. She takes us through the fascinating history of death and its depiction in art and literature, pointing to the 15th-century tradition of *ars moriendi* (a body of literature written after the horrors of the Black Plague that provided practical guidance for the dying and those attending them), as a valuable historical analogue in which a contemporary multicultural society can frame the fear of death and weigh the decision of *where* to die: at home, in a hospital, or other setting (Dugdale 2020). In the best-selling book *Being Mortal*, Atul Gawande, MD, MPH, another physician who speaks out about end-of-life issues, suggests that Western medicine treats death and aging as if it's another clinical problem to overcome, and asks us to challenge the way in which we, as a society, are living our days, including our last (Gawande 2014).

The data around people's *actual* versus *desired* location for their death to occur is compelling. A 2013 survey conducted at the University of Colorado Denver School of Medicine (n=458) showed 75% of in-patients surveyed said they'd prefer to die at home surrounded by family; but the reality is, of the 123 people who died during the follow-up period, 66% died in an institutional setting, sometimes alone without loved ones with them (Fischer et al. 2013). This and other studies suggest the concordance between *actual* and *desired* site of death is low.

While the definition of a *good* death varies widely across the times, cultures, religions, and the contexts in which we live, it's likely that pain – whether physical or existential – will make an appearance. Data show that 70–90% of people with cancer who are approaching death will experience moderate to severe pain at the end of their lives (Platt 2010). And since pain perception is subjective, any physical pain experienced in the last months and weeks of life can be amplified by anxiety, fear, and a host of unresolved emotional, spiritual, and existential issues. The idea that pain has many causes – so called *total pain* – was first introduced in the mid-20th century by Dame Cicily Saunders (founder of the modern hospice movement) who described pain as: "the suffering that encompasses all of an individual's physical, psychological, emotional, social, and spiritual dimensions" (Richmond 2005).

Within this holistic framework of pain and suffering, yoga is beautifully poised to support mind, body, and soul. By incorporating yoga and other nonpharmacologic therapies in the palliative care armamentarium, a more comprehensive and cost-effective prescription to relieve suffering can be offered to terminal patients early on – supporting their ability to self-soothe, and perhaps assigning a more circumscribed role to opioids, anxiolytics, and anti-depressants.[2] A landmark study published in 2010 in the *New England Journal of Medicine* showed that advanced lung cancer patients who received early palliative care along with standard treatment lived more than two months longer than patients receiving standard care only (Temel et al. 2010). In end-of-life work, 60 days is time cherished.

The Latin root of "inspire" – *īnspīrāre* – means to infuse life by breathing, often through divine or supernatural agency or power (Merriam-Webster 2022). Yogic philosophy recognizes this as *prāṇa*, the life-force. On the following pages, we are privy to moments of *inspiration* and grace as eight yoga therapists share tender accounts of accompanying their patients and clients across the wistful last weeks, days, and minutes of their lives on Earth. May it be that *living* their yoga supported them in *dying well*, empowering them to "lean into life, rather than simply away from it" (Wiman 2012).

As we bear witness to our colleagues and their patients, clients, and loved ones during the final stage of care, we honor their journey, and perhaps pause to

---

[2]Many cultures do not accept or encourage the use of opioids, which are commonly used for pain relief.

acknowledge our own human finitude – exploring life's bittersweet frailty and what it means to each of us as mortal beings to be *inspired*; to grieve, and to remember those who have gone before us.

5.1 *Samādhi* (oneness) meditation

Patient story: Shelly

Kelsey Kraemer, MS, E-RYT 500, C-IAYT

Shelly (she/her) is a 58-year-old White woman diagnosed with aggressive primary mediastinal B-cell (non-Hodgkin) lymphoma.

Shelly's 15-month journey began with months of a harsh multidrug chemotherapy regimen called DA-EPOCH-R,[1] then just eight months after completing treatment, the cancer returned. This time she was treated with a different chemotherapy cocktail plus radiation. But when the cancer advanced during this second line of treatment and metastasized to the liver, pancreas, and kidney, she made the difficult decision to stop treatment and transition to in-patient hospice care. She is aware of her terminal diagnosis and is in the final days, perhaps hours, of life.

Shelly and I worked together throughout her many months of chemotherapy, and I know she embraces her Christian faith. Over our 15 months of yoga therapy sessions, we often incorporated her religious beliefs into the yoga interventions – for example, using Christian-based *mantra* (spiritual word/phrase) and Christ symbolism in guided meditation. In addition to her faith, Shelly has a strong support system in her family, and this brings her joy and meaning. They have been by her side throughout her journey and continue to show their support in these final moments with the one they love so dearly.

As I enter Shelly's room for what will be the final time, the emotion within me – and within the room – is palpable. Shelly lies in bed with her eyes closed and mouth slightly open. She is on morphine, verbally uncommunicative, but appears coherent and can nod and shake her head to communicate with her loved ones. Family surrounds her. I recognize her husband and eldest daughter at the bedside. They have been by her side throughout treatment and often participated with Shelly in complementary therapies such as yoga, art, and music. Shelly's husband introduces me to their other daughters, as well as three young granddaughters. Two of the younger granddaughters play near their mother, who appears to be blinking back tears, while the third sits on her mother's lap, holding her grandmother's hand at the side of the bed. Shelly's husband stands by his wife's side, stroking her head gently. I sit on a chair, lean in close toward the bedside, and let Shelly know I am here with her.

"Hi Shelley, it's Kelsey. Can you feel your family in the room?" She gives a gentle nod of her head. We pause in silence. "There is a lot of love in here." We pause in silence. "Would you like me to guide you in one of your favorite meditations?" She nods, eyes closed, face serene.

---

[1]Dose adjusted etoposide, prednisolone, vincristine, cyclophosphamide, doxorubicin, rituximab.

I begin the mediation: "Imagine the energy of each of your family members as if they were coming together to create a golden light. The light invokes a sense of peace and comfort within you." There is a gentle softening around Shelly's eyes and a release of tension from her jaw, adding to the tranquility of her already gentle expression. "Imagine this light expanding across your body, as if to provide the love and support of your family members to every part of your being."

I continue to guide Shelly through what I call *samādhi* (oneness) meditation to invoke a sense of interconnectivity with loved ones. Shelly is invited to imagine the golden light expanding to different areas of her body, beginning with her heart center, and extending to her hands and feet, finally ending with the crown of her head. Throughout the meditation, Shelly seems to release muscular tension as each body part is acknowledged. Her husband continues to stroke her hair and the little granddaughter rests her head on her grandmother's hand.

"Now that you feel the sensation of safety and support from your loved ones, recall a happy memory with them." A few moments pass. Her family appears engaged in the meditation as well, and I imagine them recalling their own special memories.

"Are you able to identify a happy memory?" Shelly nods as the corners of her mouth turn up slightly. "Good, now remember everything associated with that memory. Imagine the memory as if it were happening right now…recall who was there, where you were, what was happening around you. Recall any tastes or smells associated with the memory, and any sensations of sight or touch. Notice any sounds from this memory. Observe any emotions that arise when remembering this time, and whether you feel them anywhere in particular in the body. Maybe a certain word or feeling arises, such as: safety, freedom, or joy. See how it is to notice that."

Again, I sense a deeper relaxation spread over Shelly, and see a gentle smile upon her face. The connection between her and her loved ones appears tangible. The family now has their eyes closed like Shelly, everyone participating in this recollection of happy times.

"Continuing to let the sensations of this memory wash over you, allow yourself to return to the present moment and the love of your family in the room with you now. Notice the feeling of your husband caressing your hair, your loving daughters at your side, and your sweet granddaughter holding your hand. Know that this love will always be with you."

The meditation ends and I let Shelly know I am honored to know her. Holding back my tears, I squeeze her hand and extend to her a blessing of peace, leaving her to spend these last precious hours with the ones she loves most.

In the final days of life, patients and families experience myriad emotions, which make emotional and spiritual support essential. Meaning-centered interventions such as meditation may enhance a patient's spiritual well-being and quality of life, as well as allow them to identify with a greater purpose (Kang et al. 2019). Focusing on meaningful relationships may also invoke a sense of self-transcendence and oneness in a patient who is dying (Clyne et al. 2019). From a yoga perspective, this connection to loved ones contributes to a sense of something greater than oneself and suggests a surrender of the Ego – an important step in the transition of the spirit from the human body. A meditation centered on supportive relationships that reflects the concept of *samādhi* (oneness) promotes a sense of eudemonia (meaning or self-realization), peace, and equanimity (Sullivan et al. 2018).

5.2 Turning inward

Patient story: Eliza

Miriam Patterson, MAT, MSJIR, C-IAYT

Eliza (she/her) is a 79-year-old Latina woman diagnosed with breast cancer that has metastasized to the brain.

Eliza was diagnosed 15 years ago with an early-stage breast cancer. She underwent a mastectomy and recovered uneventfully. Since then, she has lived a healthy and energetic life. In fact, for the last five years, she has been a regular at my community yoga classes for cancer survivors. Recently, however, she hasn't been feeling herself. After a visit to her oncologist and after a battery of tests and scans, she has learned the breast cancer has recurred and metastasized to her brain. Her daughter is supporting her through this terminal diagnosis. Together, they have made the difficult decision to forgo chemotherapy and radiation treatment due to the grim prognosis and the significant side effects of treatment, though she does take small doses of prednisone to reduce the swelling in her brain caused by the tumor. Her medical team has told her to start thinking about hospice care, but she is not yet ready to think about death, or make that decision. She is still well enough to prepare her own meals and move around a little bit using a walker, but because of dizziness, she must have her daughter or an aide by her side. She tires easily and spends most of the day in bed or on the couch. The guess is that she may live another five to six months, based on her current performance status and the usual trajectory of her disease.

Eliza and I have formed a close relationship through the years, and she wants to continue yoga with me as she approaches end of life. We decide to do one-on-one yoga therapy a few times each week in her home. At our first session, I see that Eliza has changed in the past several months since she last attended a yoga class. She now has trouble walking, prefers sitting to standing, and has trouble hearing me when I talk. She becomes vis-ibly upset and confused when too many questions are asked, or too much information comes at once. So, we go slowly. She appears to be drawing inward naturally, telling me that she cannot take phone calls, be on the computer, watch movies, or paint the way she used to.

I pull up two chairs and we sit facing each other. I invite Eliza to close her eyes and bring one hand to her chest, and to bring her awareness to the movement underneath her hand. I invite her to inhale and make a small humming sound as she exhales. We repeat this for six breaths. Eliza appears more relaxed, and her breath is smoother. She reports that the buzzing she had in one ear seems to have lessened.

Eliza asks if we can try some simple standing postures as she feels her leg strength is waning. I help her stand and get situated with her walker. Because of her fall risk, I take the utmost care to support her in all standing postures – she is always supported by both me and the wall, and she always holds on to the back of a sturdy chair (that won't move). Her trusted walker is always at her side. Once she feels secure in this set-up, she naturally stretches up onto her toes, and then back to flat feet, repeating the movements several times. I then invite her to stand tall like a mountain (*tāḍāsana* pose), hands remaining on the back of the chair for support. She keeps her eyes open for balance. Carefully, she lifts one foot, and then the other foot. Together, we slowly "march" in place as we sing a song from her past.

We then move to the floor. With my assistance, Eliza is still able to safely make the transition. Now on her hands and knees (we put pads under her knees for comfort), we chant "*Oṃ*," as she moves her hips back towards her feet. She struggles to make a loud and long sound. She is quite breathless. We slow down and rest. After a few minutes we repeat this and she is able to do it for six breaths, the "*Oṃ*" getting a bit stronger with each exhale…"*Oṃmmmmmmmm!*" Gradually, Eliza's voice gets louder, and her exhales longer. She rests. There is a sense of calm.

After gentle *āsana* (postures) and breath-work (*prāṇāyāma*) on the floor, Eliza lies on her back and rests in *śavāsana* (corpse pose). She has an essential oil diffuser in her home that she enjoys and uses every day, and I plug it in. I ask her to choose frankincense, black spruce, cypress, or lavender. Eliza's sense of smell still brings pleasure, her whole body softening as she smells the aromas coming from the diffusor. She is drawn to oils that capture the smell of Canadian forests.

One of Eliza's big complaints is that she cannot stay asleep. We talk a bit about sleep hygiene and how to create an environment conducive for sleep. I show her how to arrange her pillows to make her bed a comfortable nest for relaxation. I also give her a voice recording of a *yoganidrā* (yogic sleep), as well as a recording of a guided relaxation. She uses these recordings before falling asleep, or when she wakes in the middle of the night. Eliza reports that she uses the recordings regularly, and finds that her sleep is enhanced, and that they help to keep her calm when she is awake late at night and her mind wanders and causes her to feel anxious.

Eliza also loves classical music. Her favorites include the wistful finale of Tchaikovsky's *Sixth Symphony* and Henry Purcell's *Dido's Lament* (*When I Am Laid In Earth*, from *Dido* and *Aeneas*). We load these songs and others on her iPad and put it next to her bed for her to listen to while she looks at her family photo albums, one of her favorite activities.

Eliza's tumors are starting to cause her to withdraw from the outer world, and into herself, but the experience is enhanced, and made more intentional with the tools of yoga therapy. As her senses dull, we explore gently and intentionally bringing awareness to the senses to enhance them. Eliza finds immense pleasure in making sound, smelling beautiful scents in the diffuser, listening to beautiful music and looking at her family photo album, moving gently while breathing consciously, and resting on her fluffy pillows and allowing a gentle release into relaxation. Her practice is such an experience of opposites; she feels – and is

> A yoga therapist working at the end of life is much like a doula supporting a laboring mother. They keep their eyes on the process and search for ways to lessen suffering. On the one hand, the therapist assists a client as they prepare for death, and on the other, they work to make their client's remaining life more comfortable. Supporting a person amid this paradox is the main work of the yoga therapist working in the dying time.

deeply connected to – her senses, while at the same time, they are drifting away.

5.3 Transitioning to the light

Patient story: Karen

Kate Holcombe, MFA, E-RYT 500, C-IAYT

Karen (she/her) is a 52-year-old White woman diagnosed with lung cancer metastatic to brain.

When Karen arrives for our first session together, I greet her with a handshake and a smile. I see she is a fit and athletic woman in her early fifties, but as we sit for her intake, her head is down, and she is wringing her hands. She barely looks me in the eye and her voice is so soft I strain to hear her. She tells me that nine months ago she was diagnosed with stage III lung cancer, having undergone what everyone thought was a successful course of chemotherapy, immunotherapy, and radiation. But recently she has been experiencing dizziness and has been slurring her words. Her wife Vicky encouraged her to see her doctor immediately. After scans and blood draws last week, her oncologist told her the lung cancer had recurred and metastasized to her brain. Karen is scheduled to begin the first of twelve rounds of whole-brain radiation in a few days. Her nurse practitioner referred her to me for anxiety, hoping I could help her prepare for radiation, which involves wearing a custom-made mask during treatment to keep her head in the correct position.

After a brief silence Karen says, "I'm scared." We sit together in silence.

I talk a bit about the radiation process so she knows what to expect, then ask if she'd like to try something she can do to help her relax while waiting for her radiation sessions to begin. She says she'd love that. I invite her to lie down on her back with her hands at her sides and imagine herself lying like this for her radiation. I invite her to close her eyes. I start by guiding her through simple, relaxed diaphragmatic breathing, prompting her abdomen to gently rise on each inhale and softly fall, gently contracting, on each exhale. After a few breaths, I invite her to add another component to the breath using a technique called *nyāsam*. This is a yogic practice that involves touching various parts of the body and can include chanting a specific *mantra* (repeated word, phrase, sound). We do the practice a bit differently, substituting imagery and breath for *mantra* as we engage the fingers. With each breath, we gently slide the thumbs of each hand "up and down" each of the other four fingers (one at a time, consecutively) on the same hand. Karen tries this for a few breaths and tells me it feels relaxing. As she continues breathing comfortably, in rhythm, she gently slides her thumbs "up and down" each finger, and I invite her to visualize a light within that is pure, perfect, unchanging, and free from all suffering.

I then ask if she knows anything about the *Patañjali Yoga Sūtra-s*. She has never heard of it. I explain it's a 2,000-year-old text on yoga philosophy that describes tools and strategies to help relieve suffering. Karen's eyes light up and she asks me to go on. "There is one *sūtra*, or aphorism, I think you might particularly like," I tell her. "It's in the first chapter and speaks to a light within each of us that is free from all suffering and sorrow." We spend the rest of the session deep in conversation about yoga philosophy.

At her next appointment, I greet Karen and she looks me in the eye with a warm smile. She says the practices have been helpful and she does them before radiation, before bed, and any time she feels anxious or worried. She tells me her wife Vicky commented on how much more relaxed she seems. In our session today, we review last week's lessons, and I teach her a few gentle movements she can do lying on her back: gentle, supportive stretches coordinated with her breath. Before she leaves, she asks if it's OK for Vicky to come to the next session: "Maybe you can show Vicky some things to help her relax as well."

When Vicky arrives at the next session, I see she is more tense and worried than Karen. After checking in with Vicky to make sure she has no injuries or conditions that might warrant adjustments to a yoga practice, I invite both women to lie on their backs and join me in a series of gentle movements (*āsana-s*), breathing (*prāṇāyāma*), *nyāsam*, and meditating on the light within. By the end of the session, Vicky, too, is visibly more relaxed. Over the next several weeks they both attend weekly sessions together and then practice every day at home. They tell me it's something they look forward to, and since they can no longer take the long walks together as they used to, it is a way for them to feel connected to their bodies and feel connected to each other.

One day Karen and Vicky arrive for the session with the devastating news that the radiation isn't working. The brain tumors are spreading quickly, and the doctors expect a more rapid decline than originally anticipated. So, in our session we talk about *Patañjali* and the concept of *puruṣa* – sometimes called the witness, the authentic Self or True Self (see *Yoga philosophy* in Chapter 2). I explain *puruṣa* as being that part of us that is pure, perfect, unchanging, and always there no matter what; a part of us that is greater than the body and that can't be contained by the body. It lives on. "Like our love," Karen says to Vicky, who has soft tears rolling down her cheeks.

I work closely with the couple over the coming weeks. Each time, we review the breathing practices with the sliding fingers and the meditation on the inner light. But we also talk about love: that Karen is more than just her body and love is stronger than cancer, and love is certainly stronger than death. And even though Karen's body will die, the love they both share will never die. Remarkably, Karen remains calm and centered, and shares that when she feels anxious or worried about her impending death, she focuses on the inner light. It helps her to calm herself and to allow the light to fill her.

After Karen's death, Vicky comes back for one final session with me on her own. She is heartbroken. "To watch Karen go through that was so hard, yet I could see she truly didn't suffer. It helps me so much to know she was able to face her death with peace, grace, and acceptance. And indeed, our love lives on."

> Cancer is a family affair. A cancer diagnosis impacts not only the patient, but also their entire family, most especially their intimate partners and spouses, who often become primary caregivers. It's well documented that caregivers experience stress and grief (Alam et al. 2020). A gentle yoga practice that supports both partners can ease symptoms of anxiety and promote a deeper level of connection and intimacy that may be otherwise difficult to attain at end of life.

5.4 Terminal at diagnosis

Patient story: Ruth

Sandra Susheela Gilbert, BA, E-RYT 500, C-IAYT

Ruth (she/her) is a 52-year-old White woman with end-stage colon cancer.

Ruth had been experiencing symptoms for a year before she is rushed to the hospital with extreme vomiting, weakness, and pain. Her diagnostic abdominal surgery is scheduled for the day after Thanksgiving. She is referred to me by a family member for symptom management and holistic support. It was likely the surgery would include a colostomy. What is unexpected, however, is a finding of cancer that had spread throughout Ruth's abdominal cavity and there is no surgical possibility for complete tumor removal. Ruth is now in a situation of needing to cope with a new cancer diagnosis, a colostomy, a poor prognosis, and an awareness that her treatments will be palliative (comfort care) rather than curative. Ruth's previous tool for coping with life has been alcohol consumption, and now that this is no longer an option, another immediate stressor is added.

Within two months of her surgery, Ruth develops lymphedema of her lower extremities due to the surgical removal of several lymph nodes from her abdomen. She continues to have nausea and vomiting and eventually needs nutritional support called TPN (total parenteral nutrition), a method of feeding that bypasses the gastrointestinal tract, since she is unable to eat. She develops severe mood swings, especially following treatment which includes chemotherapy and steroids. For radiation treatment, she is transported daily by ambulance for four weeks because she is unable to walk.

During our initial meetings and interviews, Ruth has made it clear that she does not want to practice movement. One of the most important aspects of yoga therapy is the intake of information and the creation of a therapeutic relationship with the client. I explain that yoga therapy is not necessarily movement-based (*āsana*), and that our sessions could focus on contemplative practices such as meditation and mindfulness. As Ruth navigates her treatments and life choices after her colon cancer diagnosis, she finds that these opportunities to turn inward are of particular importance in helping her calm her mind and find peace. Although, as a yoga therapist, I educate Ruth on the importance of movement to help manage her lymphedema and overall health, I have the responsibility of meeting her where she is and not where I think she should be. By keeping the "shoulds" out of yoga therapy, I create trust and safety with her. I am also aware that she has a lymphedema specialist making twice-weekly visits when she is home, and we stay in touch with each other. Ruth tells me she wants to explore "who she is" during whatever time she still has. Her social network becomes her healthcare providers: her rabbi, a social worker, her family – and her yoga therapist (me). For all of us working with Ruth, the focus becomes healing versus curing, and support of her daily overall needs.

Ruth wants support from me with the nausea, anxiety, and mood swings. We begin sessions with mindful awareness to check in on all levels of her being: physical, emotional, the mind, energy levels, and the breath. From here, breath awareness leads to introductory breathing practices of gentle abdominal breathing and extended exhalation breath. This is followed with a guided relaxation combined with imagery.

Ruth has a great interest in music; her deceased husband had been in the country music business. After several sessions, we add in sound vibration in the form of the *mantra Oṃ* and a chant called *Hari Oṃ*. This leads to the practice of inner meditation with the silent repetition of the *mantra-s*. Over a period of four months, I witness Ruth take control over her physical and emotional life. She never leaves home without full makeup and dressed like she is going out to her favorite restaurant! At home, her bedroom becomes her meditation space and a place to re-center after her treatment visits, when her moods become a challenge in interactions with her partner.

There is also the challenge of the care of her ostomy bag as neither she nor her partner were ever able to navigate ostomy care, so this was left up to her caregivers. The experience of having a stoma is the cause of deep distress and loss of control for Ruth who has always taken much pride in her independence and outward beauty. During our time together, her moods express all of the levels of grief she has been working through to accept her physical reality: her ostomy will not be reversed, she cannot walk, and her length of survival is unknown. She tells me that she looks forward the most to the chanting and *mantra* in her bedroom, either alone, or with me when she returns from chemotherapy or radiation. She says it gives her a sense of peace within, though she can feel her heart racing from medication and the physical effort it takes to leave her bed. Her rabbi and social worker confirm that they are witnessing the same. We work together as a team to give her the support she wants, which is to be in control of her daily life in ways that have meaning for her. Ruth's

nausea improves and she begins spending more time in a wheelchair at home. She actually cooks several meals for her family. Ruth loves a party and during Christmas, when she returns to hospital, her room is filled with candies and pastries, with invites for all the staff.

In the spring, Ruth is hospitalized again, this time with sepsis (a systemic infection). This hospitalization, her last, is a testimony to the clear choices she was empowered to make on her own behalf in the months prior. I am with her when her physicians tell her that there is no longer any medical treatment that they can offer her. Her physician tells her that she has arranged for the family to find a hospice facility for her. Ruth is clear, firm, and to the point when she looks at her physician and says, "You are not moving me anywhere. I am going to die in this bed, in this room."

Ruth passes away a day later, peacefully, and surrounded by family, five months after her diagnosis. Her journey, that she so openly shared with her medical team and caregivers, remains a powerful example of being self-empowered through supported, personal choice.

5.5 Dancing with regret
Patient story: Mel

Doreen Stein-Seroussi, MPA, MA, E-RYT, C-IAYT

Mel (she/her) is a 45-year-old Black Latina woman diagnosed with end-stage colon cancer.

Mel has decided to end treatment for colon cancer as the remaining options offer little hope of a cure, and may only extend her life by a few months. She is referred to me by a local non-profit cancer support program. Because she is too ill to travel to see me, I am going to her home. When I enter her house, the shades are closed, and she is lying on the living room couch with her much-loved dog Gavin by her side. I can tell from her face that she is in pain, which she confirms, "I have a lot of pain and I feel like I can't breathe. I'm not sleeping because I can't get comfortable."

Looking at Mel, I can see that she's surrounded by pillows, but they're placed in a way that causes her shoulders to be pressed forward, her chest concave. With her permission, I rearrange the pillows to support her in a restorative chest-opening position. The effect is immediate, "I can relax and breathe, it's like the pressure is gone!" I give her a few minutes in quiet. I watch as her body relaxes and unclenches.

With her discomfort lessened, Mel is ready to talk about her life. Regret is a theme. "I thought I'd be married and have someone to share my life with. Instead, I pushed everyone away, including Richard, the love of my life. Better to reject than be rejected, I guess." Her career also didn't end the way she wanted. "I went to a top university, and I thought I'd have a high-power position, but it didn't turn out that way."

As we talk it becomes clear that in the last few weeks of her life, Mel wants to make amends for what she considers her failings. She'd called Richard and left a message; she'd sent another friend, with whom she'd lost touch, a note; and she sent a check to someone from her past whom she knew was struggling financially. But the emotions are tiring and draining her energy. She isn't ready to die, but the pain and exhaustion are making living difficult.

"I never thought it would be like this. You read about people having resolution in life and passing away peacefully. It isn't peaceful for me. I feel like there's so much I have to do beforehand, including arranging adoption for my sweet dog Gavin. And everyone wants something from me. I keep having unexpected visitors or people call, expecting to be invited over. This is hard work!"

Nodding, I suggest to Mel that we take a few minutes for her to pause, to notice this moment. She's eager. She doesn't want to move from the couch, so we start with some small movements and explore which ones feel good. She begins to gently circle her hands at her wrists and wiggles her fingers. Then she begins to move her feet. As she makes these small, gentle movements Mel groans with relief. "I haven't focused on feeling good.

I've spent so much time feeling bad." Soon Mel is ready to rest. I show her ways to position pillows to make herself more comfortable.

Recognizing that Mel's mind needs as much rest as her body, I ask her if she wants to try loving kindness (*maitrī*) meditation. I ask Mel to imagine herself standing in the middle of a circle of people from her life, including people from her past; they surround her with love, and I guide her to feel the love throughout her whole being. Shifting her focus from receiver to giver of love, I guide her to send love to people in her life, including those who are difficult to love, those who hurt her, and those whom she hurt. I emphasize compassion; no one, including her, is perfect. When it's over she says, "I really liked that. I feel so relaxed." At the end of the session, I help her download a meditation app to her smart phone, with similar meditations for her to use on her own.

I continue to visit Mel at home for a few weeks until her death. She never fully accepts death, but through practices she's learning to "surrender." On her last night alive, Mel tells me how she used to love to dance; it brought her such joy. Suddenly her eyes light up. "Maybe I can dance with you now?" I help her out of her bed while holding her catheter bag. Holding onto me, she leads us in a simple, slow dance. It's only a few minutes until she's tired and goes back into bed, but her exuberance is overflowing. She calls an old friend who lives in another state and says, "Guess what?! I danced!"

Paradoxical though it may sound, suffering is a condition that, to some extent, must be respected as an integral part of dying well (Hartogh 2017). The fact is, dying is not always peaceful, and many times it includes suffering. The role of the yoga therapist is not to eliminate the hard work of dying, but to assist the patient/client on their path and help lessen their suffering. *Patañjali Yoga Sūtra 2.3* acknowledges fear of death as a prime cause of suffering (Taimni 2014). Fear may become amplified as one knows death is approaching.

(continued)

(continued)
Death and dying have deep cultural beliefs attached. It is vital that the yoga therapist does not impose their belief on the client: many of our beliefs around death and dying are unconscious, and we need to do our own work (*svādhyāya*) around death before working with dying patients and their families.

5.6 Facilitating spiritual comfort at the end of life

Patient story: Paula

Jennie Lee, E-RYT 500, YACEP, C-IAYT

Paula (she/her) is a 93-year-old White woman diagnosed with stage IV ocular melanoma metastatic to liver.

When I meet Paula, she has been preparing to die for over two years. She has sold her home, made her legal arrangements, and moved in with family after choosing not to undergo treatment for stage IV metastatic ocular melanoma. But at 93 years old, she is now being taken *off* home-based hospice care because they have determined she is no longer a candidate – she still has full cognitive function, is somewhat ambulatory (though she spends most of the day in bed), and is relatively self-sufficient. Paula is refusing further medical intervention but is struggling with associated symptoms from the metastases to her liver, such as abdominal discomfort, back pain, weakness, and some difficulty breathing.

Her family calls me for yoga therapy because Paula used to attend a seniors' yoga class and enjoyed it. In addition to addressing her physical pain through yoga, her daughters think she would benefit from the therapeutic relationship, and talking with someone outside the family, as she enjoys reading and discussing philosophy.

My Mondays with Paula are rich explorations of the nature of reality, consciousness, and the spiritual questions that inevitably arise at the end of life (see Box 6.21), as she seeks assurance and meaning, particularly for why she is still living after having been pronounced "terminal" over two years prior. Some days she feels depressed, and some days angry that she is trapped in a liminal state between living and dying. Paula confides how distressing it is to "still be here." She tells me that she often wakes in the night and wonders why she is alive, in a body that isn't working like it used to, but also won't stop. She doesn't want to be a burden to her family, and she struggles with feeling any sense of purpose. She doesn't speak of being afraid to die, but I can sense her reluctance to fully let go.

Because she has spent a lot of time lying down in recent months, she is experiencing discomfort in her back, but she feels weak and dizzy if she stands for long. The cancer has not spread to her bones, but she does have diagnosed osteoporosis, so we take that into account with all movements. She enjoys very gentle supine twists (for example, Lord of Fishes pose [*suptamatsyendrāsana*]) and modified slow-moving bridge (*setubandhasarvāṅgāsana*), coordinated with the breath. When she is tired and her energy level is low, she sits on the edge of the bed and does easy neck stretches and seated cat/cow (*mārjaryāsana*) movements to ease the heart center and upper back. On really good days, she stands for a tree pose (*vṛkṣāsana*), holding her walker with one hand (see Figure 6.15).

After a bit of gentle movement, she usually wants to sit upright in bed, propped with many pillows to do some breath-work (*prāṇāyāma*). She enjoys the humming bee breath (*bhramarī*) as she finds the vibration soothing, especially if she is having a day of restless thinking or is feeling anxious or distracted. On days when fear is heightened, we do balanced breathing (*samavṛtti*) to a silent count (at her own pace) because the counting helps her shift her thinking away from fear into mindfulness of the present moment.

On days when Paula doesn't have the strength or clarity to focus on a specific breath technique, she finds comfort in following me through guided meditations. I direct her to lift her inner gaze to the point between the eyebrows, a practice called *sāmbhavīmudrā*.

Another practice she finds relaxing when fear is present is the audible repetition of a sound, the *Aum mantra*. Although her voice is weak, she says that even the smallest vibration of *Aum* makes her feel peaceful. When she tires and can no longer do it audibly, she repeats it silently with each inhalation and each exhalation.

In her last days, although she has seemingly been ready to die for a long time, she becomes quite fearful of leaving the body. I tell her that when we begin to shift away from fear, we realize that although we inhabit a body, we are the soul within. The body is not the ultimate Self, as the *Patañjali Yoga Sūtra-s* describe (PYS 2.3 and 2.47; Devi 2008). By remembering our transcendent essence, we will become unafraid to shed the mortal vehicle and return to the expansive state of pure consciousness.

I hold Paula's hand and repeat the affirmation, "You are not this body, bones, and blood. You are a spark of Spirit, filled with love and light."

This helps her quell the anxiety as she rests in the remembrance of her true spiritual nature as pure consciousness. Eventually, Paula crosses over peacefully, reunited in the awareness of her true being as part of that blissful Divine One.

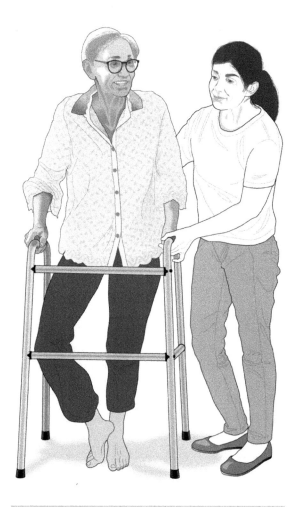

Figure 6.15
Tree pose (*vṛkṣāsana*) with support

In yogic philosophy the third eye is thought to be significant for moving toward the proverbial "light at the end of tunnel" (Yogananda 2007). This practice is said to soothe the mind, the same way concentrating on the breath calms the body – and that at the time of death, the soul passes through this portal to greater life. Sometimes she can sense this center of transcendent consciousness as an inner light, and sometimes not, but she always becomes calm while trying.

> **BOX 6.21 End-of-life practices**
>
> **Jennie Lee**
>
> There are two practices that can be very helpful at this stage. The first is initiating spiritually-focused conversation using open-ended questions to explore personal beliefs and perceptions. The second is addressing the fear of death through the teachings of the *kleśa-s* (afflictions or destructive emotions) to expand personal awareness beyond the body. Both are forms of *svādhyāya*, or reflection on the true Self.
>
> **1. Explore spiritual beliefs**
>
> To facilitate a client's exploration of their personal spiritual experience, it is essential to use inclusive language rather than religion-specific terminology.
>
> *(continued)*

(continued)

We should not introduce or impose our own beliefs, and we do not need to offer answers or solutions. Simply holding non-judgmental space and practicing loving presence and empathetic listening is enough.

Questions such as these can help people engage in gentle self-inquiry:

- Do you believe you are more than this dying body?
- What do you think is happening right now?
- Would you like to talk about your spiritual beliefs?
- Do you believe in a Higher Power and if so, what do you believe is the nature of it?
- What do you believe happens after we die?
- What gives you peace?
- What would be the most loving thought you could hold on to right now?

2. Overcoming fear through the *kleśa-s*

The *Patañjali Yoga Sūtra-s* instruct cultivating identification with pure consciousness and an awareness of our spiritual nature to dissolve the perception of separateness and the anguish it causes. There are five veils or obstructions over the perception of our true nature, referred to as the *kleśa-s* (see *Yoga philosophy* in Chapter 2). One begins to shift away from fear when we realize that although we *inhabit* a body, we *are* the soul within. The body is not the ultimate Self, as the *Sūtra-s* describe. By remembering our transcendent essence, we will become unafraid to shed the mortal vehicle and return to the expansive state of pure consciousness.

In *The Yoga of the Bhagavad Gītā*, Paramahansa Yogananda writes, "When this I shall die, then I will know who I truly am" (Yogananda 2007). This affirmation of true Self speaks to the need to practice non-attachment to – and non-identification with – the body. As we do so in life, so also at the time of death will there be less fear and suffering, and a greater ease in transition.

5.7 Healing yet not curing

Patient story: Harry

Lee Majewski, MA, PGDYEd, C-IAYT

Harry (he/his) is a 59-year-old man of Indian descent diagnosed with stage IV diffuse large B-cell lymphoma (DLBCL).

Harry travelled from Vancouver, Canada, to Lonavala, India (a hill station near Mumbai) to attend a 21-day yoga retreat, prompted by a referral from a medical doctor. He is a quiet man who underwent a stem cell transplant that ultimately failed. Two months ago, his physician told him he had six months to live. Although he is in constant pain (for which he has morphine) he is determined to attend as much of our retreat program as he can. Right from the beginning his will to live is very apparent.

Harry and seven other cancer survivors have shown up for this intensive retreat experience in which we *live* our yoga. Each daily session lasts six hours and includes discussion of yoga philosophy as well as the experiential practice of meditation, *yoganidrā* (yogic sleep), chanting *mantra* (words or sounds), *mudrā* (hand gestures), *prāṇāyāma* (breath practices), and *āsana* (postures and movement). Daily lectures describe the effect these practices have on the body and the mind. In these talks we address cause of disease, not just its symptoms. We aim to help participants recognize carcinogenic thoughts, processes, and attitudes, and explain how to effect positive change – replacing their old belief system and creating a new, healthier one. The intensity over three weeks often produces dramatic transformation in participants' lives.

Magic happens during such an immersive yogic lifestyle experience and the significance of the group setting becomes very apparent, especially during the first week. As one approaches the end of life, there is a great value in connection with others. While this can be found with close family and friends, it can also be found among strangers attending a residential retreat. Living in close proximity, they share daily experiences along with extended yoga practice. Within the first few days they build a sense of comfort, of new-found family. Participants attend yoga sessions together, eat meals together, and often spend free time together. Most importantly, they discuss what emerges from their practice and listen to each other's stirring and sometimes unusual experiences that arise in practice. Together they form strong collegial bonds and determinedly support each other in any difficulties or transformational experiences that occur in the later weeks of the retreat.

Each person, and each group, is unique, and the therapists and facilitators trust in the process of yogic practices that sometimes stir participants out of their comfort zone into unknown territory. It is the safety the participants have made among themselves that can be ultimately stabilizing. As they uncover their feelings and beliefs in their practice, yoga therapists can then guide them in a yogic understanding of human biology, functionality, and spirituality – throughout human life, and death.

On the first day of the program, each of the eight retreat participants completes the Profile of Mood States (POMS) 64-point validated survey[2] that describes feelings. Harry's results showed he has high levels of tension, depression, confusion, fatigue, and anger. He says he is filled with guilt feelings of his past actions and is very afraid of dying. His eyes reflect the pain and hopelessness he feels as he waits to die. Based on his answers and the assessment, we worked out a highly adapted *āsana* (postures and movement) protocol for Harry, noting his movements were extremely limited due to pain, and that even *yoganidrā* (yoga sleep) was difficult for

[2]POMS is a standard validated psychological test formulated by McNair et al. (1971). The questionnaire contains 64 words/statements that describe the feelings people have. The test requires a person to indicate for each word or statement how they have been feeling in the past week, including today.

him to practice because of the physical pain he felt sitting or lying down.

One day Harry asks for a one-on-one yoga therapy session. He wants to talk about his life; about those he loves, and about his regrets and the strong guilt he feels. I ask him if he'd be willing to put it all on paper to discuss at the next session. After a few days we meet again, and he reads out loud what he had written on the eight pages. He pauses frequently to hold back tears. Together we build a little fire, and he burns his words, page by page, while we hold hands chanting his favorite healing *mantra*, the *mahāmṛtyuñjayamantra*. This is commonly known as *tryámbakaṃ* or the "great death conquering mantra" (see the entire mantra on the next page). It comes from the *ṛgveda*, a collection of ancient Sanskrit hymns. This *mantra* is said to have the highest form of energy and wards off death and disease, and can, therefore, be helpful for those suffering from chronic conditions. It can also be a useful *mantra* for those suffering from fear of death, by connecting them to their soul's immortal nature. This is an important ritual in the Indian culture.

After our session, Harry then goes for dinner and shares his experiences with the group. The next day his smile is wide. "I left a lot of burden in that fire, and I feel much lighter!" Later we hear him humming a melody he remembers from his childhood.

By the end of the 21-day program, a repeat of the POMS survey confirms that Harry has improved on all fronts. Tension, depression, anger, fatigue, and confusion are drastically reduced, and vigor significantly increased. When Harry and I review the results he says, "Yes, that's about how I feel. And one more thing, when I came to the program, I was afraid of death. Now I am not. I will return to Vancouver and live as long as I can and spend as much time with my sons as possible."

Four weeks later, we all learn that Harry has passed away peacefully, surrounded by his loving wife, sons, and best friends he's known for more than 30 years. Although his cancer was not *cured*, Harry, in fact was *healed*. His fear, guilt, and anger were gone. He was serene, at peace, and accepting of his approaching death, enjoying every present moment.

Mahāmṛtyuñjayamantra

ॐ त्र्यंबकं यजामहे सुगन्धिं पुष्टिवर्धनम् ।
उर्वारुकमिव बन्धनान् मृत्योर्मुक्षीय माऽमृतात् ॥

oṁ tryámbakaṁ yajāmahe sugandhíṁ puṣṭi-vardhánam

urvārukam íva bandhánān mṛtyor mukṣīya mā 'mṛtāt

Translation by Jamison and Brereton (2014).

"We sacrifice to *Tryambaka* the fragrant, increaser of prosperity.

Like a cucumber from its stem, might I be freed from death, not from deathlessness."

Hindus believe this *mantra* is beneficial for mental, emotional, and physical health and consider it a *mokṣa* (enlightenment) *mantra* which bestows longevity and immortality. It is chanted while smearing *vibhūti* (sacred ash) over various parts of the body and utilized in *japa* (*mantra* repetition) or *homa* (religious offering ceremony).

There is a great value in being a part of a small group in a residential setting, which with time becomes a powerful support tool for each patient. They share their experiences and within the first few days they build the sense of family. That collective energy strongly supports each patient in their inner transformation and healing.

- The extended length and the intensity of yogic practices – *living* yoga – seem to create more profound spiritual and healing shifts.

- The collective energy of the group is very helpful in creating and sustaining these shifts.

- The changes depend on the individual's spiritual self-perception.

- The necessity of revival of spirituality in Yoga is illustrated by reinforcing the spiritual component of yogic practices such *yama-s* and *nyama-s* (restraints and observances), chanting, *yoganidrā* (yogic sleep), use of *mudrā-s* (hand gestures) and *bandha* (an energetic "internal lock" to control the flow of energy), meditation, as well as the understanding of philosophy through yoga courses and discussions.

- One of the reasons that yoga therapy is so effective in both preventive medicine and in assisting conventional treatment methods is because yoga addresses all aspects of wellness: the physical, emotional, mental, and spiritual. Yoga encompasses the art of self-realization, self-empowerment, self-transformation, and self-healing.

5.8 *Patañjali* saved it for last – *abhiniveśa* (fear of death)

Patient story: Laura

Jennifer Collins Taylor, MSW, CMP

Laura (she/her) is a 56-year-old White woman diagnosed with stage IV small cell lung cancer metastatic to brain.

Laura is curled up on her side, back to the door, sleeping deeply this afternoon. Outside in the hallway we stand huddled in small groups, voices hushed, several leaning heavily against the walls. Gathered are Laura's adult children, her male companion, and several grandchildren. None of us saw this coming. Laura had been in treatment for her stage IV cancer for over a year and seemed pretty stable. Then the falls, the discovery of metastases to the brain, a quick surgery, and since then the old "failure to thrive" assessment and no longer reliably communicative. The physician was due later this hour and the tension was palpable.

You see, one "camp" insisted that "she'd have wanted us not to quit." The other camp murmured, "she'd never have wanted to live like this." And a few acknowledged both camps were right. The problem? None of us ever asked Laura what she wanted, much less ever had it legally documented. Were we all in denial of this possibility? Was Laura in denial, or had she harbored a desire to talk about death, her death, and what she hoped for? Did she not want to impose on her family or her lover, or was she merely being a "good" patient and silently battling this "foe"? It appears we'll never know at this point, barring a miraculous turnaround.

Laura has a boiler plate advanced care directive that lacks specificity to provide direction this afternoon. How will we decide? What shall we say or do to support or influence the sons that share the healthcare directive duties? Does her companion voice what he thinks she'd want and risk alienating her family? Do the sons ask him? Does a social worker join the meeting as an advocate and guide? Have any of us even contemplated our own ultimate demise, or will we just be projecting our fears and needs into the process? How could we all arrive so unprepared for what of course is our only shared certainty? We will die.

Why isn't there a way we could have been prepared for today? Who could prepare us? What would it take to be prepared for the uncertainty of this certainty? Which of us need this preparation? The exhausted, harried physician? The overworked direct care staff? The family? Her lover? Laura as a human and an oncology patient?

We turn as one at the sound of the bent figure of the physician stepping off the elevator, frantically texting one-handed and running her hand back through her drooping hair.

If only…

As a social worker specializing in thanatology (death and dying) as well as a yoga therapist, I advocate for what is mistakenly seen as the far end of the cancer care continuum: death and dying. Mistakenly, because every single client is going to die, and so are we. And I'm willing to bet, at some point in every client's cancer experience, they long or need to talk about death. Every single one. Now, whether they do, can, or are given a space to do so… well, that in my experience is far less certain, but much better than it was even a decade ago. What Laura's story asks of us as yoga therapists is: is there more we can be doing to fill this void around healthy conversations and explorations of death and dying? Or have we limited yoga therapy to offering symptom management for fatigue, nausea, pain, mobility, and anxiety? Is that last *āsana* "relaxation pose" or do we call it what is? We can't say "corpse", that might be a trigger, and, and, and…Nonsense! Death is on their minds and stirring in their heart. Who will make it safe to explore that existential stirring? Trauma or not, it is time.

Ought we as yoga therapists not be the ones to bring honor and dignity to the unveiled reality that during a cancer experience, there is the unique gift of opportunity to create a safe space to explore the last of *Patañjali's kleśa-s* (causes of suffering)? It is the final and toughest *kleśa – abhiniveśa* – fear of death and fear of dissolution (see Chapter 2, *Yoga philosophy*). I know in many of the best oncology programs there are resources to support clients through psychosocial or spiritual care. Too often they are employed only reactively when there's a crisis, rather than part of a consistent full spectrum of care. Even then it tends to be the siloed support, without integration into the person's entire experience. How's that racing heart at 3:00 a.m. related to the tightness in the throat or the tapping foot in the waiting room? This *kleśa* is a master of disguise. Rarely in my experience does it march in declaring, "Hello, I'm fear of death." What skills and practices can safely unmask this *kleśa*?

The "real-ization" of impermanence and misperceptions *is* our yoga. Paradoxically, we don't have to bring up death, because it is "in" our practices, and, cultural suppression of death binds so many of us from being able to have what then are courageous conversations about death, dying, and living. Our role is to create and hold a safe space of exploration.

- First, we need to reclaim Yoga as the psychospiritual practice that it is. The modern postural yoga has denuded Yoga of its central focus as a spiritual practice.

- Then, we need to update ourselves on the evidence base of the importance and efficacy of spiritual care in palliative care, oncology, and end-of-life care.

- Finally, learning and adopting the language of our respective culture is critical for integration. The systems aren't interested in *cakra-s* (wheels of energy), *kośa-s* (layers of existence), or *duḥkha* (suffering) (see Chapter 2, *Yoga philosophy*). Rather, the burden is on us to translate for the systems to enable interprofessional collaboration.

What might that look like? Consider the following partial listing of the many resources we have within our tradition (Box 6.22). These seeds suggest how we can appropriately offer our work in a meaningful way to everyone in the vignette above. Mind you, much of this remains to be enacted.

BOX 6.22 End-of-life resources within the yoga tradition[1]
Jennifer Collins Taylor

Checklist to complete prior to serving

- Extensive preparation both professionally and personally to thoroughly address one's own personal grief and experience with loss.

- Develop a broad referral network of mental health professionals and spiritual counselors.

- Have trained in compassionate, nonjudgmental support vs. directive prescription.

- Respect all individual religious beliefs and experiences of loss, death, and dying.

Questions to invite insight/exploration

- Knowing that you will die eventually, how do you wish to live?

(continued)

(continued)

- What are the main challenges or issues in your life right now?

- What would you consider to be the main losses you have suffered?

- How would you describe the spiritual dimension of your life?

- Do you have close friends or others you can confide in?

- What do you see as ultimately most important in life?

- Do you feel you have a particular mission or vocation in life, and are you fulfilling it?

- What would you consider your philosophy of life?

Yoga practices

- *Saṅkalpa* (intention) around living and dying.

- Introspective, supported *āsana* (postures and movement).

- Simple and straightforward *prāṇāyāma* (breathing).

- *Mudrā-s* (hand gestures) to open, to receive, to ground, to pray, to offer, and to meditate.

- Skillful *yoganidrā* and *bhāvanā* (yogic sleep and meditative cultivation) practices.

- *Śavāsana as śavāsana* (corpse pose) appropriate to their comfort.

- *Pañcamayakośa* model (five sheaths of existence) translated into current language to explore the relationships.

- *Patañjali Yoga Sūtra-s* (Feuerstein translation) to include the *yama* (social restraint) of *ahiṃsā* (do no harm); *Sūtra-s I.2, 3, 18, 23, 26, 31; Sūtra-s 2.3-4, 6, 7-9*; and how *abhiniveśa* (will to live); relates to modern stages of grief, loss, and dying.

And so, we continue to create together.

---

[1]See Further reading (in References) for more resources from the author.

Section 5 references

Introduction

Center to Advance Palliative Care (CAPC), 2022. About Palliative Care. Available at: https://www.capc.org/about/palliative-care/.

Centers for Disease Control and Prevention (CDC), 2022. A Definition of Hospice Care. Available at: https://www.cdc.gov/training/ACP/page35093.html.

Dugdale, L., 2020. *Lost Art of Dying: Reviving Forgotten Wisdom*. HarperLuxe.

Eastern Cooperative Oncology Group (ECOG), 2022. ECOG Performance Status Scale. Available at: https://ecog-acrin.org/resources/ecog-performance-status.

Fischer, S., Min, S.J., Cervantes, L., Kutner, J., 2013. Where do you want to spend your last days of life? Low concordance between preferred and actual site of death among hospitalized adults. *J Hosp Med.* 8(4):178–183.

Gawande, A., 2014. *Being Mortal: Illness, Medicine and What Matters in the End*. Wellcome Collection; London, UK.

Temel, J.S., Greer, J.A., Muzikansky, A., et al., 2010. Early palliative care for patients with metastatic non-small-cell lung cancer. *New England Journal of Medicine.* 363(8):733–742.

Merriam-Webster Dictionary, 2022. Inspire. Available at: https://www.merriam-webster.com/dictionary/inspire.

National Hospice and Palliative Care Organization (NHPCO), 2022. Available at: https://www.nhpco.org.

Platt, M., 2010. Pain challenges at the end of life – pain and palliative care collaboration. *Rev Pain.* 4(2):18–23.

Prigerson, H.G., Bao, Y., Shah, M.A., et al., 2015. Chemotherapy use, performance status, and quality of life at the end of life. *JAMA Oncol.* 1(6):778–784.

Richmond, C., 2005. Dame Cicely Saunders. *BMJ.* 33:238.

Wiman, C., 2012. Dying into Life, What Faith Reveals. *Commonweal Magazine.* Available at: https://www.commonwealmagazine.org/dying-life.

World Health Organization (WHO), 2020. Palliative Care Key Facts. Available at: https://www.who.int/news-room/fact-sheets/detail/palliative-care.

Further reading

Givler, A., Bhatt, H., Maani-Fogelman, P.A., 2021. The Importance of Cultural Competence in Pain and Palliative Care. [Updated 2021 Jul 26]. In: StatPearls [Internet]. StatPearls Publishing; Treasure Island, FL. Available at: https://www.ncbi.nlm.nih.gov/books/NBK493154/.

5.1 *Samādhi* meditation

Clyne, B., O'Neill, S.M., Nuzum, D., et al., 2019. Patients' spirituality perspectives at the end of life: a qualitative evidence synthesis. *BMJ Supportive & Palliative Care.* bmjspcare-2019-002016.

Kang, K.A., Han, S.J., Lim, Y.S., Kim S.J., 2019. Meaning-centered interventions for patients with advanced or terminal cancer: a meta-analysis. *Cancer Nursing.* 42(4):332–340.

Sullivan, M.B., Erb, M., Schmalzl, L., et al., 2018. Yoga therapy and polyvagal theory: the convergence of traditional wisdom and contemporary neuroscience for self-regulation and resilience. *Frontiers in Human Neuroscience.* 12, 67.

5.3 Transitioning to the light

Alam, S., Hannon, B., Zimmerman, C., 2020. Palliative care for family caregivers. *J Clin Oncol.* 38 (9):926–936.

Desikachar, T.K.V., 2003. Sūtra I:36. In: *Reflections on Yogasūtra-s of Patañjali*. Krishnamacharya Yoga Mandiram.

5.5 Dancing with regret

Hartogh, G.D., 2017. Suffering and dying well: on the proper aim of palliative care. *Med Health Care Philos.* 20(3):413–424.

Taimni, I.K., 2014. *The Science of Yoga: The Yoga Sutras of Patanjali in Sanskrit*. Theosophical Publishing House; Wheaton, IL.

5.6 Facilitating spiritual comfort at end of life

Nischala Joy Devi, *The Secret Power of Yoga: A Woman's Guide to the Heart and Spirit of the Yoga Sutras*, (New York: Three Rivers Press, 2007).

Yogananda, P., 2007. *The Yoga of the Bhagavad Gita*. Self-Realization Fellowship; Los Angeles, CA.

5.7 Healing yet not curing

Jamison, S., Brereton, J., 2014. *The Rigveda: The Earliest Religious Poetry of India*. Oxford University Press. pp. 953–954.

5.8 *Patañjali* saved it for last – *abhiniveśa*

Feuerstein, G. *The Yoga Tradition: Its history, literature, philosophy and practice*. Arizona: Hohm Press. 1998; p294.

Further reading

Taylor, J., 2008. End-of-life yoga therapy: exploring life and death. *Int J Yoga Therap*.18(1):97–103.

Taylor, J.C., 2010. Living Life, Dying Death. Available at:https://matthewjtaylor.com/wp-content/uploads/2018/08/LLDD_DIGITAL09162010.pdf.

Taylor, J., Taylor, M.J., 2011. Yoga therapeutics: preparation and support for end of life. *Topics in Geriatric Rehabilitation*. 27:142–150.

Taylor, J.C., 2011. Courageous conversations. *Topics in Geriatric Rehabilitation*. 27:81–86.

Yoga Therapy in Oncologic Care: The Way Forward

Leigh Leibel

Well in our country, said Alice ...

Lewis Carroll,
Alice in Wonderland

The final chapter of this book is not the end, rather, it is the beginning. It is a call for our global healthcare delivery systems to prioritize the holistic well-being of all people affected by cancer and to formally integrate yoga into standard oncologic care. This call to action aligns with and supports the World Health Organization (WHO) Sustainable Development Goal (SDG) #3: To ensure healthy lives and promote well-being for all at all ages (WHO 2017).

Throughout these pages we have presented a strong evidence base that shows yoga can improve the well-being and quality of life of people with cancer, mitigate many of the physical and psychological side-effects of cancer and its treatment, and positively impact clinical outcomes. Weaving the best available empirical evidence into first-hand patient/client stories, we have illustrated the art and science of delivering safe and effective yoga to people with cancer, survivors, and their families at all stages of the care continuum, from diagnosis to end of life. With this book as a foundation, we may begin to characterize and implement solutions to advance the field of yoga therapy in oncologic care. To that point, we propose three next steps:

- Develop best practices, standards, and guidelines for the delivery of safe and effective yoga and yoga therapy for people with cancer and survivors across the care continuum. This includes people who are medically fragile and have comorbid condtions.

- Advance yoga and cancer health equity by creating a more diverse yoga therapy workforce that can better deliver accessible and culturally sensitive care to underrepresented communities and groups of people.

- Identify barriers to yoga, as well as promote its benefits as a mind-body science to all cancer stakeholders, from members of the medical team to people with cancer, survivors, families, and patient advocates.

Develop best practices, standards, and guidelines for delivery of safe and effective yoga in cancer populations

Currently, there are no universally agreed upon *best practices* and *guidelines* for the safe and effective delivery of yoga in cancer populations, nor are there *standards* in the education and training of yoga therapists and yoga professionals working in oncology. However, for yoga to be accepted as standard of care across all cancer populations, including those who are medically fragile and have comorbid conditions, yoga parameters must be identified and defined that are based on both scientific research and expert clinical experience.

In 2022, the Society for Integrative Oncology (SIO) and the International Association of Yoga Therapists (IAYT) convened a multi-institution, multidisciplinary working group of subject matter experts to begin a long-term consensus project to define yoga and yoga therapy in cancer care. The goal is to investigate yoga practices within the context of acute and longitudinal side effects of cancer and its treatment, understand how these adverse physical and psychological side effects impact a yoga practice, and make recommendations (based on research evidence and feedback from subject matter experts) for the delivery of safe and effective yoga in both clinic and community settings. These recommendations will inform the yoga and cancer teaching curricula and educational competencies; serve as practice guidelines for yoga therapists and yoga professionals working with cancer and medically fragile populations; and provide public-facing information about yoga and cancer for patients/survivors, their families, patient advocates, and healthcare providers and oncology specialists.

Advance yoga and cancer health equity

Disparity in cancer care is a critical issue facing our health delivery systems. There are many communities and groups of people who do not have access to supportive care and integrative therapies (including yoga) during their cancer treatment. SIO and IAYT are working collaboratively to address this by promoting the scientific benefits of yoga during cancer care and identifying ways to make yoga accessible to everyone. In 2022, the SIO Yoga Special Interest Group (SIG) presented a workshop *"Yoga Therapy Across the Breast Cancer Care Continuum: Creating a Safe, Inclusive, Evidence-Informed Practice"* at IAYT's Symposium on Yoga Therapy and Research (SYTAR). The workshop emphasized the need for educating yoga and yoga therapy professionals on the facts about cancer, treatment side effects, and the precautions needed to deliver yoga safely to people with cancer. A key topic of the presentation and discussion was diversity and inclusion. During the break-out groups, participants identified that "health equity, inclusion, and belonging (HEIB) covers a wide range of areas including accessibility; affordability; creating welcoming, clean, safe and brave spaces; sensitivity to language; and differences in culture and life experiences". They also identified body positivity as a standout in cancer care due to the multitude of changes that can occur over the course of the cancer care continuum. To advance cancer health equity and ensure optimal wellness for all people, the workshop findings endorsed that we must develop and support a diverse and culturally sensitive yoga workforce that more accurately represents the racial, ethnic, religious, ability, sexual and gender diversity, age, socioeconomic, and geographical distribution of people with cancer and elevates their individual and collective voices. This includes access to yoga and other integrative therapies, and representation in yoga research and clinical trials.

Educational pipeline programs for yoga and yoga therapy

One way to contribute to health equity across the continuum of cancer care is by supporting *educational pipeline programs* that create opportunities for people in underrepresented communities to enter yoga and yoga therapy training schools, so they may develop careers as yoga therapists and yoga professionals working in cancer care. Such programs play a vital role in increasing the diversity of health professions (including yoga therapy), and provide mentorship opportunities for trainees. By increasing the number of yoga professionals from underrepresented backgrounds, the roots of the social determinants of health (SDoH) that drive disparity and lead to worse patient outcomes may begin to be addressed. Working together, we can create a more culturally competent and diverse yoga workforce; promote community-based service and learning opportunities to increase lifestyle and health literacy among all people with cancer and their families; enhance patient-centered care; and ensure health equity for all people.

Identify barriers and promote the benefits of yoga in cancer care to all stakeholders: closing the gap between knowledge and practice

Despite more than a decade of research supporting the efficacy of yoga in the management of various cancer-related symptoms (and despite yoga's inclusion in the National Comprehensive Cancer Network [NCCN] guidelines for managing cancer-related fatigue and pain), patients' use of yoga for supportive care is low, ranging from 6% to 10% (Desai et al. 2021, Raghunathan et al. 2019, Rosen et al. 2013, Yildiz et al. 2013).

The reasons for low usage include a misunderstanding by people with cancer and oncologists of what yoga "is" (yoga is not a religion; yoga is not gymnastics), and a lack of awareness by all parties of the immense benefits of yoga during treatment and survivorship to help manage symptoms and improve well-being and quality of life. Other barriers are more individualized and vary from person to person.

Increasing awareness of yoga benefits among healthcare professionals

Oncologists can be a particularly effective source of information on healthy lifestyle behaviors due to reported patient trust, and the frequency of patient office visits (Hillen et al. 2012). But while 80% of cancer survivors expressed an interest in health-promotion advice (Denmark-Wahnedfried et al. 2000), fewer than half report having these discussions (Kenzik et al. 2016).

A 2019 survey of doctors (n=91) in the Midwestern United States (Stump et al. 2019), suggests oncologists rarely counsel patients on lifestyle changes that could improve their overall health and possibly reduce the risk of cancer recurrence. The study found that only 26.7% of oncologists and 9.7% of other specialists recommended lifestyle changes to their patients with cancer, whereas 90% of primary care physicians surveyed said they recommend lifestyle changes (e.g., weight loss, physical activity, and tobacco cessation) to at least some cancer survivors. All of the oncologists surveyed said that cancer control is their primary concern, with one explaining, "We're so focused on the life-or-death aspect of cancer, everything [else] falls through the cracks." When oncologists did address lifestyle factors, the subject was usually initiated by the patients.

Another survey presented at the annual conference of the American Society of Clinical Oncology (ASCO) in 2021 highlighted a significant 30% gap between oncologist (n=115) awareness of complementary medicine use in their patients (n=164) and actual patient engagement (Crudup et al. 2021). While 73% of the patients with breast cancer surveyed said they used at least one type of complementary medicine after they were diagnosed with cancer, their oncologists thought the percentage was much lower (43%). The oncologists

also said they discussed lifestyle behaviors with 55% of patients, but only 28% of patients said they had gotten their healthy lifestyle information from their physician.

These studies suggest that many oncologists may not have the time, ability, or resources to provide behavioral and lifestyle counseling to their patients, and this lack of information could impair their long-term health. Given this, an alternative suggested by the investigators is for health promotion to be delivered by survivorship clinics that provide post-treatment services to people with cancer and their families.

Increasing awareness of yoga benefits among people with cancer

We must also increase awareness among people with cancer and their families on the benefits of yoga during cancer treatment and beyond. A study conducted in 2021 on yoga awareness by people with cancer (n=857) at Memorial Sloan Kettering Cancer Center's five regional academic cancer centers in the greater New York City area found that 70% of respondents had never practiced yoga, and 52.3% were interested in practicing yoga. Among those interested in practicing yoga, half of them had no prior yoga experience. While men were more likely than women to be unaware of the yoga program (72.4% vs. 48.8%), awareness of the yoga program did not vary by age, race, education, marital status, or cancer type/stage. Of interest in this study, non-White people (67%) were more interested in practicing yoga than White people (52.2%) (Desai et al. 2021).

A 2019 study funded by the National Cancer Institute (NCI) evaluated patient awareness of a free therapeutic yoga program offered at the Abramson Cancer Center at the University of Pennsylvania. Despite a months' long promotion of the yoga program through the center's website, banners in the lobby, and pamphlets in outpatient clinics, of the 303 patients who responded to the survey, 171 (56%) said they were not aware that a yoga program was available to them (Raghunathan et al. 2019).

While larger scale quantitative studies with diverse

cancer types are needed, these two studies suggest a need for more targeted education and outreach campaigns to people with cancer and their families using appropriate marketing messages and engagement strategies to improve awareness of yoga for symptom control during cancer care and beyond.

The last word: integrating yoga in oncologic care

Yoga is a person-centered, mind-body practice that can improve the lives of people affected by cancer. To our knowledge, this is the first book of its kind that shows the evidence base and benefits of yoga at *every* stage of the cancer care continuum. Although progress is being made in some academic medical centers, hospitals, and clinics, *true* integration of yoga into standard cancer care has not yet been established. Models must be explored that:

1. Provide people with cancer, survivors, families, and healthcare professionals with equitable access to safe and effective yoga and yoga therapy.

2. Promote high-quality yoga research among all people, cancer populations, types, and stages of disease.

3. Recognize and sustain yoga therapy as a new and valued healthcare profession.

4. Provide sustainable financial compensation for yoga therapists and yoga professionals.

Working together, we can begin to create a more compassionate and equitable global community that prioritizes the holistic well-being of people touched by cancer. We enourage you to join future yoga and cancer collaborations in your local community and within larger organizations globally, with the goal of advancing yoga in cancer care and providing safe, effective, accessible yoga to the 34 million cancer survivors worldwide to improve their well-being, quality of life, and clinical outcomes across the cancer care continuum.

References

Carroll, L., 1898. *Alice in Wonderland and Through the Looking Glass*. Lothrop; Boston: 125.

Crudup, T., Li, L., Lawson, E., Dorr, J.W., Stout, R., Niknam, P.V., Jones, J. et al., 2021. *J Clin Oncol*. 39, 2021:4746712.

Demark-Wahnefried, W., Peterson, B., McBride, C., et al., 2000. Current health behaviors and readiness to pursue life-style changes among men and women diagnosed with early stage prostate and breast carcinomas. *Cancer*. 88:674–684.

Desai, K., Bao, T., Li, Q.S., et al., 2021. Understanding interest, barriers, and preferences related to yoga practice among cancer survivors. *Supportive Care in Cancer*. 29:5313–5321.

Hillen, M.A., Onderwater, A.T., van Zwieten, M.C., et al., 2012. Disentangling cancer patients' trust in their oncologist: a qualitative study. *Psychooncology*. 21:392–399.

Kenzik, K., Pisu, M., Fouad, M.N., Martin, M.Y., 2016. Are long-term cancer survivors and physicians discussing health promotion and healthy behaviors? *J Cancer Surviv*. 10:271–279.

Raghunathan, N.J., Korenstein, D., Li, Q.S., Mao, J.J., 2019. Awareness of yoga for supportive care in cancer: implications for dissemination. *J Altern Complement Med*. 25(8):809–813.

Rosen, J.E., Gardiner, P., Saper, R.B., et al., 2013. Complementary and alternative medicine use among patients with thyroid cancer. *Thyroid*. 23:1238–1246.

Stump, T.K., Robinson, J.K., Yanez, B., et al., 2019. Physicians' perspectives on medication adherence and health promotion among cancer survivors. *Cancer*. 125:4319–4328.

World Health Organization, 2017. Health is a fundamental human right. Available at: https://www.who.int/news-room/commentaries/detail/health-is-a-fundamental-human-right.

Yildiz, I., Ozguroglu, M., Toptas, T., et al., 2013. Patterns of complementary and alternative medicine use among Turkish cancer patients. *J Palliat Med*. 16:383–390.

Subject Index

Subject Index

self-care
    of caregivers 129–32
    of therapist 49–51
self-compassion 153–5
shock after diagnosis 84
small group yoga therapy sessions
    befo re the session 41–2
    check-ins 42
    check-outs 42
    client education in 42
    co-assessment in 42
    compassionate embodied inquiry 42
    end of life 213
    group witnessing 42
    notes from 42–3
    referrals to 42–3
    yoga therapist introduction 42
Society for Integrative Oncology (SIO) 78, 149, 150, 219, 220
somatic-based movement 170
spinal cord tumors 56
spiritual bypassing 48
spiritual care
    end of life 209–11
    recurrent cancers 192–5
staging cancer 57–9
stress 73, 74
suffering acknowledgement/reduction 10–11
surgery 60
Symposium on Yoga Therapy and Research (SYTAR) 1

targeted therapy 63
therapeutic principles 17–18
therapeutic relationships 25–6
TNM staging system 58–9
"toxic" positivity 28, 48
trauma
    as experience of cancer 15–16
    stewardship and advocacy for 109–12
Trauma Stewardship: An Everyday Guide to Caring for Self While Caring for Others (Van Dernoot Lipsky) 110
treatments for cancer
    adolescents and young adults 125–9
    anxiety during 103–5
    axillary web syndrome 107–9
    in Cancer Care Continuum 98–141
    and caregivers 129–32
    "chemo brain" 132–5
    chemotherapy 60–1, 122–4
    clinical trials 64
    considerations for 64
    corticosteroids 63
    disparities in 109–12
    exercise during 138–41

fatigue during 105–7
hematopoietic stem cell transplant (HSCT) 63
hormone therapy 62
immunotherapy 62
in-patient yoga therapy 137–8
lymphedema 122–21
numbers in 98
patient stories 101–3, 104–5, 106–7, 108–9, 112, 118–20, 124, 127–9, 130, 133, 135–8, 140–1
pediatric oncology 101–3
Prānic Energization Technique 132–5
radiation therapy 61–2
surgery 60
targeted therapy 63
virtual platforms 135–7
yoga benefits 98–100

uncertainty in yoga philosophy 10
Understanding Yoga Therapy (Sullivan & Hyland Robertson) 10, 20

virtual platforms 45, 135–7

Wellwood, John 48
When Breath Becomes Air (Kalanithi) 181
workplace return 157–8

Yoga of the Bhagavad Gītā (Yogananda) 211
Yoga for Grief and Loss (Helbert) 175
Yoga for Mental Health (Mason and Birch) 15, 16
Yoga nidrā 23
yoga philosophy
    awareness practice 9–10
    engagement 11
    holistic care 8–9
    impermanence 10
    interconnections in 9
    non-violence 8
    practice 11
    purposeful life 11
    returning to the present 11
    study of 7–8
    suffering acknowledgement/reduction 10–11
    uncertainty 10
yoga practices
    Accessible Yoga 22
    breath 23–4
    iRest 23
    in oncology 21–4
    Restorative yoga 23
    Yoga nidrā 23
    in yoga philosophy 11

Author Index

Author Index